W9-DJH-976

MENTAL DISORDERS IN OLDER ADULTS

MENTAL DISORDERS IN OLDER ADULTS
Fundamentals of Assessment and Treatment

STEVEN H. ZARIT
and
JUDY M. ZARIT

THE GUILFORD PRESS
New York   London

Library of Congress Cataloging-in-Publication Data

Zarit, Steven H.
   Mental disorders in older adults: fundamentals of assessment and
treatment / Steven H. Zarit, Judy M. Zarit
       p.   cm.
   Includes bibliographical references and index.
   ISBN 1-57230-368-9
   1. Aged—Mental health.   2. Aged—Psychology.   3. Mentally ill
aged.   4. Geriatric psychology.   5. Psychotherapy for the aged.
6. Neuroses in old age.   7. Depression in old age.   I. Zarit, Judy
M.   II. Title.
   [DNLM: 1. Mental Disorders—in old age.   2. Mental Disorders—
diagnosis.   3. Mental Disorders—therapy.   4. Aging—psychology.
WT 150 Z37m   1998]
RC451.A5Z374   1998
618.97'689—dc21
DNLM/DLC
for Library of Congress   98-22968
                                                                        CIP

Acknowledgments

This book has been a long time in the making and we owe a debt of gratitude to many people who have given us support and encouragement in this endeavor. We want to thank Kitty Moore, Senior Editor of The Guilford Press, who persevered when the book took longer than expected and gave us sound advice and counsel throughout the process. As was the case for the previous books that we worked on together, Kitty's efforts made this a better book. We also want to thank Judith Grauman, Editorial Supervisor of The Guilford Press, who shepherded the book through the production process. Many of our colleagues were helpful in providing insight into key issues. We particularly want to thank Dr. Heidi Syropoulos, whose comments on the manuscript were perceptive and helpful. We received excellent support in developing the bibliography from Stephanie Davey and Albert Teller. Susan Hofer did an outstanding job in producing final versions of the manuscript and bibliography. Finally, we want to acknowledge our son, Matthew, who put up with occasional late nights and fast food as his parents worked on this book.

STEVEN H. ZARIT, PhD
JUDY M. ZARIT, PhD

Contents

MENTAL DISORDERS IN OLDER ADULTS

1

Introduction: Concepts and Practice with Older Adults

The aging of the population is one of the most profound and far-reaching changes affecting contemporary society. The number and proportion of older people in the population has grown dramatically, raising concerns about the well-being of older people and their families and the economic and social health of society as a whole. For mental health professionals, these demographic and social changes mean that an increasing number of older people are seeking psychological services. There is a great need for trained mental health professionals who can provide competent evaluations and treatment for older people. Mental health treatment can address problems faced by older people and their families, including primary mental health disorders as well as the consequences of illnesses, loss, and other stresses. Mental health approaches can also play a valuable role in prevention of psychiatric disorders and in developing strategies for promoting health and functional competency, helping to make old age a productive period of life. Mental health professionals can contribute to the larger social debate about the appropriate distributions of resources and benefits in an aging society—how, for example, to provide for the growing needs of the older generation while still addressing problems of children and other segments of the population.

Despite the dramatic growth of the older population, the mental health field has been slow to respond with adequate numbers of trained professionals who have specialized training in geriatrics. Historically, older people have been regarded as uninteresting and untreatable, and they have been underserved by mental health professionals. Yet the accumulating knowledge in geriatric mental health suggests that many of the common problems of later life respond to treatment and that mental health professionals can significantly improve the functioning of patients and their families. Even in cases of untreatable disorders such as dementia, mental health interventions can have a substantial impact on the patient and his or her family. Pioneering efforts such as those of Robert L. Kahn in psychology, Alvin Goldfarb in psychiatry, and Margaret Blenkner in social work laid a foundation in research and clinical practice that has grown into a large and rich body of knowledge. Clinicians and researchers interested in specializing in geriatrics can find ample opportunities for intellectually challenging and rewarding work that pushes the boundaries of knowledge in research and clinical practice.

We have written this book for clinicians and clinical students interested in working with older people and their families. The book is designed to provide a foundation for practice with older adults and to address the main problems clinicians are likely to encounter. A major feature is the integration of clinical practice and research. A common complaint among practitioners is how frustrating it is to try to apply research findings that are based on standard protocols developed in university settings. In clinics and private practices, clients do not neatly conform to these standards, nor do they generally present with a single problem that meets the research requirements. At the same time, practice needs to be informed and guided by research so that the best methods of assessment and treatment are used. The two authors have backgrounds in both research and practice with older people but currently work in settings that emphasize these areas differently. One of us (SHZ) is in a primarily research and academic setting, and the other (JMZ) is in private practice, practicing in her office and in consultation to nursing homes and retirement communities. We believe that the combination of these perspectives helps us focus our discussions of research on practical considerations, while informing practice approaches with the practical implications of current research findings.

In writing this book we draw heavily on our own professional training in clinical psychology, but we intend it for all the mental health professions that work with older people. We emphasize psychosocial perspectives and expect the book to be most useful to psychologists, social workers, psychiatric nurses, and gerontologists. Psychiatrists and geriatricians may also find the presentation of behavioral and neuropsychological perspectives a useful complement to their biomedical approaches.

An underlying assumption of our approach is that several professional groups can make valuable contributions to mental health care of the elderly. Clinical practice is best carried out in a context of multidisciplinary collaboration, with each field contributing its special expertise. The need for a multidisciplinary approach grows out of an understanding of mental health problems of later life. Medical, psychological, and social processes are frequently entwined in later life, and an exclusive focus on one area to the neglect of the others can be detrimental. A major theme of the book is how to think about these interactions when conducting an assessment or treating an older person. As an example, a primarily medical approach to Alzheimer's disease can miss opportunities for behavioral or psychosocial treatment. Those treatments can help patients function optimally despite the disease, for example, by simplifying their environment and routines or using behavioral management skills to control problems such as agitation or depressed mood. Conversely, an exclusively behavioral approach would overlook the potential benefits of medications in the management of disturbed behavior in dementia. Collaboration across disciplines can lead to identification of the levels at which effective interventions can be made, whether medical, psychological, social, or environmental.

One of our goals is to provide nonphysicians with information on illnesses and medications in later life. By understanding the effects of medical illnesses on psychological problems in later life as well as the uses and limits of psychoactive medications, the mental health professional can be a more effective collaborator with physicians. The mental health professional should not, of course, give medical advice but can learn to make assessments and observations of patients that enable physicians to make better treatment choices.

In the current health care climate, a premium is placed on the physician's time. By contrast, psychologists and other mental health professionals are often able to spend with patients the time needed to understand and measure their strengths and weaknesses. When a good working alliance is developed with physicians, mental health professionals can complement their efforts. Development of productive collaborations depend on establishing expertise in aging and communicating findings in a succinct and jargon-free manner. Our experience shows that once physicians understand what information we can provide and how we can enhance treatment, barriers between professions fade away.

EMERGENCE OF AGING IN MENTAL HEALTH PRACTICE

There are several reasons to develop a specialization in aging. First, the growth of the older population has greatly outpaced the number of mental health professionals who are trained to work with older people and their families. A second reason is that practice with older people is intellectually challenging and personally rewarding. The process of assessment is complex and varied, involving integration of medical, psychological, social, and sometimes legal information. New and interesting assessment questions continually crop up. Similarly, older people seeking treatment are tremendously varied. Older clients are not dull or unresponsive. Instead, they bring a lifetime of experience into therapy that makes them interesting to know and that creates opportunities for interventions not available in treating young adults. Finally, the difference clinical work makes in the lives of older people and their families is gratifying.

Training programs in the mental health professions unfortunately and all too commonly do not address aging or convey only minimal or even incorrect and outdated information. Most students in clinical training programs simply do not receive exposure to geriatrics, either in their academic preparation or in supervised clinical practice. The need for knowledge and training in aging, however, is growing. Several social trends underscore the emerging importance of geriatrics.

First and foremost among these trends is the aging of the population. In 1900, only 4% of the population of the United States was 65 years of age or older. That figure has risen to 13.5% currently and is projected to increase to 17% by the year 2020 (Treas, 1995). Canada and many of the European countries have had similar patterns of growth in their older populations (Kinsella & Taeuber, 1993). This growth is largely due to increases in life expectancy. Between 1900 and 1990, average life expectancy in the United States rose from 46 to 72 years for men and from 49 to 79 years for women (National Center for Health Statistics, 1993). With so much of the population over age 65, mental health professionals with the expertise to assess and treat the problems of later life are sorely needed.

A second factor is how research has challenged many of the negative expectations and beliefs about aging and the capability of older people to respond to mental health interventions. Studies of the normal aging process have found that later life includes the possibility of growth as well as decline (e.g., Baltes, 1987, 1997). Many abilities once thought to undergo significant decline during the adult years, such as some dimensions of memory and intelligence, now appear to be stable on average or even to improve in some individuals until the 60s or 70s (Schaie, 1995). Dementia, depression, and other serious disorders typically identified with later life affect only a minority of the population and are not intrinsic or universal aspects of the aging process. Rather than characterizing aging as a period of decline, research suggests that many older people maintain their abilities as well as developing new interests and accomplishments.

People are not just living longer, they are living better longer than ever before in human history. The prospect for successful aging, that is, for older people to lead healthy, active, and fulfilling lives, has become a real possibility. Improvements in disease prevention and health promotion, the widespread availability of public and private pensions and other financial benefits, and increased educational opportunities for each successive generation have markedly improved the lives of today's older population. The next cohorts of older people will have had better education and have taken better care of their health across the life span, so their prospect of a successful old age is even greater.

Successful aging is only part of the picture of later life. The increase in life expectancy means that people are more likely to live until their 70s, 80s, or even 90s, ages when a variety of chronic illnesses and disabilities become common. Along with unprecedented numbers of vital and active old people, we have had a dramatic increase in elders with significant mental and physical problems (e.g., S. Zarit, Johansson, & Malmberg, 1995). Their complex problems are costly for society and often overwhelming for their families. This duality of unprecedented numbers of successful agers and those with significant need is a key point for understanding old age.

Fortunately, timely and well-conceived clinical interventions can make a difference. Many older people retain a resilience and can respond positively to mental health interventions. A growing body of research documents the effectiveness of psychotherapy with older people and their families (Gatz et al., in press; Smyer, Zarit, & Qualls, 1990). For disorders such as depression, response to treatment may be as good for older as for younger people (Scogin & McElreath, 1994). Even when confronted with the most devastating problems in later life, such as Alzheimer's disease, clinicians can make interventions that dramatically improve the situation (e.g., Mittelman et al., 1995; Whitlatch, Zarit, & von Eye, 1991).

Older people themselves are increasingly turning to mental health professionals for help with their problems. In the past, clinicians often remarked that older people were not interested in psychotherapy. Indeed, when we first began our practices, we found that some older clients were reluctant or embarrassed to visit a psychologist. Increasingly, however, our older clients view psychotherapy positively. Some have been in treatment earlier in their lives and do not feel the stigma associated with seeing a therapist that typified previous generations. This trend is likely to increase with future generations. The cohort of people currently in their 40s and 50s who are now consulting us about their parents will have even fewer inhibitions about seeking out appropriate mental health treatment for themselves when they are past 65.

One other major factor in the growth of clinical practice with older people in the United States is the inclusion of outpatient mental health treatment in Medicare. When Medicare was first implemented in 1965, it paid only for inpatient psychiatric treatment. Beginning in the late 1980s, however, coverage was extended to mental health services in outpatient settings and in nursing homes and other institutional settings. Although Medicare reimburses outpatient mental health care differently than other medical problems (50% of usual costs are covered, compared to 80% for most other treatments), a major financial obstacle to seeking treatment has been reduced. Increasingly, older people and their families are taking advantage of the options for mental health treatment available to them.

PURPOSE AND PLAN FOR THIS BOOK

We have written this book for the student who is exploring geriatric mental health for the first time and for the experienced professional who wants to learn the specialized knowledge and skills that are needed for meeting the growing needs of an aging population. With knowledge in geriatric mental health rapidly expanding, we have chosen to emphasize some topics and not others. Our decisions were guided by two principles. First, we wanted to write a concise introduction that provides clinicians and students with the basic knowledge and framework necessary to begin practice with older adults. We could have gone into greater depth on many topics, but instead we have focused on presenting a basic foundation for each area while providing references for readers wishing to pursue an issue in greater depth. By organizing the book in this way, we believe we have created a concise and practical introduction to practice with older adults.

Second, we have been guided by the fact that clinical practice with older people is both similar to and different from practice with other adults. Clinicians need a combination of basic clinical skills and knowledge of the specific problems and contexts of aging. In this book, we emphasize the issues and topics that are different in geriatric practice, topics that are generally not covered in general clinical training.

What constitutes essential knowledge in geriatric practice? We believe the starting point for practice with older people to be recognition of the characteristics of the common disorders of aging. While assessment is important when working with people of any age, it takes on an even more central role in practice with older people. Given the negative stereotypes and expectations for older people, there is a tendency to mislabel potentially treatable problems as irreversible aspects of age or disease. Geriatric mental health specialists must be able to make sophisticated assessments of symptoms, which, in conjunction with medical assessments, help differentiate between mild, everyday problems and the more pathological processes due to disorders such as Alzheimer's disease.

The first part of the book addresses the assessment issue. Assessment begins with an understanding of the normal psychological processes of aging and the changes in intellectual functioning, memory, personality, and other areas that are usual and expected. Clinicians need to know what is normal in order to identify problems that represent pathological changes. In Chapter 2, we review current understanding of the normal aging process and provide a profile of healthy development in later life. We next review the problems and disorders of later life. Chapter 3 focuses on disorders that impair cognition—dementia and delirium—reviewing their symptoms, prevalence, and etiology. In Chapter 4, we focus on common psychiatric disorders, such as depression and anxiety disorders. We consider how prevalent these disorders are in late life and how they are different in symptoms and etiology from the same disorders in people of younger ages.

On this foundation in normal processes of aging and psychopathology, we then present a framework for assessment. Chapter 5 presents the types of clinical information necessary for conducting an assessment, with an emphasis on differentiating dementia from other disorders. This is the most common assessment question that is raised and one that must be clearly answered before developing a treatment plan. Chapter 6 continues the discussion of assessment, focusing on the role of psychological tests and the coordination of medical and psychosocial assessments. We conclude the discussion of assessment by reviewing determination of competency.

The second half of the book focuses on treatment. We have chosen to emphasize issues in treatment that are different or unique in practice with older people. Treatment of older people with mental health problems involves a multifaceted approach. Clinicians need to draw on basic skills of psychotherapy, coordinate psychological with psychiatric and other medical treatment, and intervene at different levels, that is, with patients, their families, and other people involved in their care and by modifying the environment.

We begin the discussion of treatment in Chapter 7 by exploring basic concepts and approaches that underlie successful treatment of older people and examining differences and similarities in treatment of older clients. Among the main differences are the need to take into account the effects of medical problems and medications on psychological functioning and the frequent involvement of family in both assessment and treatment. This framework is then applied in Chapter 8 to a discussion of treatment of late-life depression. Chapter 9 introduces another key element in treatment of older people; how and when to use community-based services to help disabled older people remain at home. These services are often an important part of the treatment of older people, supporting an older person's continued independence and providing relief to an overburdened family.

Chapter 10 turns to the problem of paranoid disorders in later life. Treatment is typically different than with younger paranoid patients. We discuss approaches that combine psychotherapy, medications, and the use of supportive services. Chapters 11 and 12 look at the treatment of dementia. In Chapter 11, we focus on treatment of patients and what can be done to reduce the disability associated with this devastating disorder. Chapter 12 examines the problems encountered by families caring for someone with dementia or another chronic physical or mental health problem. We discuss the stress they experience and show how treatment can be used to alleviate stress and allow patients and their families to function as well as possible in the face of a chronic disorder.

The final focus is on two special treatment issues: consultation in nursing homes and ethical issues. One of the most important settings for assessment and treatment of older people is nursing homes. Studies have found that a majority of residents in typical nursing homes have mental health problems that often go undetected and untreated (e.g., German, Shapiro, & Kramer, 1986; Burns et al., 1993; Shea, Streit, & Smyer, 1994). Increasingly, mental health professionals are being called on to consult in nursing homes and other institutional settings. In Chapter 13, we discuss the role of the mental health consultant in nursing homes and how clinicians can apply their knowledge of assessment and treatment to assist residents, their families, and staff. We conclude the book with a chapter on ethical issues in treatment. Ethical conduct is a basic principle in mental health practice and forms a core part of clinical training. When working with older adults, however, clinicians can encounter a variety of situations that are not typically covered in general discussions of ethics. Chapter 14 focuses on three major ethical concerns in practice with older adults: confidentiality, competency, and end-of-life issues.

We undoubtedly could have included many other topics in our discussion of treatment. A chapter focused on treatment of every disorder encountered in later life would have been possible, for example, but it would quickly have become repetitive. Instead, we provide a basic framework for treatment and in-depth discussion of the three disorders—depression, late-life paranoid disorders, and dementia—that form the heart of geriatric practice. We do not discuss treatment of anxiety disorders, because the approach to treatment of depression is similar and can be applied with some minor modifications. Similarly, we do not discuss every promising treatment approach. Apart from our focus on caregiving, we do not address family or couple therapy with older adults. We believe that clinicians with a background in couple and family treatment can make the transition to working with older clients as long as they understand some of the basic diagnostic and contextual issues involved in geriatric practice. On the other hand, working with family caregivers requires some concepts and approaches not likely to have been included in the clinician's prior training. We also do not emphasize group therapy, except for discussing the usefulness of support groups for caregivers and our preference to not use therapy groups in nursing homes. There is certainly room for discussion of the use of group therapy (see, e.g., the fine book on this topic by Toseland, 1990), but we generally believe it has a more restricted than general application for older people. In the end, we tried to be concise rather than comprehensive, providing clinicians with the basic building blocks for working effectively with older adults and their families in a variety of settings.

2

Normal Processes
of Aging

Aging has two faces. One shows decline and deterioration. The other shows fulfillment and the satisfaction of continued accomplishments. There are numerous examples of great artists and writers who remained productive into very late life. Goethe completed his epic drama *Faust* when he was 80. Verdi was also 80 when he composed his comic masterpiece *Falstaff*. Picasso continued to produce innovative drawings and sculpture into his 80s. With old age having become an attainable and even expected part of the life cycle, a successful and productive old age now falls within reach of most people.

To understand the aging process, it is important to recognize this duality of productivity and decline. Both characterize late life, and set in opposition to each other they illuminate key issues for mental health professionals. A focus on the disorders of aging is central to clinical practice, but it is important for clinicians to be familiar with the normal processes of aging. By appreciating normal processes of change, clinicians can better differentiate the mild changes in functioning that normally occur in later life from the more pervasive and severe changes associated with pathology. Furthermore, an understanding of normal aging processes serves as a foundation for treatment, which can build on an older person's resources and abilities. Timely treatment of late-life problems makes it possible to extend the period of productive and independent life while minimizing morbidity and decline at the end of life.

This chapter provides an introduction to normal processes of aging. We begin by reviewing briefly the demography of aging and characteristics of the older population. Using a life-span development perspective, we then examine the processes and changes with aging in key psychological dimensions, including intelligence, memory, and personality.

CHARACTERISTICS OF THE OLDER POPULATION

As we noted in Chapter 1, the older population has grown dramatically during the 20th century, rising from 4% of the population in the United States in 1900 to a current figure of 13.5% (Treas, 1995). The proportion of elderly is higher in several European countries than in the United States, including Sweden (16.9%), Norway (15.5%), the United Kingdom (15.1%), and the parts of Germany that formerly made up the German Federal Republic (14.5%) (Kinsella & Taeuber, 1993). If current population trends hold, the proportion of older people will continue to increase to between 17% and 20% of the population in the developed countries, even without further advances in life expectancy. Developing nations typically have a lower proportion of elderly because of higher birth and mortality rates, but projections are for the numbers of older people to increase more dramatically in these countries than in the developed nations.

Two converging trends have contributed to the growth of the older population: increasing life expectancy and decreasing birth rates. Life expectancy at birth rose in the United States from 47.3 years in 1900 to 75.5 years by 1993 (Treas, 1995). People who live to age 65 can actually expect to survive beyond these averages. Life expectancy is 17.3 years at age 65, 10.9 years at 75, and 6 years at 85 (Treas, 1995). When coupled with decreasing birth rates, these changes in life expectancy have dramatically altered the number of elderly and their proportion to the total population.

The changes in life expectancy are probably not due to extension of the life span, but rather to a greater proportion of people in a birth cohort surviving to old age. Maximum life expectancy has remained roughly the same during this century and is probably determined genetically. There has been, however, a dramatic reduction of mortality earlier in life. Better treatment of infectious disease and complications of childbirth for women, as well as improvements in public health, have made it possible for higher percentages of people to survive to old age (Crimmins, 1984; Treas, 1995). Thus, for the first time in human history, later life has become an expected rather than an exceptional part of the life span.

The older population can be described along several key dimensions, including the ratio of women to men, marital status, minority group membership, health and functioning, residential arrangements, economics, and distribution of various ages. Women, for example, live longer on average than men. Life expectancy for women in the United States is currently 79 years compared to 72 years for men (National Center for Health Statistics, 1993). This gender gap in life expectancy is found in virtually every country where data are available (Kinsella & Taeuber, 1993). As a result of their greater life expectancy, women outnumber men by a ratio of 3 to 2 among people over 65. By very late life, the proportion of women to men is even greater. By age 80 there are only about 43 men for every 100 women and by

90, the rate is 33 men for every 100 women (U.S. Bureau of the Census, 1992a).

These gender differences in life expectancy affect marriage rates. Because women live longer and also marry men who are on average four years older, they are more likely to be widowed in later life. According to the 1990 U.S. Census, 42% of older women but 77% of older men are married (U.S. Bureau of the Census, 1992b). Women are also less likely than men to remarry (Treas, 1995). When one person in a married couple becomes ill or disabled, the spouse is likely to take on caregiving responsibility. Being younger, on average, than their husbands, women more often take on this responsibility. Older women often outlive their husbands, so when they need assistance for themselves, they must depend on children or other relatives.

Another important distinction is race and ethnicity. Compared to whites, life expectancies at birth for African Americans in the United States are 8 fewer years for men and 6 fewer years for women. Much of this difference is due to higher mortality rates among African Americans earlier in life, but at age 65, the difference in remaining life expectancy is still 2 years (Treas, 1995). Hispanics also have lower life expectancies than whites, but Asian Americans have higher life expectancies. The number of minority elderly is expected to grow at a faster rate than the number of white elderly in the coming decades.

Contrary to expectations, the majority of elderly are in good health. Two-thirds of older people rate themselves in excellent or good health, and 75% report no or only minor functional limitations in the ability to carry out activities of daily life (Jette, 1996).

Rates of disability, however, increase with advancing age. The percentage of older people with any disabilities in activities of daily living rises from 4.2% for ages 55 to 64 to 50% for people aged 85 and older (Jette, 1996). Despite their longer life expectancy, women have higher rates of disabilities than men at all ages.

Consistent with these figures on disability, most older people live independently. In fact, only about 5% of the U.S. population over age 65 resides in nursing homes (Treas, 1995). Among noninstitutionalized elderly, over 80% live with a spouse or live alone (Treas, 1995). Approximately 10% of older people live with an adult child, although it should not be assumed that all these situations involve caregiving.

While the number of people in nursing homes at any one time is relatively small, the risk of spending some time in a nursing home during one's lifetime is great. Kemper and Murtaugh (1991), for example, have estimated that 43% of people who die after age 65 will have spent some time in a nursing home before death, and over half of them will have lived more than a year in a nursing home. Nursing homes are an important and often underserved setting for mental health needs of older people, a point to which we will return in subsequent chapters.

Poverty among older people was once endemic in the United States, but passage of Social Security in the 1930s and subsequent improvements both in that program and in private pensions has altered the economic status of the elderly considerably. The percentage of older people below the federal poverty level has been steadily dropping in recent decades, from 38% in 1960 to around 12.4% by 1990 (U.S. Bureau of the Census, 1992a). Another 7% are considered "near poor," that is, with income levels between 100% and 125% of federal poverty levels. Poverty rates declined sharply during the 1970s following indexing of Social Security benefits to the cost of living. This change has helped older people keep pace with inflation. Despite this overall success in reducing poverty, rates remain high in some segments of the minority elderly population, women, and the very old (over age 80).

A potential source of income for older people is employment. The proportion of employed older people has steadily decreased since the 1950s (Treas, 1995), but two factors may lead to a reversal of this trend. First, mandatory retirement was eliminated for most occupations in the 1980s. This change makes it easier for people who want to work for either personal or financial reasons to do so. Although most people welcome retirement, others find that part-time or even full-time employment is a more satisfying alternative. The second factor is smaller birth cohorts of younger generations, meaning that there will be shortages of people in some portions of the labor market. Economists are worried about the decreasing dependency ratio in the population, that is, the proportions of employed and not employed people in the population. With the retirement of the baby boomers, this ratio will reach an all-time low, so there will be fewer taxpayers supporting larger numbers of people receiving government benefits such as Social Security and Medicare. Continued work participation by older people could offset the expected economic strain.

One of the most important trends within the older population is the increase in the segment of the population known as the "old old." This group is variously defined as people over 75, over 80, or over 85. The number of people age 75 and older, and particularly those 85 and older, have been increasing proportionally much faster than the rest of the population (U.S. Bureau of the Census, 1992a). These trends are expected to continue. Currently, 5% of older people in the United States are 75 and older, and this figure is expected to increase to 9% by the year 2025. Similarly, while people over 85 are currently about 2.5% of the population, they will increase to about 5% by 2025. In Sweden, which has a somewhat older population than the United States, nearly 5% are currently over 85.

Neugarten (1974) originally developed the terms "young old" and "old old" to call attention to the dramatic changes occurring in the functioning of the older population. The term "young old" denoted that many elderly lead independent and active lives that differ little from the lives of the middle aged. Their active life styles and experiences contrast dramatically to negative expectations of the elderly as dependent and in need of assistance. However, at advanced ages, rates of illness and disability increase considerably.

These trends have spawned a controversy about the significance of improved health and increased life expectancy in today's older population. Taking an optimistic perspective, Fries (1983) has proposed that factors contributing to increased life expectancy—better health care and improved nutrition and exercise—have also led to a compression of morbidity at the end of life. Fries argues that maximum life expectancy probably has fixed genetic limits, so prolonging the period of active healthy life also causes a contraction in the time of illness and decline at the end of life. Other researchers have taken the position that both life expectancy and morbidity are increasing (e.g., Verbrugge, 1984). In other words, people have a longer, healthy life *and* a protracted period of disability at the end of life. This debate has critical implications for the amount of health care and other supportive services that will be needed for the older population, particularly as the number of oldest old grows.

Regardless of how this debate turns out, it has become increasingly likely that people will have some period of morbidity before death. In the past, the main causes of death were infectious and other acute diseases. People were typically sick for short periods of time before dying. With better control of these acute illnesses, death is now more likely to be caused by chronic conditions that have persisted for many years and are associated with disability. It has been estimated, for example, that a 70-year-old who is independent can expect to live another 13.4 years, of which 10.1 will be independent and 3.3 dependent (Rogers, Rogers, & Belanger, 1989). An active 80-year-old has a life expectancy of 8.1 years, 5.2 years of which will be independent.

These findings on independent and dependent life expectancies bring us back to our characterization of the two faces of aging. Unprecedented numbers of healthy older people live independent and fulfilling lives. Older people are healthier, wealthier, and better educated than any previous generation, and these trends will continue for the foreseeable future. At the same time, the number of disabled elderly is increasing, and their need for care is placing considerable strain on society's resources.

LIFE-SPAN DEVELOPMENTAL PERSPECTIVE ON AGING

We now turn to an examination of psychological changes that occur with aging. We begin this section by examining some general concepts that are important for understanding the aging process and different methodologies used for studying aging. We then consider three central areas of psychological functioning: intelligence, memory, and personality.

A life-span developmental perspective involves a view of the aging process that helps us understand the normal changes that occur with aging (e.g., P. Baltes, 1987, 1997). From this perspective, aging is the interaction of biological, psychological, and social processes, which can have multiple effects on development. While decline occurs in some functions, growth and/or compensation can take place in other areas that enables the individual to function adequately (P. Baltes, 1997; Salthouse, 1990). Furthermore, there can be differences in the pattern and amounts of intra- and interindividual change. Intraindividual change means that a person can show stability in a particular ability while declining in another. Interindividual differences refer to variations among people in the rate and timing of change. For the clinician, this means that aging is not associated with a universal pattern of global decline. Some abilities are more likely to be affected than others, and the rates of change differ between individuals, as some people are able to delay or compensate for age-related declines.

As we grow older, we gradually experience increasing limits on our intellectual and physical performance. These limits, however, may not be important in everyday life and may not interfere with functioning. To understand the nature of these limits, P. Baltes (1987) has used the example of evaluating people while walking and running. If we compare an older and younger person walking, we will find few or no differences. By contrast, younger people can run faster and further than older people. The effects of aging, then, are not typically apparent in performing ordinary tasks, but there is a decrease in the individual's reserve capacity, so limitations become apparent under highly stressful or demanding conditions. This finding is true of intellectual abilities as well as physical performance (P. Baltes & Kliegl, 1992).

Two other propositions in a life-span developmental approach are particularly relevant for clinicians: the potential for continued growth in later life and the potential for compensation (P. Baltes, 1987). Growth in abilities in later life has been demonstrated by numerous training studies. As we will see, the results of these training studies suggest considerable plasticity in intellectual performance in later life.

A related process is the ability of older people to compensate for age-related declines in abilities. According to P. Baltes (1987), older people are able to maintain their level of performance in certain valued areas of functioning in their lives despite declines in some of the underlying cognitive abilities that contribute to performance. They do so by drawing on other cognitive resources or abilities that are not affected by the aging process. Baltes calls this process "selective optimization with compensation." One of the best examples of compensation is found in studies of expert typists

(Salthouse, 1984). In these studies, older typists were able to perform as rapidly and accurately as younger individuals, despite experiencing a slowing in reaction time, which is one of the most robust changes with aging. They compensated for slowing, however, by anticipating upcoming words in the text better than younger typists. This example suggests that older people may be able to maintain performance in valued areas of their lives by drawing on experience and abilities, such as verbal skills, that remain relatively intact with aging. The high level of expert performance maintained by older people in activities such as music, chess, and business may be due to similar compensation processes. This ability to compensate, combined with continued potential for growth in later life, means that older people can sustain performance in valued activities and can respond to treatment to help them overcome losses.

We use this framework in the following sections to examine the relation of age to the three areas of psychological functioning most relevant to clinicians: intelligence, memory and personality. Before doing so, however, it is important to consider briefly some of the methodological problems involved in studying aging, because issues such as the design of research studies affect the conclusions we make about the aging process.

Studying the Aging Process

In many ways, late life is more complicated to study than any other developmental period. The reason for this complexity is that in studying aging, we are typically trying to make comparisons over long periods of time. A developmental study of children might focus on the patterns of changes from age 2 to age 4. Following a group of children over 2 years is a relatively manageable research task to. When we study aging, however, we are often interested in making comparisons over much longer time periods. If we want to ask how aging has affected a group of 70-year-olds, for example, we are interested in comparing their current abilities with what they were like 30 or 40 years earlier. Conducting research that spans the whole of adulthood is beyond the capability of most people, though a few unique studies have done just that (e.g., Schaie, 1995; Vaillant & Vaillant, 1990).

Three research designs are primarily used in the study of aging: cross-sectional, longitudinal, and sequential. Cross-sectional designs are by far the most frequent approach. In a cross-sectional study younger and older individuals are compared to each other and the differences that emerge are assumed to be due to the effects of the aging process. Cross-sectional studies are useful particularly for exploratory research or for descriptive studies of the older population, but inherent problems in this approach suggest that results should be interpreted with caution.

The main problem with cross-sectional research is that differences between old and young may be due to other factors besides aging. Samples may not be similar in education (both number of years and quality of education) or some artifact in the research may account for the differences—for example, the younger sample may be college students who are familiar with tests and testing procedures, while older subjects experience more anxiety because of their lack of familiarity with the setting and procedures. Schaie (1967) has proposed the useful distinction between age differences and age changes. Age differences are any differences found between young and old, and may be the result of aging or of some other factors. In contrast, age changes are differences between young and old specifically due to the aging process. Cross-sectional comparisons identify age differences but do not provide sufficient information to differentiate when those differences are due to aging or to other factors.

As an alternative to cross-sectional research, longitudinal studies that follow the same people over time provide a better estimate of changes associated with aging compared to other factors. But longitudinal studies have their limitations as well. As noted already, it is very difficult to conduct studies that cover the full range of adulthood and old age. Another problem is selective attrition; people who are less able or are experiencing more decline are more likely to drop out of a longitudinal study. There can also be cohort or "generational" effects, that is, the particular cohort under investigation has a unique developmental pattern because of early life experiences or unique historical events that affected their experience. As an example, the Great Depression of the 1930s and U.S. entry into World War II have been found to have long-term influences, such as disrupted work histories and poorer health in some individuals (e.g., Elder, Shanahan, & Clipp, 1994).

Because of these limitations of longitudinal studies, Schaie (1967; Schaie & Willis, 1996) has proposed sequential research strategies, including a cohort sequential design in which several cohorts are followed over time. Using this type of approach allows for a better differentiation of cohort, historical, and age effects. For example, if two age groups (50-year-olds and 60-year-olds) differ on some ability at the initial time of measurement, and if these differences remain about the same at subsequent testing 5 and 10 years later, the pattern of results suggests a cohort difference. Period effects can be identified by comparing two or more cohorts over the same age period. For example, in the transition from age 40 to age 50, one cohort might demonstrate a high rate of midlife changes, but another generation will have a low rate in response to changed economic conditions. Age changes are identified when two or more cohorts show similar patterns of change during the same age period, for example, from age 40 to age 50. Schaie also proposes assessing the influence of attrition by drawing new, independent samples from each cohort being followed (see Schaie & Willis, 1996, for a complete discussion of various design strategies for studying development).

Due to the cost and other logistic problems of longitudinal and sequential studies, most research on aging remains cross-sectional. Nonetheless, it is important to keep in mind the limitations of cross-sectional studies. As we shall see, findings from longitudinal and sequential investigations provide a very different picture of the effects of aging than do findings from cross-sectional studies; they provide evidence for greater stability of functioning.

Intelligence and Aging

"Does intelligence change with aging?" is a key question for understanding the aging process. Can we expect older people to function competently across a range of situations, or do they lose the ability to perform some activities adequately? Should we gradually take over decision making for our parents or other older relatives in important areas, such as management of their finances or decisions about where to live, or do older people remain capable of making complex judgments themselves? While it is clear that people suffering from Alzheimer's disease and other dementing illnesses lose their ability to manage their affairs competently, what about an older person not suffering from dementia?

Regular and expected changes in the brain occur as part of the normal aging process (Scheibel, 1996). As a consequence, corresponding changes in cognitive functions can be logically expected. Historically, studies of intelligence and aging using cross-sectional research designs have reported considerable differences between old and young.

The most frequent characterization of age differences in intelligence is based on the verbal–performance split originally proposed by Wechsler (1958). Using cross-sectional data on adults who took the original or the revised Wechsler Adult Intelligence Scale (WAIS and WAIS-R), Wechsler and others (e.g., Matarozzo, 1972) have found that verbal abilities, such as vocabulary and information, are maintained relatively well in later life, while scores on performance tests, such as block design, show decline. Evidence for decline is found quite early in life (late teens or early 20s) and then continues across the adult years.

Horn and Cattell (1967; Horn, 1982) proposed that this pattern of functioning is the result of varying contributions of biological factors to verbal and performance tests. Specifically, they hypothesize that verbal tests are indicators of crystallized intelligence, reflecting knowledge that was previously acquired through education and experience. Performance tests, in turn, are considered fluid abilities that require the individual to respond in novel ways and thus are less dependent on past education and more strongly reflect underlying biological processes. P. Baltes (1987) has proposed a similar distinction between the pragmatics and mechanics of intelligence.

Pragmatics is the knowledge learned or gained with experience, while mechanics represents the underlying structure or abilities.

The verbal–performance split can be interpreted in other ways as well. From a neuropsychological perspective, lower scores on performance subscales is generally associated with right hemisphere damage. Studies of the aging brain, however, have not indicated any selective loss or damage to the right hemisphere (Scheibel, 1996). An alternate hypothesis is that verbal and performance tests vary in their degree of difficulty. Verbal tasks use relatively familiar stimuli and so pose less of a challenge to older people. The more novel performance tasks place a greater challenge on the neural resources of older people, in effect, testing the limits of performance, and result in lower scores (S. Zarit, Eiler, & Hassinger, 1985).

Another hypothesis concerns the role of speed in the performance subtests. These tests are timed, and some scales (block design, picture arrangement, object assembly) include bonus points for completing them more rapidly. In contrast, only the arithmetic subscale among the verbal tests on the WAIS has a time factor. Because reaction time is known to decline over the adult years, speed of performance may account for the verbal–performance difference. To test this hypothesis, Storandt (1977) gave the WAIS to older adults under conditions in which they had as much time as necessary to complete the performance subtests. Even when using this method, however, older people scored lower than younger individuals. It has been argued that speeded performance is an integral part of intellectual ability, although this point remains controversial (Schaie, 1990).

P. Baltes and Lindenberger (1997) have examined the role of sensory loss in intellectual functioning. They found that visual and auditory acuity were associated with decline in intelligence, particularly for fluid abilities. This link suggests a common mechanism, whereby decline in brain functioning affects both sensory abilities and cognitive processes. An alternative explanation, however, is that sensory decline makes perception more difficult, leading to an overload of attentional processes and, as a consequence, poorer performance on cognitive tasks. Whatever the mechanism, sensory loss is an important dimension to consider when evaluating functioning of older people.

In contrast to these findings, longitudinal and sequential studies paint a somewhat different picture of changes in intelligence (e.g., Cunningham & Owens, 1983; Siegler, 1983; Schaie, 1995). Principal among these investigations is the Seattle Longitudinal Study, conducted by Schaie and his associates (e.g., Schaie, 1983, 1989, 1995; Schaie & Hertzog, 1986). Initiated in 1957, this study uses a cohort-sequential design, in which a large number of individuals from different generations are followed over time. Cohorts have been added as the study has proceeded. Participants have been tested at 7-year intervals. Thurstone's Primary Mental Abilities Test (PMA) (Thurstone

& Thurstone, 1949; Schaie, 1985) was used in this study. The five components of the PMA are verbal meaning, spatial orientation, inductive reasoning, number ability, and word fluency. In contrast to the WAIS, where subtests have a complex factor structure, that is, performance is based on a combination of abilities, the PMA was designed so that component tests measure single factors or dimensions of intellectual ability. Higher-order factors corresponding to fluid and crystallized dimensions have also been found (Schaie, 1995).

Because of its cohort-sequential design, the Seattle Longitudinal Study can be used to compare people at different ages at the same time, such as would be done in cross-sectional research, or to follow people over time. Cross-sectional analyses show a similar pattern to other cross-sectional studies. Intellectual abilities peak early in the adult years and then decline. A very different picture emerges, however, from the longitudinal data. When individuals are viewed over time, intellectual ability increases into the 30s or 40s, is stable into the mid-50s or 60s, and then shows a gradual decline. Word fluency and number ability show small decrements between testing intervals beginning at age 53, and declines on other tests appear after age 60 (Schaie, 1995).

Why do the cross-sectional and longitudinal findings differ so much? Two factors are involved. First, there have been differences among generations in levels of initial ability on intellectual functions. A comparison among generations shows that more recent cohorts have done better on tests of verbal meaning, spatial orientation, and inductive reasoning. Number ability also improved in successive cohorts born up to 1945 but has been decreasing in later cohorts. The fifth PMA test, word fluency, shows no generational differences. Following cohorts over time confirms that these differences between old and young are generational. As they age, younger cohorts do not decline to the level of older cohorts; rather, they maintain their initial advantage. Thus, a cross-sectional comparison between old and young reflects, in part, differences in initial ability between generations.

The other factor to be considered in these findings is selective attrition. People who return for repeated testing in a longitudinal study are likely to have better functioning initially and to be less likely to experience a decline over time. Even after adjusting for this bias in the findings, however, cohort differences remain a much more important factor than age until the decade of the 60s or later (Schaie, 1995).

Although the Seattle Longitudinal Study shows evidence of decline after age 60, the pattern is complex. Even after 60, over 60% of participants were stable or had improved performance between assessments. The proportion of people showing a decline increases with advancing age, but even after 80, a majority of participants had stable scores between testing intervals. Additionally, when decline occurs, it is most likely to be found for one or two abilities rather than across all tests.

Another factor that may influence the relation of aging to intellectual performance is the extent to which decline is due to disuse of intellectual abilities or to other potentially reversible sources of decline. One of the most intriguing studies to use this approach was conducted by Willis, Blieszner, and Baltes (1981), who trained people in the performance of tasks of fluid intelligence. As noted earlier, these tasks are regarded as measuring biological capabilities for performance and usually show the largest age differences. Nonetheless, training resulted in improved performance. A long-term follow-up of participants revealed that training gains were maintained over time (Willis & Nesselroade, 1990). Now in their 70s and 80s, participants had higher levels of performance 7 years after cognitive training than they had at baseline.

Perhaps the most dramatic demonstration of the possibility of gains through training was a study conducted by Schaie and Willis (1986), which used subjects from the Seattle Longitudinal Study. In this investigation, people who had declined in functioning during the previous 14 years on either verbal meaning or spatial orientation were given training in that ability. The results indicated that many people were subsequently able to perform at or near previous levels on those abilities.

Several conclusions can be drawn from these studies of intelligence. Changes in intellectual performance with aging have been demonstrated, but, except for speeded tests, average declines occur relatively late in the adult years (50s or 60s). Even at advanced ages, however, there are considerable individual differences in the timing and rate of decline. Differences in performance among generations have contributed to somewhat inflated estimates of intellectual decline in later life in results from cross-sectional studies. Tasks that cause more difficulties for older adults typically involve novel or unfamiliar procedures. At least part of this disadvantage can be offset by training. These findings, of course, reflect functioning of relatively healthy individuals and do not take into account the catastrophic changes in intelligence that occur with dementia.

At a functional level, the changes associated with aging probably do not affect performance of familiar activities. Competency to perform many complicated intellectual activities in everyday life show little decline with aging (Salthouse, 1990). Age effects will be more apparent, however, when facing new or overwhelming challenges, especially at older ages (75 and older).

Finally, some individuals develop higher order conceptual skills as they age, or what is popularly termed "wisdom." Although wisdom is not a universal or normative outcome among the elderly (or in any other age group, for that matter), it represents one possible pattern of successful aging.

Memory and Aging

An older client reports having forgotten an appointment and worries, "Am I getting senile?" A colleague misplaces his glasses and says, "I must be getting old." A busy working woman stops at the grocery on the way home to pick up some items but forgets one thing she wanted to buy. She wonders if the loss of memory that happened to her grandmother is beginning to show up in her.

These examples of forgetting are very common, everyday occurrences. As people grow older, these experiences are frequently attributed to aging or the onset of dementia. Memory impairment is the hallmark symptom in dementia, and the tendency to equate senility and aging undoubtedly contributes to the expectation of decline. Healthy older people, that is, individuals without evidence of dementia or other disorders that impair cognitive functioning, also experience changes in memory, though these changes are more subtle and benign than found in dementia. Concern about failing memory is a frequent complaint in clinical settings, and the practitioner needs to be able to differentiate the mild changes typical of normal aging from more severe and persistent problems associated with dementing illnesses. An understanding of the normal and expected changes in memory with aging can be helpful both for differential diagnosis and for helping healthy older clients view their occasional lapses in memory as a minor irritant rather than a signal of impending deterioration.

There is extensive research on memory and aging, and, as in most areas of research, findings are sometimes complex and contradictory. Compared to intelligence testing, which has its origins in psychometric traditions, memory research is based primarily on experimental laboratory paradigms. This tradition affects estimates of changes in memory with aging in two critical ways. First, until relatively recently, there has been little attention to the relevance of laboratory-based procedures for everyday functioning. It was thus difficult to determine what significance, if any, was associated with age differences in performance. Use of ecologically valid test stimuli and attention to real-world tasks is now becoming more frequent (see, e.g., Poon, Rubin, & Wilson, 1989). The second consequence is the almost exclusive reliance on cross-sectional designs to examine age-associated changes. This preference is especially surprising, since memory lends itself to longitudinal investigation. Many of the questions in the current literature about the magnitude, pattern, and etiology of age-associated decrements could be addressed by examining intraindividual differences in performance over time.

Most memory research over the past 20 years has been guided by an information-processing model, which replaced older, stimulus–response approaches (Smith, 1996). From this perspective, memory is a series of interrelated systems involved in processing information: sensory memory, short-term memory, and long-term memory. Sensory memory refers to a brief holding system, which can by illustrated by the short-lived afterimage that forms after presentation of a visual image. Short-term memory comprises two related processes: primary memory and working memory. Primary memory refers to memory span, that is, the amount of information that can be actively attended to at any given time. An example of primary memory is repeating a seven-digit phone number immediately after presentation. Working memory involves the simultaneous processing and storage of information from primary memory (Baddeley, 1992). Attentional processes are a central part of working memory, and their disruption in disorders such as Alzheimer's disease may be a major source of patients' memory problems.

Information that is to be retained over a longer time must be converted from working memory into some type of permanent storage and then later retrieved. This process of storage and retrieval is long-term memory. Storage of information can be effortful or incidental, that is, the person may deliberately try to learn information for later retrieval, or the person acquires information without any deliberate effort.

Long-term memory is further divided into episodic, semantic, and procedural systems. Episodic memory describes what most people think of first as memory, the ability to remember a specific event. Semantic memory involves recall of words, meaning, and grammar. Procedural memory refers to recall of motor learning, how to perform a series of actions. Remembering how to ride a bicycle is an example of procedural memory. These distinctions reflect differences in neural organization and storage of these types of information. Most research on age differences has involved episodic memory, particularly, recall of verbal material. Attention to semantic and procedural memory, however, may be useful both in differentiating types of pathology and in planning strategies to minimize the effects of deficits. As an example, both episodic and semantic memory are affected in Alzheimer's disease, but procedural memory may be relatively unimpaired, at least early in the disease. Conversely, patients with a vascular dementia may have significant apraxias (not knowing how to do something) as an early symptom when their semantic memory is still intact.

Forgetting can occur at any point in this process. Information may fail to register on the senses, may not be processed in working memory, may not enter storage, or may decay in storage, or there may be a failure in retrieval. Much of the research on aging has searched for the main locus or source of age differences in memory, though this task has proven difficult and there probably is not one simple answer to the question of how memory changes with age (Smith, 1996).

Deficits in the brief holding system that constitute sensory memory increase with age (e.g., Walsh, Till, & Williams, 1978; Parkinson & Perey, 1980). The functional significance of this change, however, is generally considered to be minimal. Sensory memory should be distinguished from sensory functioning, that is, the integrity of sensory systems, such as vision and hearing. Deficits in senses make it more difficult for people to learn and remember because information is not perceived or is perceived inaccurately at input.

Turning to short-term memory, no age differences are generally reported for primary memory (memory span). Deficits in working memory, however, are found both in normal aging and in dementia. As examples, older people are at a disadvantage if they have to process some information while also remembering other material for a subsequent task or when they are asked to process simultaneous or competing input (e.g., Salthouse, 1994a). This distinction is best illustrated by the digit span forward and backward tasks from the WAIS. No age differences are found in digits forward, a simple task that requires minimal manipulation of the material. Digit span backward, by contrast, requires an active manipulation of the input, and marked age differences in performance are found. Age differences in working memory can be brought out when a great deal of information is presented, when the material is complex, or when subjects are required to manipulate the information in some way (Salthouse, 1994b; Salthouse & Babcock, 1991).

Age differences have been consistently found in long-term memory for a variety of task such as word pairs, word lists, and recall of text. In a classic study, Schonfield and Robertson (1966) compared performance of old and young on a word list under conditions of both free recall and recognition (i.e., choosing the correct word from among alternatives). They found age differences in recall but not in recognition, and argued that this pattern of performance suggested that older people have decrements in retrieval but not in acquisition of new information.

Subsequent research has provided inconsistent support for this hypothesis. McNulty and Caird (1966) proposed an alternative explanation to Schonfield and Robertson's proposal of a retrieval deficit. They suggested that this pattern of results could be due to differences in how well the material is learned at acquisition. If material is learned less thoroughly or adequately in the first place, it may be possible to recognize correct answers based on the partial memory traces that were formed. Students who prepare differently for multiple choice or essay examinations will immediately recognize this distinction. Whatever the primary reason for these differences, the practical implication is that older people's performance is better on recognition rather than recall tasks. This observation can be used in designing tasks to assist individuals with mild memory impairments.

The difference in performance of older people on recognition and recall tasks may reflect a larger issue, that cognitive resources necessary for processing information decline with aging. According to Craik (1994), age differences are more pronounced on tasks that provide fewer cues during learning and retrieval, or what he calls "environmental support." A recognition task provides more support, so older people perform relatively better.

Similarly, when learning a list of words, the learner receives more support when the words are grouped into categories. Older people are also less likely to provide their own supports, such as by placing words into categories or using other types of mnemonic devices (Hultsch, 1971; Witte, Freund, & Brown-Whistler, 1993). A resource deficit is also suggested by the finding that older people have more difficulty with memory tasks that require deliberate effort, such as memorizing a list of words. By contrast, they do relatively well in situations involving automatic processing, for example, remembering words that they have read but have not been told to memorize (e.g., Hasher & Zacks, 1979). Finally, increasing the complexity of the memory task places older people at a greater disadvantage (Salthouse, Babcock, & Shaw, 1991).

Speed of processing is another important source of age differences. Older people do more poorly when stimuli are presented faster or when the period allowed for recall is shorter (Salthouse, 1994a, 1994b). By controlling the speed of presentation of material and reducing time pressure for responses, age differences in memory performance are greatly reduced. Distractions also have a greater impact on older than younger people.

There have been relatively few studies of very old memories, that is, recall of events from the distant past. This is an interesting area because it corresponds to people's own conceptions of memory. Older people recall historical events as well or better than younger people (e.g., Botwinick & Storandt, 1974; Perlmutter, 1978), perhaps because they may have had greater exposure to the information in the first place. Lachman and Lachman (1980) explored recall of well-known political and entertainment figures. Older and younger subjects were asked questions with identifying information about these famous people. If subjects could not recall a name, they were asked if they had a tip-of-the-tongue response, that is, if they felt they knew the answer but could not recall it right then. When they felt they knew the answer, both older and younger subjects could pick out the correct name most of the time from a multiple choice response format. Older people had more tip-of-the-tongue responses than younger individuals, but they also had a larger total amount of knowledge. Based on these findings, Lachman and Lachman suggest that older people's efficiency in recalling old information was probably as good as younger people's, taking into account the fact that the older group had a larger store of information to sort through.

One of the most important areas of memory for clinicians is what older people say about their own abilities. This aspect of memory has been called "metamemory" and comprises people's knowledge and appraisal of memory. Consistent with findings on age differences in memory, older people report more problems and concerns about their memory (Collins & Abeles, 1996; Zelinski & Gilewski, 1988). What people say about their memory, however, may not be a reliable indicator of deficits. In samples of healthy people not suffering from dementia, the association of subjective evaluations of memory and actual performance is modest. Some people who complain about failing memory actually perform at high levels, while some who report very few problems perform at low levels. One problem in these studies is that they are cross-sectional, that is, older people evaluating their memory are making a comparison with how they functioned in the past, but the researcher has available only tests of current performance. In one of the few longitudinal studies of self-evaluations of memory (Johansson, Allen-Burge, & Zarit, 1997), a somewhat different picture emerged. In that study, how people rated their memory had a small but significant relation to how they functioned at previous assessments and how they performed in the future. People who rated their memory worse had slightly lower performance than two years earlier. They were also more likely to decline over the next two years. Subjective evaluations, however, were not a strong predictor of decline, and there was considerable overlap in objective test performance between people complaining of failing memory and those who did not.

Two other factors, depression and dementia, affect what people say about their memory. Depression is generally associated with overly negative appraisals of one's self and one's abilities. Among older people and, indeed, among some younger clients we have worked with, these negative appraisals include memory. The complaints of failing memory have usually been found to correlate with depression and not with actual deficits in memory performance (Collins & Abeles, 1996; Johansson et al., 1997; Kahn, Zarit, Hilbert, & Niederehe, 1975; Niederehe & Yoder, 1989; Zelinski & Gilewski, 1988). In dementia, there is a paradoxical relation between memory complaints and performance. People suffering from mild dementia are more likely to be aware of and to complain about failing memory, while those with more severe deficits often maintain that they have little or no trouble with memory (Johansson et al., 1997; Kaszniak, 1996; Kahn et al., 1975).

What people say about their memory is an important but not consistently reliable indicator of actual performance. The widely held expectation that memory declines with aging and growing fears about getting Alzheimer's disease make older people more sensitive about everyday instances of forgetting. They forgot names and misplaced keys in the past but did not dwell on these incidents. Now that they are older, the same events are interpreted as a sign of decline. We will return to this issue of subjective evaluations of memory when discussing clinical assessment (Chapter 5).

The nature and extent of memory changes with aging can be clarified by training older people in memory skills. Improvement of performance with training suggests that at least part of the deficit found in aging is due to reversible factors. A variety of memory training strategies have been tried, such as organizing a list of words into categories or employing a visual association strategy to link words in a list, with generally positive results (Floyd & Scogin, 1996; Meyer, Young, & Barlett, 1989; Yesavage, 1983; Hill, Sheikh, & Yesavage, 1988). Yesavage and his colleagues (1983; Yesavage & Jacob, 1984) have conducted an interesting set of experiments that suggest that combining relaxation training with instruction in mnemonic strategies has a better outcome than using either approach separately.

The most intriguing training studies have been conducted by Paul Baltes and his colleagues (e.g., P. Baltes, 1987; P. Baltes & Kliegl, 1992; Kliegl, Smith, & Baltes, 1989; Staudinger, Marsiske, & Baltes, 1995). These studies used a testing-the-limits approach that makes it possible to examine the extent of plasticity or potential for improvement among older people as well as limits imposed by the aging process. Young and old subjects learned to use a classic mnemonic approach, the method of loci, in which new material is associated with a familiar place or location. They then were asked to apply this approach to learning lists of digits and nouns. Both young and old were able to learn very long lists. When the learning conditions were made more difficult, however, such as increasing the pace of presentation of new items, younger individuals had a distinct advantage. These studies suggest both considerable plasticity in memory ability for older people—that is, they can apply cognitive resources to improve performance—and that aging also sets some limits to performance under more stressful or demanding conditions.

Memory is an important area because of its practical implications for everyday life and because memory loss is the most prominent symptom in dementia. Memory changes somewhat with aging, so healthy older people should expect not to remember a word or name or to have to take more time to learn new information. Older people can also take a variety of practical steps to improve their memory, for example, organizing information to be learned, using mnemonics, preventing distractions when learning new material, and giving themselves more time to learn and recall material.

Personality and Aging

Do we change as we age in the very core of who we are? Does our sense of self and the various traits, motives, and dispositions toward behavior and emotion change in predictable ways? Historically, aging has been associated with a variety of negative characteristics—irritability, rigidity, reactionary political and social attitudes, and self-centeredness. Competing models of personality have resulted in conflicting perspectives on the question of stability versus change with age, but most research is in agreement on a central point: in the absence of catastrophic illness like the dementing disorders, personality deterioration is not an inevitable or even common consequence of aging.

Before turning to research findings, it is worth commenting on why negative stereotypes have dominated thinking about aging, especially in Western countries. Several factors have probably contributed. First is the confusion of aging and disease. With dementia or other severe health problems, personality can deteriorate. A second factor is a failure to differentiate lifelong characteristics from the effects of aging. People with personality disorders grow older and do not generally become more pleasant or easier to deal with. Because of negative expectations about aging, their behavior may be attributed to old age rather than a lifelong pattern. Finally, Western culture prizes innovation and change. In periods of rapid social and technological change, older people may in fact be more disadvantaged and thus are perceived as old-fashioned or as blocking progress.

Early personality research usually focused on single traits hypothesized to change with age, such as rigidity, cautiousness, and defensiveness. These studies were cross-sectional and sometimes used samples of convenience, such as residents of nursing homes. More careful investigation, including longitudinal studies, have suggested that intellectual ability and generational factors play an important role in these traits. Data from the Seattle Longitudinal Study (Schaie & Labouvie-Vief, 1974) were used to examine three dimensions of behavioral rigidity: (1) motor–cognitive, (2) personality–perceptual, and (3) psychomotor speed. Cross-sectional analysis found large differences between young and old on these dimensions. In longitudinal analyses, however, only psychomotor speed showed a clear pattern of decline across the adult years. Both motor–cognitive and personality–perceptual rigidity were relatively stable, although with some evidence of decline (increased rigidity) in the oldest groups.

Older people are more cautious in test-taking style and in making personal decisions (Botwinick, 1984). On tests, they are less likely to guess than younger individuals when they are uncertain about the correct answer and, as a result, make more errors of omission. These findings have implications for testing of intelligence and other cognitive abilities, namely, that a cautious response style may lead to underestimation of performance. By changing instructions so that older people are encouraged to guess (Birkhill & Schaie, 1975) or increasing the incentives for guessing (Okun & Elias, 1977), performance is improved.

Botwinick (1966, 1969) explored willingness to take risks in response to hypothetical scenarios, such as changing jobs. As with test-taking style, differences were found in levels of cautiousness between younger and older people, with much of the difference due to the fact that more older subjects chose not to take any risk at all, even when the probability of success was high. When the task was modified so that the no-risk option was not available, age differences were eliminated. Interestingly, when older people were asked to make recommendations about a decision faced by a younger or older person, they gave cautious advice only to the young (Botwinick, 1966).

Over the past several years, findings from longitudinal studies of personality using multitrait approaches have been reported (e.g., Costa & McCrae, 1988; Haan, Millsap, & Hartka, 1986; Helson & Moane, 1987; Siegler, George & Okun, 1979). Despite differences in methods and time intervals between measurements, these studies reported considerable stability. The most extensive evidence of stability is found in the work of Costa and McCrae (1988; McCrae & Costa, 1984). Using factor analysis of personality measures, Costa and McCrae have developed a five-factor model of personality: Neuroticism, extroversion, openness to experience, agreeableness, and conscientiousness (Costa & McCrae, 1988). Findings suggest stability over time both for ratings of one's self and for ratings made by spouses.

Additional support for this position has come from behavioral genetics studies which compare twins reared together and those who were separated early in life (Plomin, Pedersen, McClearn, Nesselroade, & Bergeman, 1988). These studies have found strong genetic influences on factors similar to those measured by Costa and McCrae: emotionality, activity level and sociability. These dimensions also appear stable over time. It should also be noted that environmental factors and environmental–genetic interactions have an important influence on these dimensions.

Other studies have suggested that expression of emotions may change somewhat with aging. Specifically, both positive and negative feelings may be less intense (Filipp, 1996). This change may be the result of decreased arousal or of better control of emotions with aging. Evidence also suggests that the emotional system remains intact and that older people are able to identify and express emotions.

In contrast to these findings of stability, personality theorists have proposed models of adulthood characterized by qualitatively distinct stages (Erikson, 1950; Erikson, Erikson, & Kivnick, 1986; Jung, 1933; Levinson, 1986; Loevinger, 1976). Erikson's notion that later life involves the dichotomy of integrity–despair has probably gained more acceptance than any other theoretical proposition. Though this concept is inherently appealing, it is probably too simplistic to capture the developmental issues of later life, given the diversity of the older population and the large span of years involved (e.g., 65 to 95 or older). Clinicians should be cautioned about applying integrity–despair as a normative model of aging and about using it as a framework for successful adaptation. Undoubtedly, a sense of integrity is important in later life, as well as at other ages, but we need more careful empirical study to identify universal and normative psychological tasks in later life.

Differences in how researchers have studied personality may in part account for the controversy over stability or change. Research using measures of traits and temperament have tended to demonstrate stability. In contrast, advocates of change models have relied on clinical and/or in-depth structured research interviews (e.g., Levinson, 1986). Several proposals have been made to reconcile these positions. Lachman (1989), for example, suggests that while generalized traits and attitudes are stable with aging, domain-specific attitudes (e.g., feelings of control over health) as well as intrapsychic style (e.g., coping, mastery, defenses) may be more likely to change. Another approach has been to apply Bem and Allen's (1974) model of personality, dividing traits into salient or defining characteristics and characteristics that are less important. From this perspective, salient characteristics would be expected to be stable across situations and over time, while less important traits vary more as a result of situational factors.

One of the most intriguing studies of personality and aging was conducted by Woodruff and Birren (1972). They were able to locate and reassess a sample of people who had completed a personality inventory (California Test of Personality) 25 years earlier when they had been university undergraduates. Objective test scores showed little change over the 25-year period, but respondents indicated that they felt they had changed, becoming more self-confident and better adjusted than they had been. This discrepancy between perceived and measured change may indicate that self-report inventories of personalities capture dimensions of personality (e.g., self-concept) that are relatively stable without assessing other domains that are transformed during the adult years. More importantly, these findings also indicate that people perceive themselves as changing in meaningful ways. Regardless of whether these changes can be objectively confirmed, they represent a significant component of one's current sense of self.

The Woodruff and Birren (1972) study calls attention to another issue—cohort differences in personality. In addition to retesting the original sample, Woodruff and Birren gathered a new sample of current undergraduates at the same university. Comparing current undergraduates with the 1944 results, they found pronounced differences; in particular, the earlier cohort was better adjusted than the later one. As noted earlier, cohort differences in personality have also been found in the Seattle Longitudinal Study (Schaie, 1995; Schaie & Labouvie-Vief, 1974). In particular, extroversion has been increasing in cohorts born since World War II.

The possibility of generational differences in attitudes and personal characteristics is deeply ingrained in popular beliefs and may be a significant source of age differences in personality. Clinicians working with older clients who may be several generations removed from them need to appreciate the historical and social context in which their clients grew up and how those experiences have shaped their development. The key to overcoming a client's current problems lies not within our generational framework but in that of the client's.

Although the issue of continuity versus change cannot be resolved in a definitive way, given the varying definitions of and methods for assessing personality, some practical conclusions can be drawn. First, research provides no support for a universal pattern of deterioration on dimensions of personality. Commonplace beliefs, such as that aging involves a "hardening of the attitudes," are prejudices with little basis in fact. Second, generational differences undoubtedly influence many attitudes, beliefs, behaviors, and other dimensions of personality. Older and younger people differ in many ways, though these differences are often related to historical and cultural influences rather than aging.

Third, anecdotal and clinical evidence suggests that some individuals have significant turning points or changes during the adult years. While claims about universal stages or changes at different periods such as midlife crises cannot be supported by the available data, there are some individuals who fit this pattern. Clinicians should not become overly enamored with poetic descriptions of the life course, nor should they ignore significant turning points that some clients may experience. Finally, deterioration in personality and behavior is a prominent feature of the dementia syndrome. Understanding the etiology of these changes and, particularly, helping family members cope more effectively with them can result in important clinical gains.

CONCLUSIONS

An examination of the normal processes of aging suggests an optimistic view of old age. Today's older people are healthier and better educated than ever before, and this trend will continue as future generations reach old age. Findings from research on psychological functioning suggests both stability and change, but in the absence of dementia, decline in intelligence, memory, and other abilities is relatively mild and does not interfere with the ability to carry out everyday activities. There is also potential for improved performance through cognitive training.

These findings form a foundation for psychological intervention in later life. Decline and disability is an important aspect of later life, but aging is not just a process of unremitting decline. Rather, older people have resources and abilities that can be utilized in dealing with difficult life transitions, such as retirement, illness, or widowhood, or with other stresses and problems they encounter. When treating older clients, clinicians can build on a lifetime of learning and experiences, strengthening adaptive coping skills and helping redirect maladaptive patterns. Age is a barrier neither to leading a meaningful and satisfying life nor to successful treatment of psychological problems.

3

Disorders of Aging:
Dementia, Delirium, and
Other Cognitive Problems

In Chapters 3 and 4 we focus on the common mental disorders of aging, those that are most frequently encountered in clinical situations. The prevalence of these disorders, their characteristics, and what is known about their etiology are reviewed. Building on these descriptions, we turn in Chapters 5 and 6 to issues of assessment, in particular, how to differentiate among the common disorders in later life.

The disorders described in these chapters are listed in Table 3.1. Chapter 3 examines conditions that primarily involve impairment of cognition and brain functioning, dementia, and delirium. It also includes a section on age-related cognitive decline, a category of deficits found in late life with no known etiology. Chapter 4 focuses on disorders such as depression where cognition is usually not significantly impaired. This categorization follows the older distinction of "organic" and "functional" disorders. While it is increasingly recognized that functional disorders have biological components, it remains useful to differentiate between problems such as dementia, which involve catastrophic damage to the brain, and disorders like depression, where biological and psychosocial factors interact in both etiology and treatment.

We provide in-depth discussions of disorders such as the dementing illnesses and delirium, which are prominent in later life and are not usually covered in detail in most general courses or textbooks on adult psychopathology. For disorders such as anxiety, which receive a lot of attention in standard textbooks, our presentation is briefer, focusing on their prevalence in the older population and differences in etiology and symptoms in late life compared to younger ages. We have necessarily omitted some prob-

TABLE 3.1. Common Problems in an Aging Population

Disorders of aging: Dementia, delirium,
and other cognitive problems (Chapter 3)

Dementing illnesses
    Alzheimer's disease
    Multi-infarct dementia
    Other dementias
Delirium
Other cognitive disorders
    Nonprogressive brain injuries
    Age-related cognitive decline

Functional disorders in later life (Chapter 4)

Affective disorders
    Bipolar disorders
    Major depression
    Other depressive syndromes
Anxiety disorders
Schizophrenia
Personality disorder
Late-life paranoid disorders (paraphrenia)
Drug and alcohol problems

lems, for instance, the aging of developmentally disabled individuals, which are usually addressed within a specialized care system (see Seltzer, 1992, for a review). Our emphasis is on the disorders most frequently encountered in the general population of older people and that clinicians who work with the elderly are likely to encounter.

DEMENTING ILLNESSES

The dementing illnesses are the most feared and devastating disorders of later life. The symptoms of dementia—progressive memory impairment and deterioration of habits and personality—have been described since antiquity and have been viewed as an intrinsic part of the aging process. Fortunately, dementia is not a universal feature of aging, but it occurs with sufficient frequency to be the most costly disorder in later life, both in its human toll and in the expense of caring for patients. Nancy Reagan poignantly characterized the decline of her husband, former President Ronald Reagan, who suffers from Alzheimer's disease, as "the long goodbye" (Barrett, 1997). This phrase captures the slow, painful process of loss experienced both by patients and by their families.

We begin by describing the general pattern of symptoms of the dementia syndrome and studies of its prevalence and then discuss the more common types of dementing illnesses, such as Alzheimer's disease and vascular dementia.

Dementia Syndrome

The term dementia refers to a syndrome involving progressive decline in memory and other intellectual abilities. Dementia is a syndrome, not a disease, that is, it is a pattern of symptoms that can be caused by many different illnesses. The dementia syndrome is characterized by three key features; it is *acquired and persistent* and it involves *multiple impairments* of intellectual functioning (Cummings & Benson, 1992). Dementia, as distinguished from mental retardation, is an acquired disability. Symptoms of dementia persist and worsen over time. In contrast, people who suffer a head trauma stabilize or even improve in cognitive functioning. Cognitive symptoms in other psychiatric disorders, such as depression, tend to be transitory. Finally, dementia involves deficits in multiple cognitive functions—language, memory, visual spatial skills, and general intellectual abilities. By comparison, head trauma or stroke often involve deficits of one or two localized functions.

According to the fourth edition of the *Diagnostic and Statistical Manual of Mental Disorders* (DSM-IV) of the American Psychiatric Association (1994), three main criteria for diagnosis of dementia are (1) memory impairment, (2) cognitive disturbances in at least one other area of functioning (e.g., aphasia, apraxia, agnosia, or a disturbance in executive functions), and (3) that these cognitive impairments are severe enough to interfere with social or occupational functioning. Cummings and Benson (1992) point out that memory impairment is not always present in some dementias, for instance, in early and middle stages of Pick's disease. They suggest an alternative definition, that dementia involves impairment in at least three of the following areas of functioning: (1) language, (2) memory, (3) visual spatial, (4) emotion or personality, and (5) other cognitive abilities.

Prevalence of Dementia

How many older people suffer from dementia, and what is the risk of developing dementia at some point in the life span? Estimating prevalence is complicated, mainly because there are no definitive markers for diagnosis of dementing illnesses such as Alzheimer's. A state-of-the-art diagnosis of dementia uses behavioral, neuropsychological, and medical data (see Chapters 5 and 6). No single, simple medical or psychological test definitively detects dementia.

In order to estimate prevalence in the general population, epidemiological studies have relied on brief evaluations, such as mental status tests, that assess orientation, information, and memory or other simple cognitive tasks. These tests are useful for identifying cases of dementia, but they have limitations. First, cognitive impairment on common screening tests may be due to dementia or to potentially treatable conditions. Medical illnesses, medications, depression, and other psychiatric symptoms can lead to cognitive deficits that resemble dementia. Second, mental status tests are reliable for identifying moderate or severe cases of dementia rather than early or mild cases. The point at which mild deficits indicate early dementia as opposed to low normal functioning is not clear, and the problem is especially acute in epidemiological studies when trying to make a judgment based on only one or two tests. Mild impairment may be due to dementia or to normal variations in functioning. Longitudinal studies confirm that people who show mild impairment on typical dementia screening tests do not necessarily progress to dementia over time (Johansson & Zarit, 1997). The effect of education on screening tests for dementia is a particular problem in detecting mild cases. People with less formal education can score as mildly impaired on these tests, even when no dementia is present (Crum, Anthony, Bassett, & Folstein, 1993). Conversely, screening tests do not necessarily identify early dementia in well-educated people, who score well despite developing obvious deficits in other areas of functioning. We return to these points when discussing assessment in Chapters 5 and 6.

Given the problems in reliably detecting mild cases of dementia, it is not surprising that there is generally a consensus on rates of moderate and severe dementia but not mild cases. Most studies from North America and Europe report rates of moderate and severe dementia as ranging between 4% and 7% for the population over age 65 (Anthony & Aboraya, 1992; Canadian Study of Health and Aging Working Group, 1994; Mortimer, 1988; Kay, 1995). Similar estimates of prevalence have been found for Latino, African-American, and non-Latino white groups (Gurland et al., 1995). Figure 3.1 shows the overall prevalence and types of dementing illnesses in the population..

One U.S. study that has received a lot of publicity reported much higher rates, estimating prevalence of Alzheimer's disease alone at 10% over the age of 65 and 45% past age 85 (Evans et al., 1989). These findings, however, may be specific to the population studied, which had very low rates of formal education and included significant numbers of people for whom English was a second language. Additionally, the reported rates of dementia confounded incidence with prevalence, that is, new cases identified 18 months after the initial survey were added to the rate obtained at baseline (see Johansson & Zarit, 1995).

Turning to mild dementia, the lower reliability in identifying cases is reflected in wildly varying estimates of prevalence, from a low of 3% to as

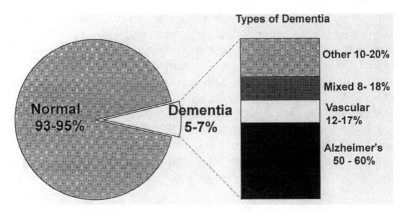

FIGURE 3.1. Prevalence of dementia at ages 65 and older.

high as 64% (Mowry & Burvill, 1988). The typical range, however, is 10% to 15%.

While estimates of prevalence in the population as a whole differ from study to study, it is clear that rates of dementia increase with age. Prevalence of dementia among people in their 60s is around 1%. It increases by the mid-70s to approximately 7% and then rises dramatically in the 80s to between 20% and 30% of the population (e.g., Canadian Study of Health and Aging Working Group, 1994; Johansson & Zarit, 1995; Kay, 1995; Skoog, Nilsson, Palmertz, Andreassen, & Svanborg, 1993).

Dementia is more prevalent among women than among men at all ages. This difference, however, may be due to women's greater longevity (Kay, 1995). Women are more likely than men to survive to the ages at which risk of dementia is greatest.

Only a few studies have used longitudinal designs to estimate incidence of new cases of dementia over time. A longitudinal approach has the advantage of clarifying the status of cases that had mild deficits or other questionable findings at the initial evaluation. Additional decline found at follow-up can confirm that mild deficits indicated early dementia. In contrast, stability or improvement in performance over time suggests that the cognitive deficits at baseline were due to other factors besides a dementing illness.

The available longitudinal studies confirm the pattern found in cross-sectional studies of increasing risk of dementia with age. For example, the Gothenberg longitudinal study in Sweden found that severe dementia rose from 1.8% at age 70 to 7.4% at age 79 (Berg, Nilsson, & Svanborg, 1988; Nilsson & Persson, 1984). In addition, 7% of women and 15% of men at age 79 were considered as having mild dementia. In another Swedish study, rates of dementia in a representative sample of the oldest old (ages 84 to 90, including people in nursing homes and other institutional settings) were found to be 31% at baseline, 40% after 2 years, and 42% after 4 and 6 years (Johansson & Zarit, 1995, 1997). Incidence of new cases was quite high (20% in the first 2 years), but this increase was offset by the fact that people with dementia had a higher mortality rate between each time of testing. The cumulative risk of receiving a diagnosis of dementia at some point before death was 55%. Similar rates of prevalence and incidence have been found in the United States (e.g., Bachman et al., 1993). These longitudinal investigations confirm the patterns found in cross-sectional research of low rates of dementia before age 70 and very high rates by the late 80s. They also indicate that cognitive deficits are a major problem for a significant proportion of the population in very late life.

Types of Dementing Illnesses

The dementia syndrome can develop from many different disorders, including some that are currently largely treatable and reversible. Cummings (1987b) identifies over 50 different disorders that can lead to dementia symptoms. Among the irreversible diseases are Alzheimer's and vascular dementia. Potentially treatable problems include metabolic disorders, infections, severe depression, and other psychiatric disorders that can present with dementia symptoms in older persons.

The particular pattern of dementia symptoms varies according to the areas of the brain most affected by the underlying disorders. Cummings and Benson (1992) distinguish among cortical dementias, subcortical dementias, and dementias with both cortical and subcortical features. Cortical dementias, such as Alzheimer's and Pick's diseases, principally result from damage in the cerebral cortex. In cortical dementias, deterioration of basic intellectual processes of memory, language, judgment, and visual spatial skills are prominent. Subcortical dementias include Parkinson's and Huntington's diseases. Symptoms in subcortical dementia include a slowing of cognitive processes and memory and an inability to spontaneously recall or integrate information. Mood disturbances and motor difficulties are also more common in subcortical disorders. Dementia resulting from vascular disease can affect both cortical and subcortical regions. Table 3.2 lists the major causes of dementia grouped according to whether damage is principally cortical, subcortical, or in both regions of the brain. Differences in symptoms for cortical and subcortical dementias are summarized in Table 3.3.

In the following sections, we discuss the most frequent types of dementing illnesses, particularly Alzheimer's and vascular dementia. For a comprehensive presentation of the full range of dementing illnesses, we recommend *Dementia: A Clinical Approach* (Cummings & Benson, 1992).

TABLE 3.2. Common Causes of Dementia Classified by Primary Site of Deficits

Cortical dementias
  Alzheimer's disease
  Frontal lobe degeneration

Subcortical dementias
  Parkinson's disease
  Huntington's disease
  Progressive supranuclear palsy
  Wilson's disease
  Hydrocephalus
  Human immunodeficiency virus (HIV) encephalopathy
  Lacunar state
  Binswanger's disease

Combined cortical and subcortical deficits
  Multi-infarct dementia
  Slow virus dementias (e.g., Creutzfeldt–Jakob disease)
  Toxic and metabolic dementias

Note. Adapted from Cummings and Benson (1992). Copyright 1992 by Butterworth–Heinemann. Adapted by permission.

TABLE 3.3. Clinical Characteristics of Cortical and Subcortical Dementias

Characteristic	Cortical dementia	Subcortical dementia
Verbal output		
Language	Aphasic	Normal
Speech	Normal	Abnormal (hypophonic, dysarthric, mute)
Mental status		
Memory	Amnesia (learning deficit)	Forgetful (retrieval deficit)
Cognition	Abnormal (acalculia, poor judgment, impaired abstraction)	Abnormal (slowed, dilapidated)
Visuospatial	Abnormal	Abnormal
Affect	Abnormal (unconcerned or disinhibited)	Abnormal (apathetic or depressed)
Motor system		
Posture	Normal[a]	Abnormal[a] (stooped, extended)
Tone	Normal[a]	Usually increased
Movements	Normal[a]	Abnormal (tremor, chorea, asterixis, dystonia)
Gait	Normal[a]	Abnormal

Note. Adapted from Cummings and Benson (1992). Copyright 1992 by Butterworth–Heinemann. Adapted by permission.

[a]Motor system impairment with increased tone and a tendency to assume flexed postures becomes evident in the final stages of the cortical dementias.

Alzheimer's Disease

Alzheimer's disease is the most common cause of dementia. This disorder was first described by Alois Alzheimer in 1907 in a 51-year-old patient. Using new staining techniques for tissue samples prepared for the microscope, Alzheimer identified the types of pathology in brain tissue that have come to be regarded as the hallmarks of the disease: amyloid plaques and neurofibrillary tangles. Because the disorder was identified initially in patients in their 40s and 50s, Alzheimer called it a "presenile dementia." In contrast, dementia after 65 was regarded as an inevitable deterioration associated with the aging process or as the result of restricted blood flow, or hardening of the arteries. Beginning in the 1960s, studies reported that many older people with dementia had similar or identical brain pathology to that of "presenile" cases (Terry & Katzman, 1983).

Recent findings, however, have suggested that the distinction between early and late onset may be worth retaining (Harvey & Rossor, 1995; Raskind, Carta & Bravi, 1995). Symptoms differ, with early-onset cases more likely to have problems associated with parietal lobe damage, such as difficulties in spatial orientation. Younger Alzheimer patients are more likely to have first-rank relatives (parents, grandparents, siblings) who also have the disease, suggesting a genetic cause, though there is now also increasing evidence of genetic influences on late-onset Alzheimer's. The disease also progresses more rapidly on average in early-onset cases (Jacobs et al., 1994). As we will see, there may be additional subtypes characterized by different etiologies as well as variations in patterns and progression of symptoms and in underlying brain pathology. Alzheimer's may be characterized best as a spectrum of diseases, rather than a single disorder (Gatz, Lowe, Berg, Mortimer, & Pedersen, 1994).

Alzheimer's disease accounts for the majority of cases of dementia in the United States and Europe (Bachman et al., 1993; Kokmen, Beard, Offord, & Kurland, 1989; Mortimer, 1988; Ott et al., 1995; Skoog, Nilsson, Palmertz, et al., 1993). Precise estimates are difficult to obtain, since a definitive diagnosis depends on postmortem examination. However, the usual rates obtained from postmortem examinations indicate that approximately 50% of cases of dementia are associated with Alzheimer-type pathologies (Mortimer & Hutton, 1985). An additional 8% to 18% of cases have characteristics of both Alzheimer's and vascular dementia (Cummings, 1985; Mortimer & Hutton, 1985). Women also have higher rates of Alzheimer's, although it is not clear if they are more at risk or are affected more due to their greater longevity than men.

Some evidence suggests that the prevalence of Alzheimer's disease may vary cross-culturally. Studies in Japan have found that the overall rate of dementia is similar to Western countries but that cases of vascular dementia are more prevalent than cases of Alzheimer's disease (Homma &

Hasegawa, 1989; Mortimer, 1988; Shibayama, Kasahara, & Kobayashi, 1986). Interestingly, Japanese American men in Hawaii have a prevalence of Alzheimer's disease similar to European and U.S. white populations and prevalence of vascular dementia only slightly lower than that found in Japan (White et al., 1996). These results suggest that environmental factors play a role in the development of these disorders.

Alzheimer's disease is characterized by an insidious onset and gradual, steady deterioration. Impairment in memory and new learning is typically noticed first, but visual spatial and language problems may also be present early in the disease. The person gradually loses the ability to perform tasks of daily life. Early in the course of the disease, the person experiences difficulties carrying out complex activities, such as work-related tasks or managing finances. Later on, people lose the ability to independently perform many basic activities of daily living, such as dressing and bathing. Personality changes may occur, including increased apathy, dependency, anger, aggressiveness, and sometimes inappropriate sexual behavior.

Patients' awareness of their condition varies. Usually, there is some recognition early on that something is wrong, although denial and covering up of problems is common. Some individuals have at least occasional recognition of their disorder until fairly late in the disease. Depression occurs with some frequency in the early and middle stages of Alzheimer's disease (Reifler, Larson, & Hanley, 1982; Teri & Wagner, 1992).

The rate of progression of symptoms can vary (Teri, Hughes, & Larson, 1990). In some cases, the patient progresses to severe disability and death in a few years. More typically, deterioration is gradual, and the patient may survive from 10 to as long as 20 years after diagnosis. Progression is more rapid among patients who are agitated, have other neurological diseases, and who abuse alcohol (Teri et al., 1990). Death is brought about by other illnesses or by complications of Alzheimer's, such as loss of the ability to swallow or greater susceptibility to infections.

The deterioration in Alzheimer's disease is sometimes described as proceeding through a series of stages. While distinct and unique stages probably do not occur, these models are useful for illustrating the pattern of decline. These models demonstrate how cognitive impairment is linked over time to an increasing inability to perform activities of daily living. Among the more widely used stage models are the Global Deterioration Scale (Reisberg, Ferris, de Leon, & Crook, 1982) and the Clinical Dementia Rating (Hughes, Berg, Danziger, Coben, & Martin, 1982).

Alzheimer's disease is identified by its characteristic brain pathology. The classic pathological features described originally by Alzheimer are brain atrophy, amyloid plaques, and neurofibrillary tangles. Atrophy is due to a loss of neurons. Damage is selective, affecting some parts of the brain and types of neurons more than others. Cell loss is most pronounced in the temporal, parietal, and anterior frontal areas of the brain (Cummings &

Benson, 1992). Damage is also extensive in the hippocampus and basal ganglia, especially the nucleus basalis of Meynert. Sensorimotor areas are relatively spared. Recently, a new type of microscopic pathology has been identified, called AMY plaques, though its role in the disease remains to be determined (M. L. Schmidt, Lee, Forman, Chiu, & Trojanowski, 1997).

Amyloid plaques (which are sometimes called neuritic or senile plaques) are accumulations of degenerative nerve endings and other material, with a core of the peptide beta amyloid. Located near synapses, plaques probably interfere with communication between neurons. Neurofibrillary tangles are twisted strands of protein found within the bodies of nerve cells. The protein that makes up the tangles, A68, is an abnormal variation of the tau protein (Lee, Balin, Otvos, & Trojanowski, 1990). The tangles probably interfere with the cells' energy metabolism and the movement of chemicals to cell endings.

Accompanying the loss of cells is a decrease of certain neurotransmitters, the chemicals that permit communication across the synapses between neurons. One of the earliest findings was a decrease of enzymes in the cholinergic system: acetylcholine, choline acetyl transferase, and acetylcholine esterase (Perry et al., 1978). These changes correspond to the loss of neurons involved in the synthesis of cholinergic neurotransmitters. The discovery of deficits in acetylcholine led to the first systematic attempts to treat Alzheimer's disease. A variety of substances that increase the availability of acetylcholine to the brain have been tried. Two of these medications, tacrine (brand name Cognex) and donepezil (Aricept), have been approved by the U.S. Food and Drug Administration for use with Alzheimer's patients. These medications have small, relatively short-lived benefits (see Chapter 11; Penn, Martin, Wilson, Fox, & Savoy, 1988; Knapp et al., 1994).

In the end, cholinergic deficits are probably only one feature of Alzheimer's disease. The disease affects other neurotransmitters, including serotonin and norepinephrine, and, in some instances, dopamine, as well as other brain chemicals. Furthermore, the deficits in acetylcholine are the result of cell loss, not the cause. Replacement of acetylcholine can, at best, offer limited symptomatic relief. A more basic approach to treatment remains to be discovered.

Much of the recent research on Alzheimer's disease has investigated genetic causes and their link to beta amyloid as the possible trigger for the deterioration process that occurs in Alzheimer's disease. The beta amyloid protein occurs normally in the brain, binding to other neurochemicals to carry out its functions. It is believed that Alzheimer's disease develops when amyloid forms into longer than normal fibers that are insoluble and toxic. The normal mechanisms that bind amyloid and render it harmless are no longer effective. These insoluble fibers form into the dense plaques that characterize Alzheimer's disease and that lead to the degeneration of brain neurons (Hardy, 1993; Lansbury et al., 1995).

Genetic investigations have been stimulated by the observation that multiple cases of Alzheimer's are found in some families. Six genetic abnormalities on five different chromosomes have now been identified as associated with increased risk of Alzheimer's disease. While it is more common to find familial patterns of inheritance in early-onset cases, genetic abnormalities have been identified for both early and late Alzheimer's disease.

The earliest investigations of genetic links focused on chromosome 21. The search for an abnormality on chromosome 21 was spurred by the association between Alzheimer's disease and Down's syndrome. Down's syndrome is a genetic disorder in which the person has an extra copy of chromosome 21. People with Down's syndrome who live to their late 40s and early 50s develop the brain pathologies (plaques, tangles) typical of Alzheimer's (e.g., Lai & Williams, 1989). Pursuing that hypothesis, St. George-Hyslop and his associates (1987) found genetic abnormalities on chromosome 21 in families with multiple cases of the disease. Moreover, these abnormalities are found in the area of the chromosome involved in the synthesis of the amyloid precursor protein (APP).

Subsequent investigations, however, found that only a small proportion of early-onset cases had this abnormality on chromosome 21 (St. George-Hyslop et al., 1990). Two other sites of genetic markers for early-onset Alzheimer's and two for late-onset cases have now been discovered. A site on chromosome 14 may be the most frequent genetic abnormality associated with early-onset cases (Schellenberg et al., 1992). A different genetic site has been identified for people descended from the Volga Germans (people of German origin who settled on the Volga River in Russia in the 18th century). The Volga Germans have maintained extensive family records, which document a pattern of inherited, early-onset Alzheimer's disease in some families. This inherited pattern of Alzheimer's disease may be associated with an abnormality on chromosome 1 (Levy-Lahad et al., 1995). Other populations have been identified with a similar pattern of early-onset Alzheimer's linked to chromosome 1 (Lopera et al., 1997).

Two genetic markers associated with late-onset cases also suggest a link with amyloid. The first pattern concerns the presence of a variation on chromosome 19. This genetic site codes apolipoprotein (Apo E), which appears to have a role in binding amyloid. Three variants of Apo E have been identified, Apo E2, Apo E3, and Apo E4. About 15% of the population carry one or two copies of the E4 allele. People with one copy of Apo E4 have two or three times the risk of developing Alzheimer's disease by age 75 than people with other types of APO E, while people with two copies of the Apo E4 gene have approximately ten times the risk (Corder et al., 1993; Holmes, 1997). Age of onset is also affected by the E4 variant. People with two copies of Apo E4 have a somewhat earlier onset than people with one copy, while late-life cases without the E4 variant have a still later average age of onset. The degree of risk may be greater for women than men. Women with one copy of Apo E4 may have the same increased risk as men with two copies (Holmes, 1997). The E4 variant may also increase risk in combination with other precipitating factors, such as head injury (Holmes, 1997).

It is speculated that Apo E4 either accelerates plaque formation or is less effective in binding amyloid than the other variants of Apo E, resulting in a buildup of the insoluble amyloid fibers that are at the core of plaques (Holmes, 1997). Apo E4 may also play a role in the development of neurofibrillary tangles.

Another genetic marker found to be associated with late-onset cases is on chromosome 14, at a different site than that for early onset. The apparent function of this gene also supports the key role of amyloid. This genetic site codes a particular peptide, ACT, which has two variants, ACT-T and ACT-A. People with the ACT-A variant, in conjunction with APO E4, have a considerably increased risk of Alzheimer's disease compared to people without these proteins (Kamboh, Sanghera, Ferrell, & DeKosky, 1995). Finally, reports have identified still another genetic site implicated in late-onset Alzheimer's, this time on chromosome 12 (Stephenson, 1997).

These diverse findings about genetic markers of Alzheimer's disease indicate that more than one cause and different genetic sites or combinations of genetic and environmental influences related to its cause (St. George-Hyslop et al., 1990). The common thread in these findings is that most of these genetic variations seem in some way to have an effect on beta amyloid. It may be possible to develop a treatment that prevents the formation of insoluble amyloid fibers, thereby blocking the developing of Alzheimer's disease. Whether or not such a treatment can be developed or will be effective with each genetic variant of the disease remains to be seen.

From a clinical perspective, the compelling evidence of genetic links means that it is important to discuss the role of inheritance with families of Alzheimer's patients. Families may already have read about genetic causes in the media and may be concerned about their own risk. Genetic testing for the Apo E4 allele is currently available, and it is likely that tests will soon be available for other genetic risk factors. With early-onset cases and an established pattern of inheritance in the family, the risk of dementia is considerable. Genetic testing, as it becomes available, may be as helpful as it has proven to be with other genetic disorders such as Huntington's disease. Counseling children of early-onset cases can address the implications of this risk to themselves and their children and the advisability of genetic testing. In late-onset cases, the risk of inheritance is usually lower, even for people with two copies of Apo E4. Given this consideration, genetic testing is not recommended for late onset cases at this time (Post et al., 1997). Counseling children of late-onset cases concerning their risk can be useful. Sessions can address planning for the possibility of one's own disability, so that it will not be an undue burden on the family and so that the person accomplishes his or her life goals well before the years of increased risk of disability.

The role of genetics and amyloid have received the most attention in research on the origins of Alzheimer's disease. Despite compelling evidence for the role of genetic factors, it is possible that other factors are involved in the development of Alzheimer's disease, either in conjunction with genetic risks or independently. Identical twins, for example, are not always concordant for Alzheimer's disease (Gatz et al., 1997). Furthermore, a high rate of Apo E4 in certain population groups, such as Finns, is not associated with greater prevalence of Alzheimer's (Holmes, 1997). These results suggest that multiple risk factors are probably involved in development of Alzheimer's disease.

Many nongenetic factors have been investigated as possible causes of Alzheimer's disease. The toxic effects of metals, especially aluminum, have been considered as a possible trigger for the pathologies found in Alzheimer's. The accumulation of aluminum as a result of kidney dialysis has been found to produce dementia (Davison, Walker, Oli, & Lewins, 1982). It remains unclear, however, if people with Alzheimer's have been exposed to excessive amounts of aluminum or have greater brain levels of aluminum than age-matched controls (Graves et al., 1990). Another hypothesis is that head injury earlier in life may contribute in some way to the etiology of Alzheimer's. Using a case–control methodology, Mortimer and his associates (Mortimer, French, Hutton, & Schuman, 1985) reported that people with Alzheimer's had a higher lifetime rate of head injury with loss of consciousness. Subsequent studies suggest that the severity of the head trauma may be a factor, with people who lost consciousness for 5 minutes or more being at greater risk (Schofield et al., 1997). Boxers frequently develop dementia symptoms later in life and have been found on autopsy to display some characteristic brain pathologies similar but not identical to Alzheimer's (see Corsellis, Bruton, & Freeman-Browne, 1973; McKenzie, Roberts & Royston, 1996).

Another important stressor to the brain is anesthesia. Onset of dementia symptoms is sometimes reported after surgery in which a general anesthetic has been used. Studies that have examined the possible association of exposure to anesthesia and Alzheimer's disease have not been able to establish a clear relation (Bohnen, Warner, Kokmen, Beard, & Kurland, 1994). An alternative explanation is that anesthesia and the other stresses of a hospital stay may uncover a preexisting dementing illness. Symptoms that were minimal and went unnoticed by the family before surgery become more pronounced afterwards. Anesthesia and other stressors usually are associated with significant declines in functioning for many people with prior diagnoses of dementia.

A recent investigation suggested that the typical brain pathology of Alzheimer's disease (amyloid plaques, neurofibrillary tangles) may not be sufficient by itself to produce dementia among some older people (Snowdon et al., 1997). In this study, a community of nuns was followed longitudinally, and autopsies were performed after death. Findings indicated that people with evidence of both Alzheimer pathologies and infarcts (strokes) were more likely to have symptoms of dementia before dying, but that people with only one type of pathology (Alzheimer or infracts) had only a slight increase in rates of cognitive symptoms and dementia.

A picture is emerging, then, of many different pathways leading to Alzheimer's disease, including genetic and environmental factors. Several factors have been identified that may be associated with lower risk, although all these findings should be evaluated cautiously. Most have not been replicated, and the mechanisms by which they are linked to Alzheimer's disease remain to be discovered. One factor associated with decreased risk among women is estrogen replacement following menopause (Henderson, Paganini-Hill, Emanuel, Dunn, & Buckwalter, 1994; Kawas et al., 1997). Estrogen is currently being used in drug trials for the treatment of Alzheimer's symptoms (Schneider, Farlow, Henderson, & Pogoda, 1996). Another possible protective factor is anti-inflammatory drugs. People using these medications for arthritis have been reported to be at lower risk of developing Alzheimer's disease (Breitner, 1996; Breitner et al., 1994). There is also some support for antioxidants as playing a protective role in preventing or delaying the onset of Alzheimer's (Sano et al., 1997).

A surprising factor reported to be related to reduced risk of Alzheimer's disease is cigarette smoking (Brenner et al., 1993). This finding, however, underscores the problem with using correlational studies for identifying risk factors. Often the investigators make comparisons of many different risk factors, raising the possibility that one or more will be significant by chance. It is also possible that some third variable may account for the association. Smoking, for example, shortens life expectancy, so people who smoke are less likely to reach the ages of greatest risk for Alzheimer's disease. Smoking also increases the risk of vascular dementia. In a risk study, someone who has already developed vascular dementia is removed from the sample. The study may then report decreased risk of Alzheimer's, not because the substance involved (nicotine, in this case) has any protective value, but because it has increased a risk of other diseases.

Finally, some studies report that better-educated people have a lower risk of developing Alzheimer's disease and other dementias (Stern et al., 1994; Liu et al., 1995). It is hypothesized that better education may be a protective factor by providing more reserve capacity in the brain, thereby delaying the onset of disease. This association may be the result, however, of greater difficulty in identifying cases of Alzheimer's disease in better-educated people or, conversely, of overestimating dementia for people with low education (Stern, Alexander, Prohovnik, & Mayeux, 1992). Substances such as nicotine and estrogen may have a similar role. Since both have a mild, stimulating effect on cognitive functioning, onset of symptoms may be delayed among smokers, better-educated people, and women taking estrogen, but these factors may not actually reduce risk.

Again, we stress these findings on risk factors for Alzheimer's disease should be viewed as tentative until definite links to the disease can be confirmed and potential third variables that might account for the observed associations are ruled out. It may be that environmental risks and exposures act in combination with genetic risk factors or as an entirely different pathway to the disease. Much more needs to be learned about Alzheimer's disease, and there may be no easy or certain answers, at least for awhile.

Other Cortical Dementias: Pick's Disease and Frontal Lobe Dementia

A significant group of patients has been found to have a pattern of degeneration affecting primarily the frontal or frontal and temporal regions of the brain and to have different neuropathology than in Alzheimer's disease. This syndrome is called dementia of the frontal lobe type (DFT). As many as 10% of dementia patients may have primarily frontal lobe pathologies (Gustafson, Brun, & Passant, 1992).

Among the disorders affecting the frontal lobe, Pick's disease is the best known. Pick's disease was originally described in 1892 by Arnold Pick. The disease is marked by extensive atrophy in the frontal and temporal lobes and the presence of characteristic neuropathologies, Pick bodies and Pick cells. Pick bodies are large, dense structures found in the cytoplasm of brain neurons in the affected regions of the brain, while Pick cells are swollen, ballooned cells. Pick's disease typically occurs between the ages of 40 and 60 but has been reported at both younger and older ages (Cummings & Benson, 1992).

In contrast to Alzheimer's disease, in which cognitive symptoms usually occur early in the disease, Pick's disease presents with personality and affective symptoms (Table 3.4). Symptoms are disinhibition of behavior, impaired social behavior and judgment, and a lack of insight. The earliest cognitive symptoms usually involve language and visual agnosias. Patients have trouble with word finding and confrontation naming, and they may use circumlocutions. A characteristic speech pattern is echolalia, that is, excessively repeating certain words or syllables. As an example, a patient who is asked, "How are you today?" might reply, "Today, today, today. . . ." As the disorder progresses, a more generalized pattern of intellectual deficits develops. Because of the predominance of psychiatric symptoms early in the course of Pick's, it is not uncommon for patients to receive a psychiatric diagnosis initially before cognitive symptoms become evident (Cummings & Benson, 1992).

Many cases of DFT involve frontal lobe degeneration but do not have

TABLE 3.4. Comparing Features of Pick's Disease and Alzheimer's Disease

	Pick's disease	Alzheimer's disease
Age of onset	45–65	>65
Presenting features		

Frontal type	Personality change
	Lacking of planning, organization,
	  etc. Antisocial behavior
	Obsessive–compulsive behavior
	Reduced verbal output
		Frontal features a late
		  development
		
		Rarely severe

Temporal type	Progressive fluent aphasia (semantic dementia) Klüver–Bucy syndrome	 Very rare
Memory	Preserved until late	Severely affected from onset
Visuospatial and perceptual skills	Preserved until late	Impaired early in course

Mental test batteries
  (e.g., Mini-Mental
  State Examination)
	Often normal	Impaired score

Imaging CT scan	Frontal and/or temporal lobe atrophy	General atrophy
SPECT or PET	Frontal or temporal hypoperfusion	Biparietal hypoperfusion

Note. From Hodges (1994). Copyright 1994 by Chapman & Hall. Reprinted by permission.

the specific neuropathology associated with Pick's disease (Mann, 1997). These nonspecific cases may, in fact, be more common than Pick's. In a series of 26 cases with primarily frontal symptoms on whom postmortem examinations were made, 4 were found to have neuropathological characteristics of Pick's disease, 16 those of DFT, 2 those of Alzheimer's, 3 those of Creutzfeldt–Jakob disease, a viral dementia, and one case had infarcts in the frontal area (Brun, 1987).

The pattern of symptoms in DFT is similar to Pick's, with changes in personality and social behavior in the early stages of the disease. Patients lack initiative, have poor hygiene, neglect their responsibilities, and engage in impulsive and socially inappropriate behavior. Mood is either blunted or slightly euphoric. Some stereotyped and repetitive behaviors may also occur. Patients are usually concrete and inflexible in their thinking and their approach to solving cognitive problems. Impairment of memory and language occurs as the disorder develops.

Etiology of these disorders is unknown, although a familial pattern is found in about one half of cases of Pick's and other forms of DFT (Mann, 1997; Neary, 1990). Links to sites on chromosomes 3 and 17 have been proposed, but like Alzheimer's, the frontal dementias may be the result of combinations of various genetic and environmental factors. In the absence of neuropathological evidence, Pick's and DFT are difficult to differentiate from one another.

Vascular Dementias

Vascular dementias are a category of disorders in which intellectual impairment is associated with damage due to vascular diseases. The most widely known type of vascular dementia, multi-infarct dementia, involves the occurrence of multiple small strokes or "infarcts" in the cerebral cortex. Other vascular dementias include lacunar states and Binswanger's disease. Vascular dementias can also be caused by brain hemorrhages. These disorders differ from one another in terms of the cause of and likely sites of damage.

The term "vascular dementia" has replaced the older concept of atherosclerotic dementia. Atherosclerosis, per se, does not result in generalized intellectual decline and dementia. Rather, pathological changes such as small strokes are the cause of the decline (Funkenstein, 1988).

The prevalence of vascular dementia has been estimated to be between 8% and 12% of cases of dementia, based on clinical investigations, and from 5% to 20% based on postmortem studies (Cummings, 1985; Peisah, Sachdev, & Brodaty, 1993). Additionally, between 8% and 20% of cases of dementia have been found to have mixed vascular and Alzheimer's pathologies. As noted earlier, some evidence of cross-cultural differences have been found, with higher rates of vascular dementia in Japan.

Similar to Alzheimer's disease, onset of vascular dementia can be as early as the fourth decade of life, though it is rare until the 50s and 60s. Prevalence increases with age, though with some decline after age 85. Life expectancy with vascular dementia is reduced, presumably because of its association with vascular disease. Within 5 years of diagnosis, 64% of cases have died, compared to 32% of Alzheimer's patients (Peisah et al., 1993). Men have a higher risk of vascular dementia than women (Barclay, Zemcov, Blass, & Sansone, 1985; Kay, 1995).

Multi-infarct dementia involves small strokes or infarcts, which occur when blood vessels in the brain are blocked. Infarcts result in the death of surrounding tissue due to insufficient blood supply. Blockages can be caused by thrombosis or embolism. Thrombosis refers to formation of a blood clot within the blood vessel and occlusion of the vessel at that point. In contrast, an embolism is a blood clot that forms at a different site and migrates to a vessel where it causes an occlusion. Dementia occurs when there is widespread damage in both hemispheres in the brain. Single strokes that occur in strategic areas of the brain can also lead to dementia (Peisah et al., 1993).

The distinction between multi-infarct dementia and stroke is a matter of magnitude. Similar mechanisms (thrombosis, embolism) can lead to a stroke. A stroke involves a single, large infarct, which results in focal cognitive deficits. In contrast, multi-infarct dementia refers to a generalized pattern of intellectual decline usually associated with lessor damage at multiple sites. It can be brought about by a number of larger, focal infarcts, by many small infarcts widely distributed in both hemispheres, or by a single infarct in a strategic region. Some patients have typical symptoms of stroke (unilateral motor weakness, aphasia), but others do not. Another pattern is transient ischemic attacks (TIAs), which are brought about by brief blockages of vessels. Loss of consciousness and temporary motor, language, and sensory changes can occur.

Another type of vascular dementia involves lacunar states. Lacunar states are caused by small infarcts in the basal ganglia and thalamus (Cummings & Benson, 1992). Symptoms of dementia and Parkinson-like motor deficits are typical. Binswanger's disease involves multiple infarcts in the white matter of the brain near the ventricles. There may also be infarcts in the basal ganglia and thalamus, as in lacunar states (Román, 1987; Cummings & Benson, 1992). Symptoms are similar to lacunar states, involving motor impairment and dementia. Changes in mood and behavior, including a trend toward apathy and urinary incontinence, are also common. Some postmortem investigations suggest that evidence of infarcts and other changes typical of Binswanger's disease may be quite common (Román, 1987). Risk factors include heart and vascular disease and diabetes.

A finding of white matter lesions or hyperintensities in the brains of older people is quite common with magnetic resonance imaging (MRI) (Wahlund, 1994). Small amounts of white matter hyperintensities do not usually result in dementia but are associated with subtle changes in cognitive functioning, especially on complex reaction time tests (R. Schmidt et al., 1993). White matter hyperintensities are common in both Alzheimer's disease and vascular dementia (Peisah et al., 1993). Nonetheless, a radiological finding of white matter hyperintensities is not in itself sufficient for the diagnosis of dementia without other evidence of brain damage or of clinical evidence of dementia (Wahlund, 1994).

The symptoms of vascular dementia are variable because the sites and extent of damage can differ. Typically, both cortical and subcortical damage is involved (Cummings & Benson, 1992). Impairment usually occurs in memory, abstract thinking, and language, though deficits in other neuropsychological functions such as visual spatial ability can also be found. Depression, anxiety, emotional lability, and psychotic symptoms such as paranoid delusions are common in vascular dementia, perhaps occurring with greater frequency than in Alzheimer's disease (Cummings, Miller, Hill, & Neshkes, 1987; Sultzer, Levin, Mahler, High, & Cummings, 1993). Neurological symptoms such as rigidity, altered gait, dysarthria, and dysphagia are also frequently found.

Brain scans such as MRIs can identify infarcts and other damage typical of vascular dementia. The increased use of MRIs and other advanced imaging procedures as part of diagnosis is probably leading to more frequent diagnosis of vascular dementias.

One of the most reliable indicators of multi-infarct dementia is the history of onset and progression. Onset is usually sudden, and decline often occurs in a stepwise fashion. Patients are stable for periods of time and then experience a sudden drop in functioning. Not all people with vascular dementias, however, follow this pattern.

Several risk factors have been identified for vascular dementia. These include hypertension, atherosclerosis, diabetes, inflammatory diseases (e.g., systemic lupus erythematosus), and conditions that can produce embolisms, such as a heart attack and plaques in the aorta and carotid arteries (Cummings, 1985; Skoog, 1994). Cigarette smoking and obesity are also risk factors. There may be genetic influences as well in development of vascular dementia.

The role of hypertension may be especially important for cognitive impairment and dementia. Chronic hypertension has been linked to cell loss in the brain, particularly in the temporal and occipital lobes (Strassburger et al., 1997). Complicating this situation is the fact that some of the antihypertensive medications can affect cognition, producing symptoms that mimic dementia. As is typical of drug side effects, these changes may be reversed by discontinuing the medication.

Parkinson's Disease

Parkinson's disease is the most common subcortical disorder that can lead to dementia. Parkinson's disease is generally identified by its characteristic motor symptoms, such as rigidity and tremor. Most Parkinson's patients, however, also have some intellectual impairment, due, at least in part, to a slowing of thought processes and motor impairment that interferes with performance of some cognitive tests. A full-blown dementia, however, is found in significant numbers of cases. Typical estimates of dementia in Parkinson's have ranged widely, between 10% and 80% (Brown & Marsden, 1984). Summarizing results from several ongoing studies, Kay (1995) estimates the cumulative incidence of new cases of dementia in Parkinson patients as ranging between 19% and 65% over a 5-year period.

The primary site of brain damage in Parkinson's disease is the substantia nigra, a small region in the brainstem. Neurons in the substantia nigra are involved in the synthesis of the neurotransmitter dopamine, and the loss of these neurons results in significant dopamine deficits. Deterioration, however, can extend to other areas of the brain. The main pathological feature in Parkinson's disease is the presence of Lewy bodies. These structures are insoluble filaments of protein that have a dense core, and they are found in the bodies of neurons or adjacent to them in affected parts of the brain.

At least two patterns of pathology are associated with dementia in Parkinson's disease. Postmortem examinations have revealed that some Parkinson's patients with dementia have Alzheimer-type changes in the cortex (Boller, Mizutani, Roessmann, & Gambetti, 1980). In the second pattern, dementia was associated with extensive neuronal loss in subcortical nuclei as well as frontal and temporal regions but with no evidence of Alzheimer's pathology in the cortex or hippocampus (Double et al., 1996). Additionally, a minority of patients with Alzheimer's disease, estimated variously at between 10% and 45%, have been found to have Parkinson types of pathology (e.g., Lewy bodies, cell loss in the substantia nigra) and to have Parkinsonian symptoms prior to death (Ditter & Mirra, 1987; Leverenz & Sumi, 1986; Schmidt, Martin, Lee, & Trojanowski, 1996; Liu et al., 1997).

The characteristic features of Parkinson's disease are difficulty initiating movements, rigidity, and tremors in the arms and/or legs. Because of rigidity of facial muscles, patients appear expressionless. They can no longer swallow spontaneously, and so saliva accumulates in their mouths and they may drool. Speech is usually abnormal as a result of these motor problems. Depression is common.

Because of these deficits in motor functions and speech, evaluation of cognitive functioning is difficult. Impairment is pronounced on tests that are timed or involve motor performance. In most cases, at least some cognitive impairment is found that appears independent of motor deficits and response speed, including deficits in memory and visuospatial performance (Pirozzolo, Hansch, Mortimer, Webster, & Kuskowski, 1982). The distinction between Parkinson's with and without dementia is based primarily on functional grounds. More extensive memory, intellectual, and behavioral impairment results in patients needing greater amounts of assistance and more stress on family caregivers. The clinician assessing a patient with Parkinson's should be less concerned with whether testing meets the criteria for a diagnosis of dementia than with the problems that the patient's motor and cognitive deficits cause for everyday activities.

Parkinson's patients can benefit from treatment with levodopa. This substance is a precursor of dopamine and is utilized in the brain to synthesize dopamine, thus partly offsetting the deficits brought on by the disease. Relief of motor symptoms occurs in perhaps 60% of patients (Cummings & Benson, 1992). Intellectual performance also improves with treatment. Treatment of depression can also be useful for improving patients' functioning. The benefits of levodopa are short-lived, however, and symptoms worsen again in 1 to 4 years. New medications are becoming available that are increasing treatment options.

A related syndrome has recently been described, which has been called variously "diffuse Lewy body disease," "senile dementia of the Lewy body type," and "Lewy body variant of Alzheimer's disease" (Cercy & Bylsma,

1997; Kosaka, Tsuchiya, & Yoshimura, 1988; McKeith, 1997). In this disorder, Lewy bodies are widely distributed in the cortex, but there is little involvement in the substantia nigra. Correspondingly, symptoms include cognitive and behavioral impairments but only mild motor deficits. Diffuse Lewy body disease is characterized by a progressive decline in cognitive functioning, with attention and visuospatial abilities most likely to be affected. Memory impairment may not be present early in the disorder but becomes prominent over time. Psychiatric symptoms such as hallucinations and delusions are common (Klatka, Louis, & Schiffer, 1996).

These findings suggest that Parkinson's and Lewy body disease are part of a spectrum of disorders (Raskind & Peskind, 1992). Lewy bodies can be concentrated in the substantia nigra and associated regions, with or without Alzheimer's pathology. They can also be widely distributed throughout the cortex. Symptoms vary depending on the site and extent of Lewy bodies.

Patients with Lewy body disease may be more likely than Alzheimer's patients to respond positively to cholinergic agents such as tacrine (McKeith, 1997). Treating behavioral symptoms of both Pick's disease and Lewy body disease with neuroleptics is problematic, as a common side effect is Parkinsonian-type symptoms.

Other Dementing Illnesses

As we noted earlier, a variety of disorders can result in dementia. Among the most important from a public health perspective are those due to viral infections. Acute viral infections typically have a rapid onset and course, with partial or complete recovery of intellectual functioning among survivors. Slow-acting viruses, by contrast, can produce mental status changes that develop gradually over a period of months or years.

The most common of viral dementias is HIV encephalopathy, or AIDS dementia. While estimates vary, symptoms of dementia affect between 6% and 14% of AIDS patients (Bacellar et al., 1994; McArthur et al., 1993). Symptoms are more common when the full AIDS syndrome has developed, but some people with HIV infection but not AIDS have mental status changes. Symptoms resemble those of a subcortical dementia and include forgetfulness and poor concentration (Holland & Tross, 1985; Cummings & Benson, 1992). Memory impairment and other cognitive problems increase over time. The HIV virus affects the white matter of the brain and subcortical areas, including the basal ganglia. Postmortem studies suggest brain infection eventually affects nearly all AIDS patients (Holland & Tross, 1985).

Differential diagnosis of mental status changes in AIDS patients is important. Early symptoms of HIV dementia can resemble depression. In turn, depressive and other psychiatric symptoms are common in AIDS and should be treated (Holland & Tross, 1985). Cognitive impairment can also be caused by disorders that are secondary to HIV infection, such as various opportunistic infections (Cummings & Benson, 1992). Thus, mental status changes in HIV-infected individuals should be evaluated carefully to differentiate among psychiatric symptoms, secondary brain disorders, and primary infections of the central nervous system.

Another form of viral dementia is Creutzfeldt–Jakob disease (sometimes called Jakob–Creutzfeldt). This rare disorder may be caused by a virus-like substance known as a prion (DeArmond & Prusiner, 1995). Prions are implicated in a progressive dementia known as kuru, found mainly in New Guinea. They are also believed to be similar to the viral agent that causes scrapie in sheep and bovine spongiform encephalopathy (BSE), better known as "mad cow disease." Following the infestation of British cattle with BSE, there were reports of increases in cases of Creutzfeldt–Jakob disease, but confirmation that the disease can be transmitted from cattle or other animals to humans remains controversial (MacKnight & Rockwood, 1996). There may also be an inherited form of Creutzfeldt–Jakob disease.

Reversible or Secondary Dementia Syndromes

One of the most important yet poorest described phenomena is dementia due to reversible causes. Dementia symptoms have been associated with a variety of illnesses and other disorders (National Institute of Aging Task Force, 1980). These disorders do not necessarily cause diffuse damage to the brain, except when left untreated. Timely treatment results in considerable improvements in cognitive functioning. Despite their importance, little systematic research has been conducted on these dementias, including such issues as prevalence and presenting symptoms (see, however, Cummings & Benson, 1992, for a comprehensive review of these disorders).

Maletta (1990) proposes using the term "secondary dementia" rather than reversible or treatable dementia. He points out that the distinction between reversible and irreversible dementia is inaccurate. Cases of secondary dementia due to causes such as excessive exposure to heavy metals may not be completely reversible, while primary dementias such as Alzheimer's may have treatable components. The central issue for clinicians, however, is that the search for possible reversible aspects must be part of the evaluation of anyone with dementia.

Maletta (1990) identifies three groups of disorders that fall under the rubric of secondary dementias. First are cognitive disturbances that develop rapidly in relation to acute medical or psychosocial stressors. The psychiatric classification for these disorders is "delirium," though neurologists and other physicians and health professionals sometimes refer to them as a "reversible dementia." Delirium is described in the next section.

The second group of secondary dementias have an onset and symptoms similar to the primary dementias. A wide range of illnesses and problems can lead to the secondary dementias. Among the most frequent causes are nutritional deficits, such as vitamin B12 deficiencies, chronic hypothyroidism and other endocrine disorders, exposure to heavy metals, and normal pressure hydrocephalus. Medications acting singly or in combination can result in dementia symptoms. Chronic alcoholism can also produce dementia, which may partly reverse with treatment.

A third group of secondary dementias is associated with psychiatric disorders, particularly depression. This pattern of symptoms has been called a number of different names: pseudodementia, depressive pseudodementia, and reversible dementia. According to Caine (1981), pseudodementia involves intellectual impairment that resembles dementia but is reversible. Examination of the patient reveals other psychiatric symptoms but no evidence of a primary neurological disorder. Estimates of prevalence of pseudodementia have ranged between 2% and 32% of cases of elderly presenting with cognitive symptoms (Cummings & Benson, 1992), with the variation due to different methods of defining this syndrome.

The earliest reports on pseudodementia (e.g., Kiloh, 1961; Roth & Myers, 1975) emphasized the role of depression. As noted in Chapter 2, depressed older people frequently complain of failing memory and may have some cognitive impairment associated with aging and/or related to depression. Subsequent studies of pseudodementia (Wells, 1979; Caine, 1981) have confirmed depression as the most frequent pattern but have also identified a variety of other psychiatric problems that can present with cognitive impairment in older people. In a sample of 10 patients meeting criteria for pseudodementia, Wells reported extensive depressive symptoms among 7. He also found evidence of personality disorders, particularly dependency, among the entire group. Caine identified 11 patients with cognitive deficits resembling dementia that were subsequently found to be treatable. Of the 11 cases, 6 met criteria for a diagnosis of major depression, while the others had other psychiatric diagnoses. Both Caine and Wells reported that some cases had subtle signs of neurological abnormalities, which may have contributed to their cognitive impairment.

In contrast to the pseudodementias in which psychiatric problems present with cognitive symptoms, we should note that the opposite happens—primary dementias sometimes present with psychiatric symptoms, as is frequently the case with frontal dementias. Depression is frequently an early symptoms in both Alzheimer's and vascular dementias.

People with a primary dementia can also have secondary problems that worsen their symptoms. As an example, an Alzheimer's patient who is depressed or has a nutritional deficit will functions more poorly than if the patient had Alzheimer's alone. Treatment of these secondary problems often improves functioning. The overlap of psychiatric disorders such as depression and primary dementia is a central diagnostic issue to which we will return in subsequent chapters.

DELIRIUM

An 80-year-old man returned home from the hospital following minor surgery. He had been prescribed an anti-inflammatory medication to aid the healing process. Waking up in the middle of the night, he called his children on the telephone. His children quickly realized that he did not know what time it was, that his thoughts were disorganized, and that he reported the events of a dream he had had as having actually happened. He seemed fearful and agitated. Prior to the hospitalization, he had been functioning well, although with occasional memory lapses, especially in unfamiliar surroundings, but he had never had symptoms like these. His children were concerned that he was becoming senile and consulted with one of us. On hearing the sequence of events, we encouraged the children to involve their father's physician and to review the medication that had been prescribed following the surgery. The physician agreed that the medication was a possible cause of the patient's difficulties and discontinued it. In a few days the symptoms subsided, and the man was able to function independently again.

This sequence of events is very common. An older person who has been functioning adequately suddenly develops global impairment in intellectual functioning. The onset of symptoms can occur in a few hours or a few days. Changes may include impaired perceptions, delusions or hallucinations, altered mood that can range from euphoria to fear, impaired ability to attend or focus on events, very high or very low levels of activity, and other disruptions of thinking and behavior.

These symptoms characterize delirium. While delirium can occur at any age, it is most frequent among older people. It results from a disruption of brain metabolism or an alteration in levels of certain neurotransmitters (Lipowski, 1990). Delirium can be brought about by many different factors acting singly or in combination. Many illnesses, medications, and stressors have been associated with delirium. Often the causes are treatable and the outcome positive, as in the example. In that instance, the likely causes of delirium were the medication acting in conjunction with stress associated with surgery. The mental symptoms usually remit when the precipitating causes are identified and treated.

All too often, however, delirium goes unrecognized or is misdiagnosed as dementia or a psychiatric disorder (e.g., Farrell, & Ganzini, 1995). We have frequently encountered situations where an older person with a delirium has been mislabeled as having dementia or Alzheimer's disease, and the family has been advised that nursing home placement is needed. Even more serious is overlooking the causes of a delirium. Untreated, these causes can lead to permanent brain damage and death. There is probably no more important clinical skill than being able to recognize a delirium.

A major factor contributing to the problem in identifying a delirium is terminology. Many different terms are used to refer to delirium, such as acute brain syndrome, acute confusional state, and, as we saw earlier, reversible dementia. The confusion over terminology has been compounded by vague and inconsistent definitions. "Delirium" replaced "acute organic brain syndrome" from earlier editions of the *Diagnostic and Statistical Manual*, because the latter was not widely recognized or used outside psychiatry.

Delirium is most likely to be encountered in an acute hospital, where the problems that led to hospitalization and the stressors encountered in the hospital can combine to produce the syndrome. Estimates of delirium range from 11% to 26% of older inpatients (Inouye & Charpentier, 1996; Levkoff, Cleary, Liptzin, & Evans, 1991; Pompei et al., 1994). These rates are much higher than found in a review of medical charts alone, indicating that underdetection of delirium continues to be a problem (Levkoff et al., 1991). Delirium rates are even higher among some selected groups of inpatients. Estimates of delirium after surgery range widely, from 7% to 52%. The risk associated with certain kinds of surgery seems especially high; delirium has been reported for between 28% and 52% of people having orthopedic surgery for hip fractures and for approximately 30% following heart surgery (Levkoff et al., 1991; Tune, 1991). Patients who develop a delirium in the hospital stay longer and have a higher mortality rate (Pompei et al., 1994). Surprisingly, many acute hospitals are unprepared to deal with delirium when it develops and may even adopt a punitive attitude toward the patient and his or her family.

Nursing homes are another setting where a delirium is likely to be encountered. While there are few studies to date, one report suggests that between 6% and 12% of residents of a nursing home may develop a delirium during a 1-year period (Katz, Parmalee, & Brubaker, 1991). Prevalence among community populations is low, given that the symptoms often result in hospitalization. Nonetheless, one epidemiological survey estimated the rate of delirium at approximately 1% among community-living people over the age of 55 (Folstein, Bassett, Romanoski, & Nestadt, 1991).

Efforts to clarify and improve criteria for diagnosing delirium have been made in recent years. DSM-III provided the first operational criteria for diagnosis. These criteria were subsequently revised in DSM-IV. Several research instruments and structured interviews have been developed to assist in diagnosis (Levkoff, Liptzin, Cleary, Reilly, & Evans, 1991). A thorough discussion of delirium is found in Lipowski (1990).

The pattern of onset of symptoms may be the most distinctive feature of a delirium. Onset is typically rapid, occurring over a period of a few hours or days, and represents a dramatic change in a person's level of functioning. A delirium often develops at night. Wakiing from a dream, the person may mix the content of the dream with reality. Symptoms fluctuate over the course of the day, often with a worsening toward evening.

Changes in attention are a frequent part of the delirium syndrome. Patients have difficulty focusing and sustaining or shifting attention. Disorders of thinking and perception may be the most prominent feature of a delirium. Someone who had been functioning well may suddenly become illogical or incoherent. Thinking may be characterized by a dreamlike quality with some merging of content from dreams with reality. Delusions, hallucinations, and illusions are very common with delirium. Both auditory and visual hallucinations can occur. Rates of hallucinations between 40% and 75% have been reported (Lipowski, 1990).

Three patterns of delirium, having to do with the level of arousal and activity, have long been recognized (Lipowski, 1990; Ross, Peyser, Shapiro, & Folstein, 1991). The first type is characterized by hyperalertness and hyperactivity. Patients are restless, agitated, and vigilant. In contrast, the second type involves hypoalertness and hypoactivity. Patients are quiet and subdued. They may be drowsy and difficult to arouse. The third pattern involves fluctuations between the other two types.

In the effort to develop more precise operational criteria for delirium, the DSM definition has eliminated two terms that have long been associated with delirium: clouding of consciousness and confusion. While both terms are graphic, they also have vague and overlapping definitions. Critiquing the term "clouding of consciousness," Lipowski (1990) points out it was used to refer to many different features of delirium, including drowsiness, a reduced awareness of self and surroundings, deficits in short-term memory, disorganized thinking, deficits in perception and misperceptions, and impairment in new learning. Confusion has similarly been used to describe many different features of delirium. In fact, confusion is one of the most overused terms in geriatrics; it lacks any degree of specificity or precision. It is used variously to refer to behaviors of people with delirium, dementia, schizophrenia, and other disorders. Some of the different meanings ascribed to confusion have been lack of orientation or disorientation, inability to think clearly or coherently, poor contact with reality, and reduced awareness of the environment (Lipowski, 1990).

The main problem with the imprecise terms clouding of consciousness and confusion is that they do not facilitate differentiation of delirium from dementia or other disorders. Replacing these global terms with more specific descriptions of behavior will lead to greater reliability in identifying delirium. More precise criteria can also improve communication among professionals. While a term like confusion can be interpreted in different ways, precise description of the patient's behaviors allows each clinician involved in the case to reach a similar understanding of the situation.

Many different conditions can produce a delirium (Table 3.5). In fact, a report by a National Institute of Aging (NIA) Task Force (1980) stressed that any disruption of the internal environment of an older person can bring about a delirium. The more factors to which someone is exposed, the greater the likelihood of a delirium.

TABLE 3.5. Common Organic Factors Precipitating Delirium

1. Intoxication with medical drugs: anticholinergics, sedative–hypnotics, diuretics, digitalis, antihypertensive and antiarrhythmic agents, cimetidine, lithium, hypoglycemic agents, levodopa, nonsteroidal anti-inflammatory drugs, narcotics, cancer chemotherapeutic drugs

2. Alcohol and sedative–hypnotic withdrawal

3. Metabolic disorders: fluid and electrolyte imbalance; endocrine disorders; renal, hepatic, and pulmonary failure; nutritional (including vitamin) deficiency; hypothermia and heat stroke

4. Cardiovascular disorders: myocardial infarction, congestive heart failure, cardiac arrhythmias, pulmonary embolism

5. Cerebrovascular disorders: stroke, transient ischemic attacks, subdural hematoma, multi-infarct dementia, vasculitides, orthostatic hypotension

6. Infections, notably pulmonary and of urinary tract, bacteremia, septicemia, tuberculosis, meningitis, encephalitis

7. Neoplasm: intracranial, systemic

8. Trauma: head injury, burns, surgery

9. Epilepsy

Note. From Lipowski (1990). Copyright 1990 by Oxford University Press. Reprinted by permission.

Among the elderly, the most frequent precipitating factor for delirium is medication reaction, either to a single medication or to the interaction among drugs. Medications are not metabolized or excreted as quickly on average by older compared to younger people (Beizer, 1994). As a result, medications can build up to toxic levels if not monitored carefully. Adding to this problem is the fact that many older people take multiple prescription medications. Over-the-counter drugs can also contribute to a delirium. Common over-the-counter medications such as antacids can on rare occasions cause cognitive impairment and other delirium symptoms. The risk is greater, however, when over-the-counter drugs are used in combination with prescription medications that add to or potentiate their effects.

As noted earlier, surgery with general anesthesia is another common cause. Infections, metabolic and endocrine disorders, and fractures can also trigger a delirium in an older person. Sometimes the first symptoms that are noticed are mental changes associated with the delirium syndrome rather than physical symptoms or complaints. Delirium can also indicate the presence of a brain disease. Focal events such as a stroke or transient ischemic attack or more pervasive disorders such as a rapidly growing tumor or infection can produce symptoms of delirium. A delirium can also follow a head injury.

A frequently overlooked precipitant is alcohol. Alcoholic intoxication is itself a form of delirium. Alcohol can also interact with medications an older person is taking, resulting in a delirium. Alcoholism has been found to be a frequent cause of delirium among older hospitalized patients (Pompei et al., 1994). Older people who abuse illegal drugs or psychoactive medications are also at greater risk of suffering delirium or cognitive impairment.

Lipowski (1990) proposes a useful distinction of predisposing, facilitating, and precipitating factors for delirium. Predisposing factors increase susceptibility for delirium. These factors include increasing age and brain damage, either due to focal damage or a progressive disease like Alzheimer's. People at highest risk of delirium are dementia patients. Facilitating factors can contribute to the development of a delirium or can worsen or prolong its course. Facilitating factors include psychological stress, sleep deprivation, sensory deprivation or overload, and immobilization. While relatively rare, a delirium can develop following the death of a spouse. Moving to a new location is frequently associated with a delirium, especially for someone with dementia. Precipitating factors are the immediate medical conditions involved—the medications, illnesses, and other problems that lead to the delirium.

Many of the conditions that produce delirium can also lead to a reversible dementia, the difference being in the types of presenting symptoms. With a reversible dementia, memory impairment is a prominent symptom, while in delirium, fluctuations in attention and alertness and a greater likelihood of delusions and hallucinations are characteristic. How the underlying physiology differs is not known.

The outcomes of delirium are variable, depending on the course and treatment of precipitating factors. Complete recovery is the most common outcome (Lipowski, 1990). It occurs when the factors precipitating the delirium are treated or run their course, for example, in the aftermath of surgery or relocation. Recovery may be relatively rapid, for instance, in about a week, or it may be more gradual. Conversely, delirium can progress to a coma and death or to irreversible brain damage. Patients who develop a delirium in the hospital have higher mortality than those who do not (Levkoff et al., 1991). Delirium patients who survive are more likely to stay in the hospital longer and to go to nursing homes on discharge. With the current pressure to keep hospital stays brief, a patient who develops a delirium may be more likely to be misdiagnosed as demented and discharged to a nursing home.

People often have amnesia for the events and experiences they had during delirium (Roth, 1991). Sometimes, however, a patient remembers a hallucination or delusion and is convinced that it actually happened. Even long after the delirium has cleared, some people persist in the belief that the imagined events actually took place.

The main approach to a delirium needs to be a vigorous search for the cause combined with a calming and reassuring environment. A thorough medical evaluation, including a review of medications, is essential. Major tranquilizers are often prescribed for managing the more disruptive symptoms in a delirium, but they often worsen the situation. We have observed many patients who have paradoxical reactions to the neuroleptics, that is, they become more rather than less agitated. Tranquilizers can be helpful in certain situations, but they should be monitored closely.

Cutbacks in nursing staff in many hospitals and the trend toward shorter hospital stays make it more difficult to identify, treat, and care for patients with delirium. There is an increasing tendency just to throw medications at the problem, rather than to identify the cause or provide the type of supportive environment that can calm patients down. Families are an invaluable resource for providing information that helps differentiate between delirium and dementia, but they are often overlooked in the hospital setting. An important role for the geriatric mental health specialist is to identify delirium and advocate for its proper treatment.

OTHER COGNITIVE DISORDERS: NONPROGRESSIVE BRAIN INJURIES

With the attention given to dementia and, to a lesser extent, delirium in older populations, other sources of brain damage are sometimes overlooked. Accidents that involve head trauma can lead to both transitory and permanent cognitive deficits. Another important source of cognitive disorders is surgery. In addition to the risk of delirium in the period immediately following surgery, some people experience permanent cognitive deficits. Loss of oxygen during the surgery, the occurrence of a stroke, or other changes can lead to significant cognitive changes. It is estimated, for example, that 3% of people who have coronary bypass surgery suffer complications that lead to decreased cognitive functioning (Roach et al., 1996).

The importance of differentiating these causes of brain damage from dementia is that they have very different consequences and prognosis. Often, the deficits caused by the damage are focal, not global. There are, as a result, more opportunities for compensation and rehabilitation. These conditions are also not progressive and do not result in the type of catastrophic decline found in dementia.

AGE-RELATED COGNITIVE DECLINE

Aging is associated with changes in memory and other intellectual functions, as well as an increased rate of subjective complaints about failing memory (see Chapter 2). Over the past decade, there has been particular interest in people who have mild deficits in memory or other cognitive abilities but who do not meet criteria for dementia or another psychiatric or neurological condition. This group may include people in the earliest stages of dementia. More effective detection of the earliest symptoms of dementia is important because any new treatments are likely to be maximally effective before an accumulation of damage. Conversely, if a pattern of cognitive decline can be identified that is distinct from dementia, it may also be possible to improve functioning with medications, cognitive stimulation, or other means.

In 1986, a task force of the National Institute of Mental Health proposed the term "age-associated memory impairment" (AAMI) (Crook et al., 1986). AAMI was defined by subjective complaints of failing memory and objective test performance that falls at least one standard deviation below the mean for tests of memory. Following up on this work, DSM-IV includes a diagnosis of "age-related cognitive decline (V780.9)" under the category "Other Conditions That May Be a Focus of Clinical Attention." People with age-related cognitive decline do not meet diagnostic criteria for dementia or other disorders, but they do have cognitive problems. DSM-IV specifically notes difficulties in remembering names or appointments and in solving complex problems. Since difficulty in remembering names is nearly universal, the diagnosis is quite inclusive. The criteria for AAMI are much more explicit and useful.

There have been attempts to clarify the significance of mild cognitive deficits. While some studies suggest an increased risk of dementia, other research has found that many of the people with mild deficits remain stable (Hänninen et al., 1995; Johansson & Zarit, 1997). One potential complicating factor is education. Older people who meet the criteria developed for AAMI are likely to have less education. If test scores are adjusted statistically for education, the number of people who meet the criteria for AAMI is greatly reduced (Goodman & Zarit, 1994).

More work is needed to clarify the significance of these mild deficits. In the meantime, the DSM-IV category of Age-Related Cognitive Decline provides clinicians with a diagnosis to be used in cases where a wait-and-see attitude is needed to determine if problems worsen into dementia (see Chapter 6). It is also useful to explore the extent to which excessive anxiety over failing memory might contribute to these problems. Reassurance and teaching practical memory strategies can sometimes be very helpful. Chapter 2 describes some promising approaches. It is especially important to recognize that many of the memory problems that concern older people, such as forgetting a name, can occur at any age. Just as at any age, these problems are often due to inattentiveness and inadequate learning rather than a lack of ability to learn and remember. Often, the reattribution of everyday instances of forgetting as a normal and expected problem can allay an older person's anxiety.

CONCLUSIONS

The syndromes of dementia and delirium are, in many ways, the most important mental health problems of the elderly. Dementia is a devastating problem that involves the gradual loss of the person. Delirium is usually of short duration but is frequently misidentified and mistreated. In this chapter, we have provided definitions and descriptions of these syndromes and their prevalence and etiology. We have also considered other types of age-related cognitive decline. We return to these disorders in Chapters 5 and 6, where we examine assessment approaches and criteria for making a diagnosis, and in subsequent chapters that focus on their treatment in community and institutional settings.

4

Functional Disorders
in Later Life

In this chapter, we examine the most common functional disorders that occur in late life: depression, anxiety, adjustment disorders, alcoholism, schizophrenia, late-life paranoid disorders, and personality disorders. Our main focus is on how these disorders differ in presentation and symptomatology when they occur in old age. We review the incidence and prevalence of these disorders and factors associated with their etiology in later life.

Perhaps the most central distinction is whether a problem has its onset in later life or is a recurrence of a disorder from earlier in the life span. Many older clients suffer from disorders that had their onset earlier in life. Recurrence of a disorder in old age usually is embedded in long-standing patterns of functioning. In those cases, the gerontological issue is to identify what new factors in the person's life might be contributing to the current episode. Knowing that a problem is recurrent is also important for planning treatment, since approaches that were successful earlier in life may continue to be effective in old age. Alternatively, older people can experience a problem for the first time in old age. An important consideration is whether the late-life form of a disorder represents a significant variation or subtype of that problem and therefore if treatment should differ. A related concern is whether the presentation of symptoms in late-onset cases differs from presentation in people who had onset earlier in life.

We have necessarily limited the range of problems that are examined in this chapter. An older person may suffer from virtually any disorder listed in DSM-IV. People with mental disorders earlier in life grow older, and sometimes their problems remain unchanged. In effect, the psychopathology of aging is a psychopathology of adulthood, encompassing the full range of mental health problems. We feel that a comprehensive review of all the disorders that are found in the older population is beyond the scope of this book, so we concentrate instead on providing a gerontological perspective on the problems that occur most frequently in later life.

We also want to note that how frequently a clinician encounters any of these problems is a matter of practice setting. In an outpatient private practice, the most common problems are depression, anxiety, and adjustment reactions, sometimes complicated by a long-standing personality disorder. An acute inpatient unit is likely to see a more severely disturbed range of patients. Similarly, an outpatient clinic tends to have more patients with chronic and severe disorders, such as schizophrenia or alcoholism. It is important to keep in mind that patients seen in any particular setting are not representative of the general population. It is easy to become pessimistic about the treatment potential of older clients if one works only with the chronically mentally ill. In those cases, however, the limited response to treatment is due to the chronicity of the disorder, not to the person's age. Conversely, clinicians can become too optimistic about treatment possibilities if their clients are high-functioning individuals. The diversity of late life includes both people whose problems are largely intractable and those who respond positively to appropriate treatment.

DEPRESSIVE DISORDERS

Depression has long been regarded as a defining characteristic of later life. The view that the elderly are more prone to depression goes back at least to the second-century Roman physician Galen, who described a link between melancholia and aging (Jackson, 1969). In contemporary society, older people are frequently portrayed in the media as sad and withdrawn. It is assumed that their depression is due to the losses they experience, their exclusion from positions of influence and importance in society, declining health, or because of fears of impending death. Like most popular stereotypes, these images contain both elements of truth and distortions. Nonetheless, depression is probably the most important and frequent problem that clinicians encounter in their older clients.

Rather than being an intractable problem embedded in the aging process, depression often improves with treatment. Modern geriatric mental health owes its origins in large part to a classic study by the British psychiatrist Sir Martin Roth. In a landmark 1955 paper, "The Natural History of Mental Disorder in Old Age," Roth examined the outcomes of geriatric patients with a variety of disorders who were seen as inpatients in an English mental hospital. He described the prevailing pessimism about treating older patients and the belief that any mental disorder that occurred in later life was a manifestation of brain disease. Not much was expected of older patients except further decline. What Roth observed, however, was quite different, namely, that recovery depended on the presenting problem, not the patient's age. In particular, people who were hospitalized with affective disorders were much more likely to be discharged as recovered and to have higher survival rates at 6 months and 2 years than people with symptoms of dementia. This positive finding, during an era when treatment for severe depression was relatively limited, spurred interest in identifying treatable mental health problems in later life.

The term depression refers, of course, to both symptoms and disorders. This duality introduces some confusion into discussions of depression and, as will be shown, into estimates of the prevalence of depression. The primary diagnostic categories in DSM-IV are major depressive disorder (MDD), dysthymic disorder, and adjustment disorder with depressed mood. Depression can also be a feature of bipolar mood disorders. Depressive symptoms are a defining feature of these disorders, but depressive symptoms can occur with some degree of severity and regularity among people who do not meet criteria for diagnosis.

Besides these primary diagnoses of mood disorders, depression can be a prominent feature of other illnesses and psychiatric disorders. Koenig and Blazer (1992) distinguish three patterns of comorbidity in the elderly. The first pattern is depressive symptoms that are psychosocial in origin but occur in reaction to medical illnesses and disability. Second, depressive symptoms can be caused by a variety of illnesses and medications. For example, depression is a common feature of Parkinson's disease. Of course, a Parkinson's patient may be depressed because of disease-related changes in levels of dopamine *and* because of his or her growing disability and poor prognosis. The third pattern is called "masked depression": patients who are depressed present primarily with medical complaints that have no organic origin. Masked depression differs from hypochondriasis in that the patient's cognitions involve depressive themes: hopelessness, helplessness, and worthlessness. One additional pattern is that depressive symptoms can be a part of other psychiatric disorders.

The overlap of depression and medical problems constitutes a major diagnostic issue. Depressed people often have somatic complaints such as poor sleep and appetite, fatigue, and muscle or skeletal pain. In a younger patient with few medical problems, it is often easy to establish that these complaints are part of the depressive disorder. The situation is frequently more ambiguous among older people who may suffer from one or more chronic health problems that could be the source of the symptoms or where symptoms are sometimes due to the effects of aging. There is no easy formula for differentiating chronic illness from depression in the elderly; rather, clinicians must evaluate each case carefully, considering the possibility of comorbidity, while making sure that clients are receiving appropriate treatment for somatic ailments.

Rates of Depression in Community Populations

Estimates of rates of depression among the elderly vary considerably from one study to the next, largely due to the use of different assessment and diagnostic criteria. Studies in the United States that have used DSM criteria for diagnosis have generally reported paradoxical findings, that is, high rates of depressive symptoms but generally low rates of diagnosed disorders. The major investigation of rates of mental illness in the United States is the Epidemiologic Catchment Area (ECA) study, which examined prevalence of disorders at five sites across the country. The ECA investigations used a structured interview (Diagnostic Interview Schedule—DIS) and operational criteria for diagnoses to identify prevalence of various disorders. A rate of 2.5% (0.7% for major depressive disorder and 1.8% for dysthymic disorder) was found among community-dwelling people 65 years of age or older (Weissman et al., 1988). The prevalence for women was about twice as high as for men at every age. Compared to younger people, however, prevalence of depression was much lower among the 65-plus age group. For example, MDD had a prevalence of 3% among adults aged 25 to 44 and 2% for adults aged 45 to 64. In a detailed analysis of findings from one ECA site (Piedmont), Blazer, Hughes and George (1987) reported rates of MDD and dysthymic disorder that were similar to the other research sites and also that another 27% of the sample had prominent depressive symptoms but did not meet diagnostic criteria for a depressive disorder.

An earlier study, conducted in New Haven, Connecticut, by Weissman and Myers (1978), used DSM-III criteria for diagnosis but had a different assessment instrument (the Schedule for Affective Disorders and Schizophrenia, or SADS). They found somewhat higher rates of depressive disorders among a community sample of elderly: 5.4% with MDD and 2.7% with minor depression (a category similar to but not identical to dysthymic disorder). As with the ECA studies, however, rates of depressive disorders were higher among younger age groups.

Several studies have used different diagnostic criteria than the DSM for determining prevalence of late-life depression. The foremost example is the work of Gurland and his colleagues (1983). Using structured ratings from a clinical interview, the CARE, they established a reliable diagnostic category of pervasive depression, which identifies people with clinically significant depressive symptoms. This diagnostic system has been used in research in New York and in several studies in Great Britain and Australia. Rates of pervasive depression among older people have ranged between 12.4% to 17.3% (Gurland et al., 1983; Kay et al., 1985; Livingston, Hawkins, Graham, Blizard, & Mann, 1990; Lindesay, Briggs, & Murphy, 1989). In the Hobart study in Australia, people were classified using both DSM-III criteria for MDD and the criteria for pervasive depression (Kay et al., 1985). It was found that 10.2% of people aged 70 to 89 had MDD and 16.1% of the cases were categorized as pervasive depression (Kay et al., 1985). The rate of DSM-III-diagnosed depression was much higher in Hobart than in other studies, but it was still lower than prevalence of pervasive depression.

Blazer (1994) also made similar estimates of prevalence of depression in community populations. Using a classification system similar to Gurland's category of pervasive depression, he estimated the rate among older people as ranging between 8% and 15%.

These findings have several possible interpretations. It may be that DSM-III (and probably also DSM-IV) criteria are too restrictive and yield rates of MDD that are low. When applying criteria for pervasive depression, the prevalence of depression among community-dwelling older people is markedly higher. Depression may also be manifested in a more muted way in later life than at younger ages. An alternative explanation is that older people are *less likely* to suffer from severe depression but experience frequent, minor, but troublesome depressive symptoms. Blazer (1994) proposes adoption of the term "minor depression" to identify elderly people with clinically significant symptoms who do not meet DSM criteria for MDD.

Two other possibilities should be considered. First, there may be generational differences in rates of depression. How people label feelings of distress is in part cultural, and it may be more acceptable for younger people to express their emotional state as "depressed." In turn, older cohorts may find it more acceptable to express distress indirectly or as physical symptoms. Evidence indicates differences in presentation of symptoms in other cultures, where depressed people may have cognitive and somatic symptoms typical of this syndrome but may not complain of depressed affect (Caine, Lyness, King, & Connors, 1994). Another possible explanation involves selective survival. Suicide rates are higher among people with severe depression. The lower rate of MDD among older people may reflect that some people with severe, recurrent depression do not survive to old age.

These hypotheses concerning rates of depression cannot be sorted out until we have better criteria for identifying depressive disorders and a better understanding of the significance of varying types and severity of depressive symptoms in older people. From a practical standpoint, epidemiological research indicates that depressive symptoms have a considerable prevalence but that rates of the more restrictive category of MDD are relatively low. Many of the people with significant depressive symptoms but who do not meet the criteria for MDD undoubtedly benefit from treatment.

Prevalence of Depression among Medically Ill Elderly

Depressive symptoms are common among people with medical illnesses. Treatment of depression often facilitates recovery from medical illness because of better compliance with medical regimens or improved participation in rehabilitative procedures. Rates of MDD among older hospital patients vary considerably from one study to the next, ranging from 6% to 44%, with an average of about 12% (Koenig & Blazer, 1992). Rates are higher among people with more severe illnesses, such as cancer, or with greater functional disabilities. Other depressive diagnoses (dysphoria, adjustment disorders) have been found in 18% to 26% of patients (Koenig & Blazer, 1992).

Rates of depression among specific outpatient samples are also considerable. As an example, in one study 36% of people with aging-related vision loss had significant depressive symptoms (Horowitz, Reinhardt, McInerney & Balistreri, 1994). Depressive symptoms are common in dementia (Reifler, Larson & Hanley, 1982; Logsdon & Teri, 1995) and in Parkinson's disease (Cole et al., 1996). Table 4.1 summarizes the common medical conditions associated with depression.

A recent concept that has been gaining considerable attention is that of subsyndromal depression (Mossey, Knott, & Craik, 1990). This term describes hospital patients who experience significant depressive feelings but do not meet diagnostic criteria for depression. People who fall into this category have many of the same negative outcomes in health and other areas of functioning, albeit to a lesser extent, as do people who receive a depression diagnosis (e.g., Judd, Rapaport, Paulus, & Brown, 1994; Mossey, Knott, & Craik, 1990). Appropriate treatment of depressive symptoms in these patients improves their health and functional performance.

One of the populations at highest risk for depressive symptoms is nursing home residents. In perhaps the most complete study of depression in this population, Parmalee, Katz, and Lawton (1992) reported that 15.7% of residents of long-term care facilities met criteria for MDD and another 16.5% had significant depressive symptoms. A 1-year follow up on this sample indicated a 5.6% incidence of new cases of MDD and a 6.3% incidence of minor depression. About one half of people with either MDD or depressive symptoms at baseline were still symptomatic a year later.

TABLE 4.1. Common Medical Problems Associated with Depressive Symptoms

Alzheimer's disease	Lupus
Cancer	Nutritional deficits (e.g.,
Cardiac illness	B12 deficiency)
Cerebrovascular accidents	Parkinson's disease
Chronic pain	Vascular dementia
Endocrine disorders	Vision loss
(e.g., hypothyroidism)	

To summarize these findings on rates of depression, severe depression, as indicated by a diagnosis of MDD, is less common in the elderly in community populations than in younger age groups. MDD is, however, prevalent in specific groups, such as hospitalized elderly, people with chronic illnesses, and nursing home patients. Depressive symptoms that do not meet diagnostic criteria for MDD are quite prevalent in community and institutional populations. Treatment of these mild depressive symptoms may help medically ill patients respond more positively to medical treatments or rehabilitation.

Does Depression Differ in Later Life?

Is depression different in later life, and do clinicians need to take different approaches in its diagnosis and treatment? These questions have been partly addressed already in three ways: in the elderly, (1) rates of MDD are fairly low, (2) rates of depressive symptoms are relatively high, and (3) comorbidity of depression and medical problems is quite common.

This question can be approached in two other ways: (1) examining people with the first onset of depression in late life, and (2) evaluating how depression symptoms change with aging for people with recurrent episodes. Little information is available on changes in symptoms as people with recurrent depression age. Several differences have been noted, however, when the onset is after age 60 (see Koenig & Blazer, 1992, and Caine et al., 1994, for reviews). These differences include (1) more frequent occurrence of psychotic or delusional symptoms (Meyers & Greenberg, 1986), more hypochondriacal symptoms (Brown, Sweeney, Loutsch, Kocsis, & Frances, 1984), and less frequent evidence of a family history of affective disorder (Alexopoulos, Young, Abrams, Meyers, & Shamoian, 1989). Some of these differences may be due to the fact that depression is sometimes the first observed symptom in dementia. If cases with cognitive impairment are eliminated, late-onset depression actually has a better long-term prognosis than recurrent depression (Cole, 1983).

An interesting series of studies by Peter Lewinsohn and his colleagues (Lewinsohn, Fenn, Stanton, & Franklin, 1986; Lewinsohn, Hoberman, & Rosenbaum, 1988; Lewinsohn, Rohde, Fischer, & Seeley, 1991) evaluated how age and age of onset affected depression symptoms. Depression symptoms did not vary with age, though there was a trend suggesting that symptoms decline up to the late 60s or early 70s and then gradually increase. Depression, but not aging, was associated with a variety of psychosocial variables, including greater life stress, less social support, reduced social interaction and social skill, engagement in fewer pleasant activities, and higher levels of depressive cognitions. Contrary to expectations, a later age of onset was not related to greater duration of depressive episodes. In a short-term (8 months) longitudinal panel, younger people had a greater likelihood of developing a new episode of depression.

Comparisons have also been made on whether the types or patterns of depressive symptoms differ between older and younger people. Using a community sample of people aged 20 to 98, Gatz and Hurwicz (1990) looked at the relation of age to four dimensions of depression: depressed mood, psychomotor retardation, lack of well-being, and interpersonal difficulties. These factors were derived from a commonly used screening instrument, the Center for Epidemiological Studies Depression Scale (CES-D) (Radloff, 1977). Younger people had higher scores on the depressed mood subscale, while older respondents reported lower rates of positive feelings. Surprisingly, older people did not report higher rates of somatic symptoms on the psychomotor retardation subscale. Similar findings are reported by Newmann, Engel, and Jensen (1991). In a longitudinal panel of older women, classic depressive symptoms involving mood tended to decrease with advancing age, while symptoms reflecting lack of well-being increased with age.

These studies provide a partial answer to the question of how depression changes with aging. Some differences in the pattern of depressive symptoms over time and in late-onset cases have been identified. As we see below, however, there may be multiple etiologies for depression in later life and, as a result, multiple patterns of symptoms.

Etiology of Depression in Later Life

Depression has been linked to many different processes. Biological influences, early life experience, stressful events, cognitive style, and loss of reinforcement are among the most prominent theories. With the exception of theories involving early childhood losses, each of these approaches would predict an increased vulnerability to depression in later life. We have seen, however, that prevalence does not increase, at least of severe depression. As we review possible etiological factors, we should also consider ways in which older people may compensate and adapt to threats to their well-being. We can learn a lot from healthy older people about adaptation in later life that can be incorporated into prevention and treatment programs.

Before discussing specific theories, we want to stress the importance of avoiding simple dualities, such as whether biological or psychosocial factors cause depression. Biological, psychological, and social processes occur simultaneously, with complex interaction and feedback among them. As an example, learning has biological, psychological, and social components and can be investigated at each of these levels. Discoveries about the biological correlates of depression are often interpreted as giving primacy to that domain, yet findings do not pin down whether biological differences in depression are the cause or outcome of behavioral or cognitive patterns. Furthermore, even if one domain has a primary role in etiology, successful treatment may occur in any domain. For example, treatments that emphasize learning new patterns of behavior may be effective, because changes in overt behavior are accompanied by modification of the underlying biological processes. Even biological treatments are heterogeneous, that is, drugs acting on different neurotransmitters have similar outcomes in relieving depression symptoms. As Akiskal and McKinney (1973) proposed in their classic paper, depression is likely to be is the common outcome of many different pathways, with biological, psychological, and social processes contributing in varying degrees.

Important discoveries of the role of neurotransmitters in depression have given biological theories of depression considerable prestige. Several neurotransmitters have been implicated in depression, notably, serotonin and norepinephrine, but other neurochemicals such as dopamine, histamine, gamma-aminobutyric acid (GABA), glutamate, glycine, and acetylcholine may play a part (Shuchter, Downs, & Zisook, 1996). Antidepressant medications block the reuptake of serotonin and norepinephrine by brain neurons or, in the case of monoamine oxidase (MAO) inhibitors, block the chemical that deactivates norepinephrine at uptake at nerve endings. The result is to increase the levels of these neurotransmitters available for brain cells.

Significant age changes have been found in the neurotransmitter systems associated with depression (see Ferrier & McKeith, 1991, and Morgan, 1992, for reviews). Serotonin receptors are estimated to decrease by 20% to 40% in later life. Norepinephrine levels decrease with aging because of increased MAO activity. Dopamine also has a similar reduction with advancing age. It has been speculated that both the amounts of various neurotransmitters as well as the balance among them contribute to depression (Cohen, 1992). Besides the identified neurotransmitters, other neurochemicals may be involved in the etiology of depression.

Another biological indicator of late-life depression is anatomical changes in the brain. Several studies have reported brain abnormalities in older depressed patients, including enlargement of the ventricles, changes in white matter, and other alterations (Alexopoulos, 1994; Alexopoulos, Young, & Shindledecker, 1992; Leuchter, 1994). Ventricle enlargement in depressed patients has been found to be associated with poorer performance on neuropsychological tests (Abas, Sahakian, & Levy, 1990). These findings suggest that brain abnormalities may have a role in the etiology of at least some cases of late-onset depression. These types of abnormalities may also indicate the presence of Alzheimer's disease or vascular dementia. Depression is a frequent, early symptom in dementia, and so these findings of brain abnormalities are at least partly due to inclusion of people who have early dementia and comorbid depression.

Many different psychosocial theories have addressed the etiology of depression. We wish to comment on three theories, which, in varying degrees, have been applied to the study of late-life depression: (1) stressful events as a trigger, (2) behavioral theories concerning loss of reinforcers, and (3) cognitive theories of dysfunctional thought patterns that predispose people to depression.

Stressful life events have long been regarded as a precipitant for depressive episodes (e.g., Paykel, 1974, 1979; Brown, Bifulco, & Harris, 1987). Rates of depression increase in the 6 months following negative life events (Paykel, 1979). The number of stressful life events and daily hassles has been found to be related to depression in samples of older people (Lewinsohn et al., 1991).

The psychological, social, and biological implications of stress and loss may result in increased vulnerability to depression. Nonetheless, the role of stressful events as a precipitant is complex. On the one hand, most depressed people identify negative events as precipitants. At one time, it was considered that a more biological (endogenous) form of depression did not have environmental precipitants. But individuals with so-called endogenous depression were more severely depressed and were poor reporters of their past history. More careful interviewing of these individuals has led to identification of triggering events (Goodwin & Bunney, 1973). But many people who experience negative life events do not become depressed. Specific losses, such as retirement, loss of friends, and particularly death of a spouse, can be very stressful but do not necessarily lead to depression. Stressful events, then, may create a vulnerability to depression, which then unfolds depending on other factors, such as biological predisposition, the meaning of the loss to the person, social support, and coping resources.

Early childhood loss is another type of stressful event that has been evaluated as a risk factor for depression, but empirical findings are mixed. Some studies suggest increased lifetime rates of depression among people who lost a parent early in life, while other studies have found no association (Paykel, 1979; George, 1994). George reports that separation or divorce, but not death of a parent during childhood, are associated with subsequent risk of depression. She speculates that disruptions in a child's life due to dysfunctional family relationships are more important than loss in producing a vulnerability to depression. The effects of losses and other childhood events may also depend on other factors, such as how the loss is handled, coping resources, and biological vulnerability.

Behavioral theories of depression have been developed by Ferster (1973) and Lewinsohn (1975) and elaborated in a series of classic papers by Lewinsohn and his associates (e.g., Lewinsohn, Biglan, & Zeiss, 1976; Lewinsohn & MacPhillamy, 1974; Lewinsohn et al., 1991; Teri & Lewinsohn, 1982). This approach begins with careful observation of the behavior of depressed people. Depressed people engage in lower rates of behavior and receive lower levels of positive reinforcement. The key to depression is a loss of reinforcement, which can occur as a result of losses of significant people in one's life, erosion of positive exchanges with other people, or because the depression-prone individual has fewer skills to elicit positive responses from other people (Lewinsohn et al., 1976). Decreases in positive reinforcement then set up a vicious cycle: the person decreases the output of behavior, which further reduces the amount of reinforcement, which lowers mood, behavior output, and so forth. From this perspective, people who experience common losses in later life, such as becoming widowed or disabled, are at risk for depression because of decreased opportunities for obtaining positive reinforcement.

To examine the relation of depression and behavior, Lewinsohn and his colleagues developed the Pleasant Events Schedule, an instrument that assesses the extent to which people engage in behaviors that are reinforcing or enjoyable to them (Lewinsohn & MacPhillamy, 1974). As might be expected, depressed people engage in fewer pleasant activities and find fewer activities potentially enjoyable. This pattern has been found for both younger and older depressed people. A version of the Pleasant Events Schedule has been developed specifically for use in assessment and treatment of older people (Teri & Lewinsohn, 1982).

Lewinsohn's group has also described specific deficits in social skills, that is, behaviors that elicit positive responses in social situations (Lewinsohn et al., 1976, 1991). Examining social skills in group situations, they found that people who receive fewer positive reinforcements from other people are less active, less likely to respond quickly to other people, are sensitive to an aversive person in the group, give fewer positive reinforcements to other people, and do not direct their behavior evenly to the members of a group (Lewinsohn et al., 1976). Social skills deficits are also central to the interpersonal theory of depression (Klerman, Weissman, Rounsaville, & Chevron, 1984).

A cognitive model of depression has been developed by Beck and his colleagues (Beck, 1976; Beck, Rush, Shaw, & Emery, 1979). As with behavior theories of depression, the cognitive model begins with observation, in this case, of what depressed people think. Depression has been found to be associated with specific patterns of thinking, in which people hold exaggerated, negative views of themselves, other people, and the future. As a result of negative appraisals of themselves and their experiences, people feel depressed. They may not, however, be aware of these negative beliefs. In fact, these cognitions are termed "automatic thoughts" because they constitute rapid and habitual ways of evaluating information.

A key feature of the theory is that these cognitions are distortions produced by faulty logical patterns that emphasize the negative features or implications of any event or experience. These logical errors cause events to be interpreted consistent with a core set of beliefs about the self as worthless, unlovable, incompetent, and so on. The therapist's role is to help patients identify and question their automatic thoughts and develop alternative ways of looking at themselves and the world that do not result in depression.

As with other theories of depression, the cognitive theory would predict increased rates of depression in later life. Old age is associated with a variety of negative stereotypes and expectations, as well as real losses. The extent to which people incorporate negative cultural views of aging into their self-image and the extent to which losses activate negative belief systems are associated with increased depression. One of the keys to becoming an effective cognitive therapist is to be able to identify the distortions in a person's thought processes. With an older client, that means being able to differentiate realistic appraisals of negative events in later life from exaggerated cognitions, a point we will return to when discussing treatment of depression (Chapter 8).

There is considerable overlap in theory and practice between behavioral and cognitive approaches to depression. Similar features can also be found in other approaches, such as the interpersonal theory of depression (IPT) (Klerman et al., 1984) and Seligman's theory of learned helplessness and depression (1975, 1991). Although emphasizing cognitions, behavior, and social relationships to varying degrees, each approach incorporates all these dimensions. Lewinsohn's behavioral theory includes negative thought patterns and social behavior as important dimensions. Similarly, Beck's cognitive theory emphasizes behavioral tasks as a useful way to generate and challenge negative cognitions. IPT uses behavioral and cognitive strategies in building improved social behavior and social relationships. These approaches share a focus on the specific behaviors and cognitions that are associated with depression. They emphasize immediate and habitual patterns of response and implement strategies in a direct manner to change one's usual reactions. The result is a highly effective set of approaches that have outcome rates similar to antidepressant medications with younger patients (Robinson, Berman, & Neimeyer, 1990) and that have all been found to be effective in controlled trials with older adults (Gallagher-Thompson & Thompson, 1996).

In summary, depression is probably the most frequent problem that clinicians encounter in the elderly. Although estimates of depression vary, there is considerable consensus that depressive symptoms are a frequent problem in later life. Depression is particularly prominent in certain populations, notably people with medical illnesses and in nursing homes. Depressive symptoms are best viewed as the outcome of multiple processes involving biology, behavior, and cognition. As we will see in Chapter 8, interventions can be made at any of these levels and can result in considerable improvement for older depressed people.

Related Disorders

Bipolar Disorders

Before leaving depression, we want to discuss briefly two related phenomena, bipolar disorders and suicide. Bipolar disorders are rarer in later life than at younger ages (Koenig & Blazer, 1992). Onset is usually earlier in life. Some research suggests that onset occurs by about 20 years of age (Loranger & Levine, 1978), while other studies suggest a somewhat later average age of onset (see De Leo & Diekstra, 1990). Onset of bipolar disorders in later life has been reported, but it is infrequent. The rates of bipolar disorders in later life are also low because of a tendency for manic depression to become diminished with aging (Koenig & Blazer, 1992). Nonetheless, some people with bipolar disorders continue to have significant mood swings in later life. Thus, the possibility of a bipolar disorder needs to be considered during an initial assessment of an older client. Depressed patients should be evaluated for a history of mood swings. When manic symptoms are encountered, a differential diagnosis should include consideration of the possibility of delirium.

Suicide

Evaluation of suicide risk is a necessary consideration when working with older adults. Older adults commit suicide at a much higher rate than any other age group. The rate for suicide in the United States is about 12.2 cases per 100,000 of the population; for the elderly, the rate is 20.1 per 100,000. Though they make up only 13% of the population, older people account for 20% of all suicides (McIntosh, Santos, Hubbard, & Overholser, 1994; Conwell, 1994; Mościcki, 1995).

The increase in suicide rates in later life is due solely to the high rates found among older men. Women commit suicide at a lower rate than men at every age. The rate for women reaches a peak in the decade of the 50s and then declines slightly thereafter. Men, on the other hand, have a dramatic increase in suicides beginning at around age 60, with the highest rate found among men over age 85. The difference in rates of male to female suicides has continued to grow, increasing from 3.1 to 1 in 1979 to 4.2 to 1 in 1990 (Mościcki, 1995). Some differences are related to race and ethnicity. Rates of suicide increase with age for white, Japanese, Chinese, and Filipino American males. For African Americans and Native Americans, however, the peak for suicides occurs at around age 35, with a decline at later ages (McIntosh et al., 1994). Similar effects of culture and ethnicity are found in other countries as well. In Great Britain, for example, older English-born white men have an increasing rate of suicide with aging, but male immigrants from the Indian subcontinent do not (Dennis & Lindesay, 1995).

Suicide attempts, compared to completed suicides, follow a very different pattern with age. Young adults attempt the most suicides and the rate of attempts declines with advancing age (Bille-Brahe, 1993). Women also make more attempts than men at every age, though the differences have narrowed both in young adulthood and again after age 65. These findings suggest that older men are more likely to make suicide attempts with more lethal means and greater intent to end their lives.

In contrast to rates, the methods of suicide do not vary much with age (McIntosh et al., 1994). The most common method is use of firearms, followed by hanging. Use of gas or poisons (including medication overdose) is the third most common method. Women are less likely to use firearms than men and more likely to use poisons, but firearm use by women is increasing.

A related problem is self-destructive behavior. Examples include inappropriate use of prescription medications or alcohol, delaying medical treatment for a life-threatening condition, or risk-taking behavior such as driving recklessly. There is little systematic information available on this type of indirect suicide. Estimates suggest that self-destructive behaviors are more common at younger ages, although that finding might partly reflect the reluctance of physicians or medical examiners to subject the families of an older person to an extensive and potentially embarrassing inquiry about cause of death (McIntosh et al., 1994). The methods of self-destructive behavior the elderly use may also be more subtle than those chosen by younger people—for example, taking too much of a prescription medication or taking none at all.

There are several risk factors for suicide. The two foremost risks are physical illness and depression, typically in combination (Conwell, 1994; Heikkinen & Lönnqvist, 1995; McIntosh et al., 1994). There is some indication that depression plays an even greater role in suicides of older people than younger (Conwell & Brent, 1995). Somatic illnesses that lead to suicide may or may not be life-threatening. Typically, they involve pain or discomfort. They also tend to have a poor prognosis, that is, the condition will only get worse, not better. Widows, widowers, and divorced men are more likely to commit suicide than married persons, especially if they have a weak social network (Conwell & Brent, 1995; McIntosh et al., 1994). Other factors associated with increased risk include alcoholism and recent losses. Retirement does not have a direct relation to suicide but the long-term social, emotional, and economic consequences of retirement may contribute to some suicides. Finkel and Rosman (1995) suggest that knowing someone who committed suicide may be an important predisposing factor.

An illness not related to higher risk of suicide is Alzheimer's disease. As a result of their cognitive deficits, people with dementing disorders are limited in their ability to formulate or follow through on a suicide plan

(McIntosh et al., 1994). As with any other client, however, dementia patients should be assessed for suicide risk and appropriate precautions taken when suicidal ideation or behaviors are identified.

Assisted suicide is more likely to be an issue for dementia patients. Suicide pacts and double suicides by older couples get considerable media attention. The typical pattern is for one person to kill the other and then him- or herself. The motivation usually involves preventing further suffering, for example, when the husband of an Alzheimer's patient kills his wife and then himself. When working with couples on issues of chronic illness or disability, clinicians should assess if there is a suicide or homicide–suicide risk.

One of the most important factors for identifying risk is a history of prior suicide attempts. Older suicides, however, are less likely to have made prior attempts or to have talked about committing suicide (Carney, Rich, Burke, & Fowler, 1994; Conwell, 1994). Many, however, have made visits to health professionals in the immediate past. In one large sample of older suicides, over one half had seen a health professional in the past 30 days (Carney et al., 1994). Similarly, Conwell, Olson, Caine, and Flannery (1991) reported that 7 of 18 suicides had seen their primary physician in the preceding week. The medical visits may have triggered feelings of hopelessness over their medical condition. Whether the health professionals involved might have been able to detect indirect evidence of suicide risk in the patient's behavior or demeanor or if inquiry into the patient's mood might have identified the suicide risk cannot be determined. These findings, however, underscore the importance of monitoring older clients for suicidal thoughts, especially individuals in high-risk groups—men, depressed, chronically ill.

We also want to note that some suicides occur in nursing homes and other institutional settings (McIntosh et al., 1994). It is usually difficult to gain access to the means to commit suicide in a nursing home, but some patients are able to develop and carry out a plan. As with other suicides, these patients tend to have better cognitive functioning and no dementia. A case in point is the psychologist Bruno Bettelheim, who ended his life in a nursing home by taking an overdose of medications and tying a bag over his head (McIntosh et al., 1994). Anticipation of being placed in a nursing home or any other unwanted move can also increase risk of suicide.

One consequence of suicide may be feelings of embarrassment and shame among friends or relatives. Close relatives of older people who commit suicide may have greater difficulties in grieving and resolving their grief than if the person died of natural causes. They also may receive less social support in the period following their relative's death than do mourners of elderly whose relative died of natural causes (Farberow, Gallagher-Thompson, Gilewski, & Thompson, 1992).

ANXIETY DISORDERS

Anxiety disorders in later life have not received as much attention as depression, but findings from the ECA studies have suggested that the prevalence of anxiety is actually higher than depression. The ECA studies found anxiety disorders, including phobias, panic attacks, and obsessive–compulsive disorders, to be the most common psychiatric diagnosis in the adult population (Regier et al., 1988), with a 1-month prevalence of 7.3%. Prevalence was lower among people over age 65—5.5%—but anxiety was still the most common problem among older people except for cognitive impairment. Rates of anxiety disorders were almost twice as high among women as men at every age.

To some extent, these findings may be an artifact of how depression and anxiety were determined. As noted previously, rates of diagnosed depression in the ECA studies were low, while depression symptoms were common. Because depression and anxiety symptoms frequently occur together, the decision to classify a patient in one category or the other becomes problematic. Whatever the true rate of anxiety disorders in later life, however, the implication of the ECA studies is that clinicians should be aware of the possibility of anxiety symptoms in their older clients.

As with depression, the term anxiety describes both a syndrome and symptoms. When examining anxiety symptoms, several surveys have found increases with age, particularly for somatic symptoms such as shortness of breath or rapid heart rate (Himmelfarb & Murrell, 1984).

As was the case with depression, anxiety symptoms in older people generally occur in conjunction with other psychiatric and medical disorders (Gurian & Miner, 1991). Symptoms of anxiety and depression frequently coexist, and anxiety can be a concomitant of many other psychiatric disorders. Anxiety is associated with many different medical problems. Table 4.2 lists medical disorders and medications commonly accompanied by anxiety symptoms. Anxiety may also be a feature of brain disorders including Alzheimer's and Parkinson's diseases (Cohen, 1992). It is a common symptom with hearing and vision loss. Of course, anxiety symptoms can be part of the psychological reaction to illness and hospitalization. Anxiety may also present solely in terms of somatic symptoms that have no underlying medical cause (Gurian & Miner, 1991). An older person may complain of headaches, chest pains, fatigue, or gastrointestinal symptoms that are primarily psychological in origin. As in depression, clinicians need to be able to differente the causes of anxiety symptoms as medical or psychological or an interaction of both.

Only a little information is available on the age of onset of anxiety symptoms or its life course. The available evidence, however, suggests that anxiety usually develops earlier in life (e.g., Blazer, George, & Hughes,

TABLE 4.2. Medical Disorders Associated with Anxiety

Cardiovascular/respiratory	Neurological
Asthma	Epilepsy
Cardiac arrhythmias	Huntington's disease
Chronic obstructive pulmonary disease	Multiple sclerosis
Congestive heart failure	Dementia
Coronary insufficiency	Delirium
Hypertension	
	Substance related
Endocrine	Intoxications
Cushing's syndrome	Anticholinergic drugs
Hyperthyroidism	Aspirin
Hypothyroidism	Caffeine
Hypoglycemia	Cocaine
Menopause	Hallucinogens
	Steroids
	Sympathomimetics
	Withdrawal syndromes
	Alcohol
	Sedative–hypnotics

Note. Adapted from Raj and Sheehan (1988). Copyright 1988 by *Psychiatric Annals*. Adapted by permission.

1991). Older people who are anxious usually have a history of similar symptoms that have recurred during their adult years. We have, however, observed the onset of anxiety symptoms, including phobias and generalized anxiety, in later life.

There is also not much known about the specific etiology of anxiety in older people, apart from its occurrence as a primary or secondary symptom in a variety of illnesses. People have often speculated that fears about death and dying might play a part in anxiety reactions. Fears about the circumstances of how one might die, for example, dying alone or being put through painful medical procedures, can trigger anxiety or depression in an older person. In general, however, fear of death is not more common among the elderly than in other age groups and may lessen with advancing age (see Gurian & Miner, 1991, for a review).

At a biological level, epinephrine and norepinephrine are critical in anxiety reactions, while some features of serotonin function increase and others decrease. The pattern of changes in these systems with aging probably do not place older people at increased risk of anxiety (Sunderland, Lawlor, Martinez, & Molchan, 1991).

SCHIZOPHRENIA

Schizophrenia in later life has two distinct patterns. First, many people who develop schizophrenia earlier in life continue to be symptomatic in old age. Second, there is a pattern of late-onset paranoid disorders that often meets diagnostic criteria for schizophrenia. These late-onset cases have been considered as a variant of early-onset schizophrenia and as a problem that is distinct from it (Roth, 1987). Whatever the classification, the distinction between early- and late-onset cases has considerable importance for clinical practice, since approaches to treatment vary depending on age of onset.

Prevalence of schizophrenic disorders is low in later life. Combining all schizophrenic disorders, the ECA studies found rates of 0.1% among people over age 65 compared to rates of 0.8% for 18- to 24-year-olds and 1.1% for 25- to 44-year-olds. There are several reasons for this low rate. First, the ECA study examined community populations. At least some people with chronic schizophrenia are likely to reside in institutional settings—particularly in nursing homes, since the advent of deinstitutionalization of long-term patients from mental hospitals (e.g., Meeks et al., 1990). Gurland and Cross (1982) estimated prevalence of schizophrenia in nursing homes at 12%. Second, late-onset cases usually involve paranoid symptoms and suspiciousness. These people are likely to refuse to be interviewed in a community sample. Third, as we will see, there is evidence of remission of symptoms with aging.

Early-Onset Schizophrenia

Let us first examine the course of early-onset schizophrenia over the life span. Despite progress in its treatment, schizophrenia remains the most devastating and intractable disorder of the adult years. Symptoms interfere with relationships and work and push many chronically ill individuals to the margins of society.

In his classic work on schizophrenia, Kraeplin (1971) believed it had an unremitting, deteriorating course. This view was reinforced by experiences with chronic mentally ill patients who grew old in mental hospitals. There is, however, increasing evidence that at least some people experience partial or complete remission of symptoms over time.

Several longitudinal studies have tracked the lifetime course of schizophrenia. These studies vary on key methodological questions, such as how the diagnosis is confirmed and the method and frequency of follow-up, but they provide a consistent picture of long-term outcomes. Many people diagnosed with schizophrenia earlier in life show improvement over time (e.g., Ciompi, 1987; Clausen, 1986; Harding, Brooks, Ashikaga, Strauss, & Brier, 1987; Strauss, 1987; Tsuang, 1986). It is estimated that between one third and one half of people with a documented schizophrenic episode recover completely or have only minimal and occasional symptoms in later life. Improvement may occur in one area of functioning, for example, work or social relationships, but not in other domains (Strauss, 1987). Some people, however, have little or no remission of symptoms over time.

The results from a particularly well-conducted study in Lausanne, Switzerland, illustrate these outcomes (Ciompi, 1987). In this study, people who had been hospitalized for schizophrenia 30 to 40 years earlier were interviewed. Hospital records were evaluated to confirm that they met current diagnostic criteria for schizophrenia at the time of the hospitalization. Age at follow-up ranged between 65 to 97. Higher mortality was found for the original cohort of hospitalized patients compared to the normal population. Among survivors, 20% had been free of symptoms for a period of at least 5 years, and another 43% were markedly improved compared to earlier functioning.

In a critique of schizophrenia outcome studies, Cohen (1990) has argued that some problems have been emphasized and others ignored. Grouping symptoms into three broad categories—psychopathological symptoms, organic factors, and social functioning—Cohen reviewed evidence of changes with aging for each domain. Psychopathology, including both positive and negative symptoms, diminishes with aging. In contrast, organic factors, including cognitive deficits and ventricular enlargement, increase with aging, possibly due to normal age effects. Results for social functioning are more complex. Schizophrenics generally have smaller social networks than other people, and their networks have a higher proportion of kin than nonkin. These trends are accentuated in older patients, though that may reflect age-related factors rather than schizophrenia. On the other hand, improvement may occur in other social domains, including quality of relationships and vocational activities.

A significant proportion of early-onset schizophrenics continues to be troubled by recurrent symptoms, such as hallucinations, delusions, apathy, and impaired social functioning. As they age, family support remains critical, although their social network may erode somewhat (Meeks et al., 1990). They may also suffer from neurological side effects of neuroleptic medications, especially tardive dyskinesia (Jeste & Wyatt, 1985). These chronically ill individuals are disproportionately represented in single-room-occupancy hotels, among the homeless, and in nursing homes. Some mild cognitive dysfunction also appears to be associated with chronic schizophrenia, though the extent of disability is milder than found in dementia (Heaton et al., 1994; Goldstein, Zubin, & Pogue-Geile, 1991).

Late-Onset Paranoid Disorders

Late-onset paranoid disorders, often defined as development of symptoms after age 45, are considered a form of schizophrenia, although symptoms can have other etiologies as well. Various terms have been used to describe these disorders including "late-life paraphrenia," "late-life paranoid disorder" and late-onset schizophrenia. Late-onset paranoid disorders are both similar to and different from early-onset cases. Hallucinations and delusions are more florid in late-onset cases, that is, they tend to be vivid and dramatic. Late-onset cases also have less evidence of a thought disorder or flattening of affect. As an example, Rabins, McHugh, Pauker, and Thomas (1987) described symptoms in a series of older patients meeting DSM-III criteria for schizophrenia. All patients had delusions, 69% had auditory hallucinations, 29% had visual hallucinations, and 26% tactile hallucinations (some had more than one type of hallucination).

Roth (1987) proposes that onset typically occurs in two stages. During the first stage, which may last for a period of 6 to 18 months, there is a gradual increase of suspiciousness, irritability, and hostility. During this period, people become more reclusive, develop ideas of reference about other people, and may begin making frequent complaints to the police or other authorities. The second stage involves the eruption of visual and auditory hallucinations. This second stage may be precipitated by stressful life events, but often the events are of a trivial nature. Patients, however, regard these events as highly significant, interpreting them within the framework of their delusions.

Two predisposing characteristics have been identified in late-onset paranoia. First is a pattern of a lifelong history of marginal adjustment, particularly in the area of interpersonal relationships (Kay, Cooper, Garside, & Roth, 1976; Post, 1966, 1980; Rabins, 1992). These individuals may have been employed but either did not marry or had brief, unsuccessful marriages. Symptoms are sometimes precipitated by an increase in social isolation, such as following retirement or the loss of a key family member or friend. This pattern occurs more frequently among women than men. In the second pattern, sensory loss plays a central role in the development of symptoms. People with hearing loss, particularly bilateral hearing loss that develops in midlife, are prone to development of paranoid disorders. Some association with vision loss has also been reported (Cooper & Porter, 1976). There are fewer predisposing personality factors in paranoid patients with sensory loss compared to those without (Cooper, Garside, & Kay, 1976).

The following example illustrates a common pattern of a late-onset paranoid disorder. The client, Miss Thorpe, was a woman in her early 70s who sought help at an outpatient program serving the elderly because she believed that her landlord was stimulating her sexually by means of extrasensory perception (ESP). Miss Thorpe provided a detailed life history. She was the unwanted, only child of older parents. She described an upbringing devoid of attention. Her mother raised her with an odd set of beliefs, which combined psychoanalysis and astrology in an idiosyncratic way and emphasized that sex and elimination were disgusting processes. Miss Thorpe still maintained these beliefs. She married at age 40, shortly after her mother's death. Almost immediately after the marriage she had a hysterectomy. She and her husband soon drifted apart, though she maintained occasional contact with him. During her adult years, she worked continuously as a salesperson in department stores. She had never had a psychiatric hospitalization, but she described one apparent psychotic episode 20 years earlier. This incident occurred in a dentist's office, during which she felt sexual feelings toward him or he made sexual advances toward her. This story, however, was jumbled, and it was not possible to tell what had happened. It is possible there were other, similar episodes, but she did not volunteer information about them. Since she retired a couple of years earlier, she lost contact with the few friends she had at work and lived a largely isolated life.

Miss Thorpe's current symptoms had begun a few months earlier. She lived in a small apartment building built around a courtyard and could see her landlord's apartment from her window. She had been friendly with him, conversing with him when they met in the courtyard. One time she invited him to dinner, but he responded with a noncommittal answer. She concluded that he had signaled her that he was coming to dinner by moving the venetian blinds in his window in a particular way. When he did not show up for dinner, she became very upset. She confronted him, but he treated her in a dismissive way. After that incident, she began experiencing sexual discomfort at night which she believed was caused by ESP. Her symptoms included both revulsion at being violated and attraction toward her landlord.

This case is typical of many late-life paranoid disorders. Miss Thorpe had functioned adequately during her adult life, with possibly only one previous psychotic episode. Symptoms developed following a period of increasing social isolation and after an incident where she felt rejected and humiliated. Her symptoms were dramatic and florid. Despite these symptoms, she was continuing to function adequately and did not exhibit any other obvious problems.

In cases involving sensory loss, symptoms often revolve around the disability. People with hearing loss may fill in what they think others are saying. They assume people are talking about them, saying negative things or making threats. In cases where vision loss is involved, visual sensory input can be distorted, for example, seeing a threatening stranger in the mirror or believing someone is coming into the house and stealing things or rearranging the furniture.

Other patterns of late-life paranoid symptoms do not meet diagnostic criteria for schizophrenia. One such pattern involves a single, encapsulated symptom. The older person may believe that a light is being shined in on him while he sleeps or may hear sounds or may feel discomfort in a part of the body.

Paranoid symptoms can be associated with delirium and dementia. Patients with a delirium may have hallucinations and paranoid delusions, which resemble a late-life paranoid disorder. As an example, a patient who was in the hospital began refusing food and medication because she believed staff were trying to poison her. Dementia patients may fill in the information they have trouble processing or remembering. Common complaints in dementia include someone stealing the patient's wallet, purse, money, or other valuables or an intruder who breaks into the patient's apartment and takes things. Some patients have an imaginary companion, often a child, who may or may not be threatening. Late in dementia, patients may experience illusions, especially in situations where there is low illumination. They may be watching television in a dimly lit room, for example, and report seeing small animals running across the room. The onset of paranoid symptoms with delirium and dementia needs to be clearly differentiated from late-onset schizophrenia.

Studies have investigated the relation of late-onset paranoid disorders to organic causes. Delusional symptoms, for example, are more common in people with evidence of small cerebral infarcts (e.g., Cummings, 1987a). Most patients with late-onset schizophrenia, however, do not progress to dementia (Roth, 1987).

PERSONALITY DISORDERS

There is little systematic knowledge about personality disorders in late life, but practicing clinicians can attest to the enduring and disruptive effects that a personality disorder has on the patient's life and on the therapeutic relationship. As at earlier ages, the persistent problems of the client with a personality disorder absorb a disproportionate amount of a clinicians's time and energy. Adding to the usual difficulties in dealing with patients with a personality disorder are age-related issues, such as coordinating with health care providers over treatment of chronic health problems. Therapists often find themselves having to repair disrupted relationships between the patient with a personality disorder and other professionals and instructing clients on how to present themselves to health professionals in ways that assure that care is given, rather than withdrawn in angry reaction to the patient's typical interpersonal style.

DSM-IV defines personality disorders as personality traits that are rigid and inflexible and that lead to functional difficulties and intrapsychic distress (American Psychiatric Association, 1994; Tyrer, 1995). Personality disorders are difficult to diagnose reliably at any age. One source of unreliability is that diagnosis depends, in part, on making inferences about personality structure underlying overt behavior (Sadavoy & Fogel, 1992). Another problem in developing reliable diagnostic criteria is the various types of overlap in the disorders; patients often have characteristics of two or more disorders (Tyrer, 1995; Widiger & Sanderson, 1995). An alternative classification scheme, a dimensional model, is based on scores on standardized personality assessments (Widiger & Sanderson, 1995). From a dimensional perspective, personality disorders represent a blending together of traits in unique patterns, which are captured only in part by current diagnostic categories. As yet, this type of dimensional approach is still in early stages of development.

The difficulties in establishing diagnosis are reflected in estimates of the prevalence of personality disorder, which vary widely from study to study. Surveys of community populations have found prevalence to range from less than 1% to around 13% of the population (see Girolamo & Reich, 1993). The ECA main studies included only one category of personality disorders, antisocial personality (Regier et al., 1988). A rate of 0.5% was reported for the adult population. Younger men were most likely to have this diagnosis, with the rate dropping to 0.1% for men over age 65 and to virtually zero for older women. In a subsequent study conducted at the Baltimore ECA site, specific assessments were made using DSM-III diagnostic criteria to identify personality disorders (Samuels, Nestadt, Romanoski, Folstein, & McHugh, 1994). A rate of 5.9% of personality disorders was found in that sample. Including people with a provisional diagnosis of personality disorder increased the rate to 9.3%. Comparing older (55 and over) and younger (18–54) people in that sample, it was found that personality disorders were less common in the older sample (6.6%, compared to 10.5%) (Cohen et al., 1994). Focusing on specific diagnoses, older people were much less likely to have antisocial or histrionic disorders than younger people. Older people also had lower rates of maladaptive personality traits.

Despite the limited information available on personality disorders in late life, some impressions of the natural history of these disorders emerge from the available clinical literature. By definition, personality disorders have their onset in adolescence or early adulthood (American Psychiatric Association, 1994), so older clients with a diagnosis of personality disorder typically have a long history of symptoms and problems. There are, however, two exceptions to this pattern. First, a personality disorder may be "uncovered" by a loss or other change in later life (Sadavoy & Fogel, 1992). As an example, a woman with a dependent personality may have functioned adequately because of the efforts made by her husband, but after he dies, she is unable to cope with even elementary tasks in everyday life. A careful history reveals features of personality disorder that have been consistent throughout adulthood but that were contained by social support or work routines. A second pattern is that personality traits may be exacerbated by other psychiatric problems such as depression or brain disorders. In these cases, the patient may meet most of the criteria for a personality disorder, but these symptoms are secondary to another problem. Using current criteria, personality disorder should not be diagnosed in these instances.

How do personality disorders change with aging? Because of the virtual absence of longitudinal data, we do not know if there are predictable changes in symptoms as people age or a tendency to move from one disorder to another. It is also not known if the course of a personality disorder is characterized by gradual improvement or deterioration with aging. Patients with diagnoses that involve dramatic and emotional symptoms (e.g., antisocial, borderline, histrionic) have been reported to improve as they age (Tyrer & Seivewright, 1988). Improvement may be due largely to a decrease in activity level and impulsivity. Case examples also suggest that personality disorders can be exacerbated by losses associated with aging. For example, a person concerned with issues of trust who experiences losses may brood excessively on them and become increasing isolated, suspicious, and paranoid. Clinical observations also suggest that features of a personality disorder can shift with age toward somatic and depressive preoccupations and conflict with children or other close relations (Sadavoy & Fogel, 1992).

The absence of more information is regrettable but understandable in light of continuing controversies over diagnosis and conceptualization of personality disorders. Nonetheless, older people with personality disorders are likely to present considerable challenge to clinicians, just as they do at earlier ages. Their relationships with family, friends, physicians, and the other people in their lives are likely to be complex and problematic. Their own emotional distress is prominent and difficult to change. And their relationship with the therapist will be stormy, challenging, and ultimately a significant drain on time and energy, which is not offset frequently enough by signs of improvement. Personality disorders can be especially disruptive in institutional settings such as hospitals and nursing homes, taking up disproportionate staff time and involvement. The clinician's role is varied, sometimes consisting of providing treatment, frequently consisting of stepping in to prevent things from getting worse.

ALCOHOL AND SUBSTANCE ABUSE

Alcohol and substance abuse constitutes another of the hidden problems of later life. Many people cannot conceive that older people would abuse drugs or alcohol and so ignore the signs and symptoms of a problem. Even professionals in the substance abuse field sometimes mistakenly believe that these problems burn out before old age or that abusers die before reaching old age. Another barrier to recognition of this problem is that older people with drinking problems often do not fit the stereotype of the down-and-out alcoholic. Instead, they may come from middle-class homes and communities and have a history of stable functioning. As a result, professionals are sometimes reluctant to look for and identify substance abuse problems (Atkinson, 1990). Another problem in recognition of substance abuse among older patients is that symptoms can be wrongly ascribed to aging or senility. Falling, depression, slurred speech, poor memory, or a decline in personal hygiene and self-care are all common symptoms of dementia and other age-related problems, so the role of drugs or alcohol can be easily overlooked.

Substance abuse rates are lower in old age compared to earlier periods of adulthood. Nonetheless, abuse, especially of alcohol, is a significant problem. Reviewing prevalence studies on alcohol abuse in later life, Atkinson, Ganzini, and Bernstein (1992) reported that rates of heavy drinking (that is, greater alcohol consumption than normal but without adverse consequences at present) ranged between 6% and 24% for community-dwelling men and between 1% and 2% for women. For problem drinking, that is, where there were adverse social, behavioral, or health consequences, estimates for older men ranged between 1% and 12%, while for women the rates were 0.01% to 1%. These rates are lower than for other age groups, in part because of the difficulties detecting older alcoholics that were noted earlier and in part due to the lower life expectancy for heavy drinkers.

The proportion of alcohol problems is higher in certain populations, including hospital and psychiatric patients (Curtis, Geller, Stokes, Levine, & Moore, 1989; Mangion, Platt, & Syam, 1992). In outpatient mental health programs, alcohol problems have been found to be involved in 10% of geriatric cases (Reifler et al., 1982). A study of consecutive admissions of older people to a hospital emergency room identified 14% who were currently alcohol abusers (Adams, Magruder-Habib, Trued, & Broome, 1992). Their most common medical complaint was gastrointestinal problems. Physicians detected only about one fifth of people with alcohol problems.

High rates of alcohol use have sometimes been reported in retirement communities. A careful analysis of these findings suggests that many residents drink moderately but that heavy drinking is rare (Adams, 1995). Heavy drinking may be more common among the young old than people age 75 and over. Finally, the possibility of alcoholism among residents of nursing homes and other congregate living situations should not be overlooked. Although they may have limited access to alcohol, nursing home patients may be able to obtain sufficient amounts from family or friends—or even staff—for it to be a problem.

Two distinct patterns have been identified among older alcoholics (Atkinson et al., 1985; Atkinson, Tolson, & Turner, 1990; Mishara & Kastenbaum, 1980). First are the lifelong drinkers, people who have been either regular or intermittent abusers of alcohol all their adult lives. This group constitutes about two-thirds of older alcohol abusers. The other third of older problem drinkers are people who increased their consumption of alcohol in later life, usually following a stress or loss. A common pattern is for an older man who becomes widowed to drink more heavily as a way of dealing with loneliness and social isolation.

One key aspect of alcohol use by the elderly is that they are more sensitive to its effects, as they are to the effects of most drugs (DeHart & Hoffman, 1997). Older people can develop adverse effects with lower rates of consumption than younger problem drinkers. As an example, even moderate amounts of alcohol can lead to mild cognitive impairment among older people (Atkinson & Kofoed, 1982). A person who always drank moderately with little or no adverse consequences may begin having problems in functioning in later life without any increase in alcohol consumption.

The role of alcohol in development of dementia is controversial. Some studies, however, have found that alcohol plays a role in the etiology of dementia in 20% to 24% of cases (Carlen et al., 1994).

A summary of common presenting symptoms of alcoholism in the elderly is shown in Table 4.3. Many of these symptoms can be mistakenly attributed to age or other illness and the alcohol problem overlooked.

Alcohol interacts with many medications (Adams, 1997). Even people who drink moderately may develop problems due to the interaction of alcohol with prescription medications they are taking. Some medications can increase the impact of even small amounts of alcohol. In turn, alcohol may block the effects of certain medications or the combination may produce significant adverse effects. Some of the common drug–alcohol interactions are shown in Table 4.4.

Small amounts of alcohol can have positive effects, including decreasing latency to sleep, sedation, and improved digestion. Mishara and Kasten-

TABLE 4.3. Clinical Clues to Active Alcoholism in the Older Patient

- Therapy is not working for a normally treatable medical illness (e.g., hypertension).
- Insomnia or chronic fatigue related to poor sleep.
- Diarrhea, urinary incontinence, and weight loss or malnutrition.
- Cognitive deterioration, including confusion and memory loss.
- Complaints of anxiety (related to undiagnosed withdrawal), with frequent use of or requests for anxiolytics, sedatives, or hypnotics.
- Unexplained postoperative agitation, anxiety, and confusion, or new-onset seizures (suggesting withdrawal), especially in patients without known cerebrovascular disease.

Note. From Egbert (1993). Reproduced with permission from *Geriatrics*, Vol. 48, No. 7, July 1993, pp. 63–69. Copyright by Advanstar Communications Inc. Advanstar Communications Inc. retains all rights to this article.

TABLE 4.4. Potential Drug–Alcohol Interactions

Clinical effect	Drugs involved	Comments
Increased blood alcohol levels	Cimetidine, ranitidine, aspirin levels even with moderate drinking	This interaction can cause significant elevation of blood alcohol.
Increased metabolism of drug (chronic heavy alcohol use)	Benzodiazepines, warfarin, tolbutamide, propranolol, isoniazid use	Chronic heavy drinkers require higher doses of these drugs. This effect may last for a few weeks after cessation of alcohol.
Increased hepatotoxicity (chronic heavy alcohol use)	Acetaminophen, isoniazid, phenylbutazone	Heavy drinkers can experience liver necrosis even with therapeutic doses of these drugs.
Decreased metabolism of drug (acute alcohol use)	Narcotics, barbiturates, benzodiazepines, chloral hydrate, warfarin	Binge drinkers can develop toxicity from usual doses of these drugs during binges.
Increased bleeding time	Aspirin, NSAIDs	Can occur with moderate use.
Gastrointestinal inflammation and bleeding	Aspirin, NSAIDs	Can occur with moderate use. Binge drinkers are probably most at risk of hemorrhage.
Sedation, psychomotor impairment	Benzodiazepines, narcotics, tricyclic antidepressants, antihistamines, barbiturates	Degree of central nervous system impairment depends on doses of alcohol and drugs as well as individual tolerance.
Disulfiram-like reactions	Oral hypoglycemics (tolbutamide, chlorpropamide), antibiotics (metronidazole, sulfonamides, griseofulvin, cefoperazone), phenylbutazone, nitroglycerine	All patients who take these drugs should be warned about the interaction, but heavier drinkers are at the highest risk.
Interference with effectiveness of drugs	Antihypertensives, antidiabetic drugs, drugs for congestive heart failure, gout, ulcer disease	When these drugs do not have their expected effect, be alert to possible heavy drinking.
Hypotension	Reserpine, aldomet, hydralazine, nitroglycerine	Heavy and binge drinkers are most at risk.

Note. Adapted from Adams (1997). Copyright 1997 by Springer Publishing Company, Inc. Reprinted by permission.

baum (1980) suggest that small amounts of alcohol can benefit older people in various settings, including nursing homes.

Drug abuse is much less of a problem for older people than is alcohol abuse and usually involves misuse of legal rather than illegal drugs. This situation may change, however, as cohorts of people who had greater exposure to illegal drugs grow older. Currently, the main type of drug abuse involves minor tranquilizers (e.g., Ativan, Valium) (Finlayson & Davis, 1994; Task Force on Benzodiazepine Dependency, 1990). Abuse or dependency on tranquilizers is found in some depressed older people. In these cases it appears that physicians prescribed the medication for complaints of anxiety and insomnia but failed to detect underlying feelings of depression (Finlayson, 1997).

Dependency on tranquilizers can develop even at low dosages, due to decreased rates of metabolism and excretion of medications in the elderly. The major consequences of dependency include falls and fractures, depression and memory impairment (Ancill, Embury, MacEwan, & Kennedy, 1987). As noted earlier, these problems can incorrectly be ascribed to aging rather than drug dependency.

Finally, we want to note that a variety of over-the-counter medications, commonly consumed substances (nicotine, caffeine, vitamins), herbs, vitamins, and other nutritional supplements can result in problems for older people. In sufficient quantities, these substances can lead to health symptoms or may interfere with therapeutic regimens of prescription drugs.

ADJUSTMENT DISORDERS

Adjustment disorders, especially when they involve a depressed, anxious, or mixed affective state, are probably the most frequent diagnoses for older clients seen in a private practice. These problems have milder symptoms than affective or anxiety disorders and occur in reaction to specific life events. Adjustment disorders can develop following the major losses that older people experience, such as death of a spouse or child, chronic illness, retirement, or taking care of a severely disabled spouse.

There has been little systematic investigation of adjustment disorders as a category in the elderly. Many of the topics reviewed earlier in this chapter pertain to adjustment disorders, for example, depressive symptoms that do not meet criteria for major depression and comorbidity of depression and anxiety with medical illnesses. Specific epidemiological data on incidence and prevalence of adjustment disorders in later life are not available.

There has also been little attention to differentiation of normal grieving processes from situations in which older people might benefit from clinical intervention. A certain amount of grief is normal following a loss, and so clinicians must differentiate between the normal grieving process (which is a V code in DSM-IV) and people whose symptoms become more pronounced and disabling. Both major depression and subsyndromal depression are prevalent among widows and widowers in the first two years following the death of a spouse (Zisook, Shuchter, Sledge, Paulus, & Judd, 1994).

Clinicians can use common sense for determining whether someone needs treatment. Interventions are warranted when grief reactions are unusually pronounced or disabling in the period immediately following a loss or when symptoms of anxiety and depression persist or worsen rather than diminish over time. The person who is having persistent difficulties adjusting to everyday life more than three months after a loss should be considered for treatment. A similar approach can be taken to reactions to other late-life transitions, such as retirement.

CONCLUSIONS

In this chapter we have introduced the major functional disorders that affect older people. For the sake of economy, we have not presented every potential problem. Since people with mental disorders grow older, and many chronic problems are unabated with the passage of time, it is possible to encounter virtually any type of pathology in an older population. We have, instead, concentrated on the more frequent problems.

Several conclusions can be drawn from this survey. First and foremost, there is only the beginnings of a true developmental perspective on mental disorders, which examines age of onset and the course of symptoms over time. In later life, we encounter clients with varying developmental histories and patterns. Some have problems with early onset, some have late-onset disorders, and some have had fluctuating or changing patterns of symptoms over the years. The practical significance of these differences in history are not fully understood at this time.

Another consideration is the overlap of symptoms among the various syndromes we have described. Depression, for example, frequently coexists with anxiety and other disorders found in later life. Comorbidity is important when planning treatment. In the case of someone suffering from dementia, depression symptoms represent a potentially treatable part of the problem, which may result in clinically significant improvements for the patient and the patient's family. The frequent coexistence of anxiety and depression suggests that treatment should address both types of symptoms.

The overlap among syndromes calls attention to the limitations of current classification systems for mental disorders. These systems have been developed largely on the basis of patterns of symptoms found among younger people. A reliable classification system for disorders of late life has not been developed. It may also be that psychiatric disorders would be better described as falling along a continuum or multiple continua based on different symptom or problem groups, rather than falling within categories. At least some part of the spectrum we call anxiety and depressive disorders are probably better described that way, as are the personality disorders. In any event, current classification schemes provide a framework that, as experienced clinicians know, is useful but could be improved.

Finally, we want to reiterate that mental disorders can be encountered in any of the settings where older people live. The ECA studies emphasize prevalence in community populations of older people. Nursing homes, however, have become the mental hospitals of the 1990s. It is not unusual for more than one half of residents of nursing homes to have mental health problems, although often these symptoms are unrecognized and untreated. Problems include not only dementia and its consequences but also schizophrenia and personality disorders. Other settings, such as retirement communities, assisted living, and board and care homes, also have significant numbers of residents with mental health problems.

The disorders of aging, then, represent a complex array of problems that are found in many different settings. Chapters 3 and 4 describe the characteristics of the most frequent disorders. The next chapters build on these descriptions to describe the process of assessment and how late-life disorders can be accurately diagnosed.

5

Clinical Assessment

Assessment is the most important clinical skill in practice with older people. As a fundamental part of practice, clinicians need to know how to assess for dementia, delirium, depression and other common disorders of later life, and to differentiate these disorders from normal aging. This process combines knowledge of normal aging and disorders of aging with knowing how to conduct a structured and multifaceted evaluation. It also involves being able to navigate between the excessively negative expectations about aging that are sometimes held by physicians, families, and older people themselves and the very real, catastrophic problems that can occur.

Psychologists can play a unique role in this process. Diagnosis of the major disorders of late life depends to a considerable extent on evaluation of behavior and cognition. With their training in testing and other systematic approaches to assessment, psychologists are well prepared to conduct the type of assessment that can clarify current symptoms and problems. The use of normed and standardized tests makes it possible to evaluate older clients' symptoms in light of objective indicators of their overall functioning. By combining the results of psychological testing with information from structured clinical interviews, it is possible to determine whether behaviors and cognitions meet criteria for a particular diagnosis or if they fall within the boundaries of normal aging.

Over the years, we have seen many avoidable errors in diagnosis, such as labeling someone as demented who is not and failure to detect a delirium. These errors are often made by busy physicians or other professionals who make their assessment too quickly or casually, drawing on snapshot impressions that are gathered during a rushed office visit. Physicians usually do not have the time to conduct the thorough evaluation of behavior and cognition that is needed to complement the medical components of an assessment. That can be done by a psychologist.

Given the importance of assessment and the breadth of information available, we have divided the assessment material into two chapters. In the present chapter, we develop a foundation for conducting clinical assessments with older adults. The chapter begins by examining basic considerations when evaluating older adults and then focuses on the first steps in making a differential diagnosis: evaluating symptoms, taking a history, and testing mental status. The discussion of differential diagnosis continues in Chapter 6, where the focus turns to psychological testing, integrating information from psychological assessments with medical examinations, and differentiating among different types of dementia. We conclude Chapter 6 by examining assessment of competency.

These chapters on assessment are organized around the issues of differential diagnosis and competency evaluations. Many textbooks address assessment differently, either by discussing diagnostic features disorder by disorder or by including a chapter that presents information on tests and other assessment tools in a general way without focusing on how to make clinical decisions. We present the material in these chapters to reflect the decision-making process we go through when conducting an assessment, because we believe that it is reasoning, rather than the use of any particular test or procedure, that leads to sound clinical decisions.

Assessment, of course, can serve other important functions, particularly, treatment planning and evaluation. We address those issues in the chapters on treatment.

BASIC CONSIDERATIONS IN ASSESSMENT

It is important to set the stage carefully when assessing an older person. Poor performance can be caused by an underlying brain disorder, but it can also be caused by such things as evaluating a patient too quickly or in a noisy or poorly lit setting. Assessment and testing of older adults should be conducted under optimal conditions in order to minimize the effects of noncognitive influences on performance. In particular, evaluations should attend to the following: (1) developing rapport with the patient, (2) monitoring fatigue, (3) noting the time of day the evaluation is made, (4) evaluating the role of time pressure on performance, (5) identifying sensory problems that could affect performance, (6) minimizing test anxiety, and (7) weighing how the setting in which the assessment is conducted might affect performance.

Developing Rapport

The starting point for any assessment is to put the client at ease and to establish rapport. Throughout an evaluation the clinician should monitor the client's anxiety, providing reassurance when needed and conducting the assessment in a supportive way. Even in the face of obvious deficits, the clinician can be encouraging and positive. One strategy we have found useful to head off anxiety over making incorrect responses is to begin the session by explaining that the purpose of the tests is to analyze the patterns of errors. We tell clients that in other settings, getting everything right might be desirable, but here tests are designed so that it is impossible to get everything right, and it is only from the type of errors that someone makes that we can get an idea what the problem might be.

Monitoring Fatigue

Fatigue should be monitored closely among older clients, especially when evaluation sessions are long. Splitting up long assessments into two or more days, taking breaks, and generally monitoring the client's fatigue can address this concern. Having a snack during a long testing session may also help. Sometimes an individual is simply unable to continue because of fatigue. It is advisable to stop testing well before that point is reached in order to assure that the tests best reflect the client's ability and that the client will agree to return to complete the evaluation.

Time of Day of the Evaluation

A related issue is the time of day the older person is evaluated. Most older people function better in the morning. If the goal is to determine the highest level of function, then the assessment should be conducted in the morning. In some cases, however, the presenting problem may have to do with fluctuations in a client's functioning from one part of the day to the next. In these cases, we recommend conducting the assessment twice, once in the morning and again during the period of the day when the client is reported to have problems.

Reaction Time and Performance Speed

Reaction time and speed of performance decline with age and must be taken into account during testing. Performance suffers if clinicians read the instructions too quickly or do not give clients an adequate amount of time to respond. Clinicians who are used to evaluating younger people need to adopt a completely different pace so as not to rush through tests or press older clients for quick responses in untimed tests. If a clinician hurries through an assessment or tries to do it at the same pace as with younger people, the results will clarify only how an older person responds to time pressure, not what typical functioning might be.

A related issue is allowing an older person to complete a timed test even after the allotted time has expired. Although the test should be scored in the standard way, giving no credit for answers made after the allotted time has elapsed, the clinician can note that the client was able to complete the task successfully. That allows clinicians to distinguish between people who cannot do a task at all and someone who can perform adequately, albeit very slowly.

Sensory Problems

Vision and hearing problems can interfere with test performance in pronounced ways. To the extent possible, the assessment should differentiate between decrements due to cognitive as opposed to sensory problems. From a functional perspective, both can be debilitating, but there are more opportunities for correcting or compensating for sensory deficits.

For that reason, testing should be conducted under optimal conditions. Background noise and poor acoustics make hearing problems worse. Similarly, glare and low illumination hamper visual functioning. To reduce vision problems, lighting should be adequate and focused on the test materials that the client reads. Clients should be seated so that they are not looking directly into a window or strong light. When evaluating a client with hearing loss, talking loudly does not help. Instead, clinicians should speak in a clear and distinct manner, using complete sentences. Background noise should be reduced to a minimum.

An important step is to remind older clients to bring eyeglasses, other vision devices, and hearing aids to the testing session. Clinicians should check that the client has brought along the appropriate aids. We have found it better to reschedule an assessment than to try to conduct it when the client does not have eyeglasses or a hearing aid.

In addition to determining if the client has brought sensory aids, the clinician should inquire about everyday visual and hearing function, for instance, difficulty hearing ordinary conversation or hearing what people say on television or difficulty reading newsprint and headlines.

The following example illustrates how sensory loss can complicate an assessment. An 84-year-old woman was brought to an outpatient clinic by her son and daughter-in-law for an evaluation so that they could develop plans to care for her adequately. The older woman had been living in another part of the country until the death of her husband of 50 years. Following his death, she had become deeply depressed and began not caring for herself. She was hospitalized in an inpatient psychiatric facility for a 2-week period. The staff reported to her family that she was "hopelessly senile" and recommended that they should arrange for nursing home placement. Following her discharge, her son and daughter-in-law brought her across the country to live with them.

The assessment was begun with all three people present. The son and daughter-in-law began by reviewing the history. They indicated that the client actually functioned quite well in their home and did not have memory problems, but they were concerned that she did not have many activities. Her son was also concerned that her smoking would be harmful to her health. It immediately became apparent in the interview that the client was very hard of hearing. She could not answer to even simple mental status questions when administered orally. When the questions were written down for her to read, however, she responded quickly and accurately. She performed well on other visual tasks. When discussing her situation, she expressed sadness over her loss and gratitude that her family had taken her in. Rather than managing her "senility," the goal that emerged was to identify activities she would enjoy and to explore ways of minimizing the communication problems caused by her hearing loss.

Further confirmation of her good cognitive ability came from an incident that took place at the end of the interview. At the beginning of the evaluation, the client's daughter-in-law had taken her purse from her and placed it alongside the chair she was sitting in, outside the older woman's sight. At the end of the session, the daughter-in-law got up to leave without taking her mother-in-law's purse. The mother-in-law, however, reminded her daughter-in-law that she had put the purse alongside her chair. Consistent with everything else that occurred during the assessment, this type of recall indicated normal cognitive functioning.

The diagnosis of dementia in this case had clearly been erroneous. In retrospect, staff at the psychiatric hospital had probably failed to identify the client's profound hearing loss and mistook her lack of responsiveness as dementia rather than sensory loss that was compounded by depression following the death of her husband.

Test Anxiety

Lack of familiarity with testing and test anxiety can also interfere with performance. Older people who have not had to perform a structured cognitive task, such as arithmetic or block design, for some time may have difficulty because of not being familiar with testing procedures or strategies. Tests that allow for a certain amount of practice can be useful; evidence of improvement over several trials may be a better indication of the older person's functioning than a summary score. Another strategy is to administer tests that use familiar stimuli and tasks that are ecologically valid. For example, recall can be tested by asking people to place familiar objects into the model of an apartment and then to recall each object and where they placed it (Johansson & Zarit, 1991; Johansson, 1988–1989). Money can be used for simple mathematical operations (Johansson & Zarit, 1991). Similar to everyday situations, these tasks can engage people's interest in situations and with stimuli with which they are familiar.

People may also have anxiety over what a test will show. Establishing good rapport before starting an assessment and conducting the testing in a supportive and encouraging manner go a long way to reducing anxiety.

Setting of the Assessment

The setting in which an assessment takes places can influence performance. When an assessment takes place in a hospital or other setting that can be viewed as threatening, the clinician should make sure that everything has been done to make clients comfortable and relaxed before beginning. Even when an assessment is conducted in a private office, the client's fears could adversely affect cognitive performance and behavior. The advantages of a familiar setting were demonstrated by a study that compared mental status test performance at a clinic and in the client's home. Scores on the Mini-Mental State Examination were 1.5 points higher at home than in the clinic (Ward et al., 1990). While we do not advocate routinely conducting psychological testing in the home (and indeed some people would experience home visits as intrusive and upsetting), we cite this example to indicate how the test setting can affect performance.

There are times, however, when a home visit should be part of the assessment. Home assessments should be conducted when there is a question about the competency of a person to remain in the home. A dementia patient, for example, may have a great deal of difficulty functioning in an unfamiliar setting but may still be able to perform everyday activities in a familiar setting. A good informant may obviate the need for a home assessment, but in some cases, the information about how a client actually carries out activities and interacts with other people at home may make a home visit worth the effort.

The following example illustrates the value of a home assessment. An older man had suffered a mild stroke while in the hospital, which left him incontinent and with limited speech. Staff were very concerned that he would not be able to function at home but were willing to give it a try. A nurse who accompanied him to his home to observe him described his adjustment this way: "He walked in, looked at the open fire, and said, 'Oh, isn't that nice?' He saw the cat and said, 'Oh, there is Whiskey,' and took the cat on his lap. He sought out the toilet when he needed it. He was a completely different man in the afternoon from what he had been in the morning" (Glasscote, Gudeman, & Miles, 1977, p. 140). Of course, not everyone responds so positively to being at home, but when there is a question about a client's ability to function at home, the best assessment is one that includes a home visit.

An older person's functioning, then, can be affected by many different factors. As a result, an important question is whether the goal of an assessment is to identify optimal or typical functioning. When there is a question of possible dementia, it is important to make testing conditions as favorable as possible. In that way, the clinician can first identify what level of functioning the older person is capable of. There are quite different implications of suffering from dementia compared to having difficulty performing optimally when there is time pressure or because visual conditions and acoustics are not ideal. Once a client's optimal level of performance is determined, the clinician can then evaluate possible sources of variability in everyday functioning. Some of the factors related to variability in performance may be modifiable. For people suffering from sensory loss, for example, many different approaches can enhance vision and hearing, including the use of aids and modifications in the environment.

DIFFERENTIAL ASSESSMENT

Process of Differential Assessment

We begin with a discussion of general principles that guide the process of differential assessment. Given the prevalence of cognitive disorders in later life, the first and most basic question in an assessment is to determine if an older person is having significant cognitive problems and what the probable cause is. Whenever there is any indication of a possible dementia or delirium, whether from the client's own reports, from information obtained from family or the referral source, or from direct observation, the initial focus of the assessment should be to differentiate cognitive from noncognitive disorders. This type of assessment is, in many ways, the hallmark of practice with older people.

Some clinicians would argue that a thorough assessment of cognition should be undertaken at the outset for any older client. This approach is warranted in certain settings. In a teaching clinic or hospital, for example, it is very useful for interns or postdoctoral fellows to conduct at least some minimal cognitive screening tests on every client in order to learn to differentiate normal and impaired patterns of performance. Likewise, screening every referral in a nursing home is helpful, because the rates of dementia can be quite high and questions about cognitive functioning are usually part of the reason for conducting an evaluation in the first place. The issue is less clear-cut when an older person seeks psychotherapy in a private practice setting and presents no complaints or problems that might indicate a cognitive disorder. In this situation, the risk of not conducting an assessment has to be weighed against the cost of doing so in fiscal expense, the client's time and energy, and the age-ist implications of presuming that the person has a cognitive deficit. When no cognitive problems are indicated, the clinician can proceed by evaluating the client's presenting problems and gathering other information necessary for planning treatment.

When there is a possibility of a cognitive disorder, delaying an assessment could have detrimental effects. For example, we were asked to consult on a case of an older couple who had been seen in marital therapy by another therapist for about 1 year. From the beginning of treatment, the wife had complained about her husband's forgetting. The therapy sessions were not very productive, and the man's memory problems contributed at least in part to the lack of progress. Finally, out of frustration, the therapist asked for a consultation. The assessment indicated that the man had some specific memory deficits but no other problems that indicated dementia. The etiology of the memory problems was unclear. This problem, however, could have been identified a year earlier without putting the couple through a long, frustrating treatment. Once the nature of the memory problem had been more thoroughly identified, treatment that focused on the couple's relationship proceeded more productively by finding ways of compensating for the husband's difficulty with memory.

Differential assessment is complex but not overly difficult. The assessment process involves hypothesis testing. There are no definitive markers of dementia, delirium, depression, or other disorders in later life. Rather, signs and symptoms overlap, and the clinician must go through a process of evaluating the evidence to determine the most likely explanation for current symptoms. We approach this task by gathering information from several sources—interview, reports from informants, observations and psychological testing—and then deciding among competing possibilities. We continually ask if the pattern of symptoms, test results, and other observations is more like one disorder or another. The results of this process are then examined in light of medical findings. In the discussion that follows, we present the decision-making process we use in clinical situations, emphasizing the types of information that are most useful and the reasoning used in reaching decisions.

An older person who is referred for an evaluation could be experiencing any of a wide range of disorders. Symptoms may result from a recurrence of a disorder first experienced earlier in life, with an overlay of age-related issues, or from a new disorder. Given the many different disorders that can occur in later life, the clinician should start with a broad outlook and then narrow down the choices as information is gathered. It is important not to reach a conclusion prematurely, because that could lead to overlooking some important evidence that suggests a different outcome. At the end of the evaluation process, the clinician then weighs the evidence for and against competing hypotheses about the diagnosis. Although the symptoms of the various disorders of aging overlap, a diagnosis can be established by a preponderance of evidence, which points toward one disorder and away from others. If no firm conclusion can be reached, then the clinician should consider doing other assessments that might clarify the situation, as well as conducting another evaluation at a later date to determine if the client's problems are stable or worsen.

Another important principle is to take a systematic approach to assessment. Clinicians should use a comprehensive battery of tests and other assessment procedures, without skipping tasks that they believe might be irrelevant. As a result, a more complete picture of the client will emerge. Clinicians can make better comparisons across clients if they gather comparable information on each. They also become more skilled in interpreting the results from that battery of tests, including the kinds of subtleties that are involved in making assessments of difficult cases.

When possible, the clinician should use tests that have age norms that extend past 65 (see Chapter 6). The availability of norms is very helpful for identifying what is expected with aging and what might be different with dementia (e.g., Kaszniak, 1990). Norms should be interpreted, however, in light of probable individual differences in prior functioning. A person's current performance needs to be evaluated against expected performance, given past education and history. It can be difficult to assess people at the high and low end of the spectrum of abilities, because their performance differs more from norms. A person with prior high levels of intellectual ability may still perform above the norm for his or her age, yet be experiencing early dementia symptoms. Conversely, low performance in a person with a history of poor functioning may indicate continuity rather than change.

One way of estimating prior performance is with years of education. While this approach can be helpful, years of formal education does not tell the whole story for today's cohort of older people. Many older people had only limited opportunities to get a formal education but had work and other life experiences that allowed them to function at a much higher level. Both education and life achievements need to be weighed when evaluating test performance, a point to which we will return in Chapter 6.

The problem of determining if a change has occurred would be simple if prior testing were available. On occasion, a client may have been evaluated previously, and the information from that session can serve as a baseline. We once saw a 50-year-old man who sought help for coping with Alzheimer's disease, which had been diagnosed a year earlier. The history and current symptoms indicated that he had been depressed, and while he reported some episodes of forgetting, his cognitive functioning seemed stable. Psychological testing had been performed a year earlier at the time the diagnosis was made. Records of that testing were obtained and the tests were repeated. Results of the new testing indicated that performance had not changed, which meant that he was unlikely to have a degenerative disorder such as Alzheimer's. Furthermore, performance at both times of testing was generally good, and the original psychologist who saw him thought he did not have Alzheimer's. The diagnosis had been made by a neurologist, based on complaints of forgetting. The ability to compare new tests with previous tests confirmed the impressions of the original psychologist. In other cases, we have found evidence for deterioration where testing and other observations were initially inconclusive. In those instances, repeated testing is strong evidence of a degenerative disorder.

When no prior testing is available, the clinician must estimate what the client's previous functioning might have been. Some clients may have developed specific abilities to high or expert levels. Decline may occur later in these well-practiced abilities. An accountant, for example, may still have high levels of performance on arithmetic tests, despite early dementia. On the other hand, decline can be indicated by small errors that would be normal for most people but represent a change for the person being tested.

As there is no definitive sign or symptom for a diagnosis of Alzheimer's disease or dementia, the potential for an incorrect diagnosis is always present. When the evidence is not conclusive, it is always better to err on the side of diagnosing a treatable disorder. If, for example, the clinician suspects that a client is depressed but is concerned about findings that suggest the possibility of early dementia, it is better to treat the depression first. The minimal cognitive changes may be related to the client's mood and may clear up with treatment. In the event that the case turns out to involve dementia, however, no real harm will have been done. In fact, people with early dementia often respond to treatment for depression. The biggest error we have seen over the years is to make a diagnosis of dementia in a cavalier way, without sufficient evidence. This can be devastating to a client who becomes depressed in response to the diagnosis. Similarly, if there is any evidence of delirium or any other potential treatable cause of cognitive symptoms, those possibilities should be explored first before assuming that the case involves dementia. When evidence points at least in part to the possibility of a treatable disorder, the clinician's bias should clearly be toward diagnosing that disorder.

The following example illustrates the importance of identifying potentially treatable causes of cognitive symptoms. Mr. Smith was referred by a geriatrician for a neuropsychological evaluation. Mr. Smith had been the geriatrician's patient for about a year and a half and had been noted to have mild memory impairment. He had had a cerebrovascular accident (stroke) twenty years earlier with full recovery and heart bypass surgery 4 years earlier. He was otherwise in excellent health, maintaining a healthy weight and walking 5 miles per day. His son had taken Mr. Smith to the geriatrician because he was concerned about his memory problems. In the physician's office, the complaints seemed vague and not out of line with the previously noted memory impairment. But the son's concern prompted the physician to refer the patient for a more thorough evaluation.

Mr. Smith was 85 years old and had been retired from an accounting position for 20 years. Careful interviewing of his son revealed that Mr. Smith, who had always managed his own investments and finances, had suddenly become unable to balance his checkbook. He asked his son for help, and the son was alarmed by the tangled mess in the checkbook. Also, Mr. Smith's handwriting had become micrographic (very tiny). Because of the ominous suddenness of these changes, the evaluation was done immediately. The Wechsler Memory Scale—Revised was given, as well as the WAIS-R. Massive deficits were found on all tests, particularly on calculations. The geriatrician was called and a thorough medical examination was begun. Mr. Smith's left carotid artery was found to be 99% occluded and the right carotid was 75% occluded, placing Mr. Smith at high risk for another stroke. An MRI revealed several new areas of small infarcts, which accounted for the specific deficits seen. A carotid endardectomy was performed, and Mr. Smith recovered fairly well. He most likely could not return to his baseline functioning before the carotid occlusion because of the infarctions he suffered. Still, if his memory problems had been ignored, he would have suffered either a massive cerebral vascular accident or such significant anoxia (lack of oxygen to the brain) that he would have been much more severely impaired. As it was, he continued to live independently with his wife in an apartment in a retirement community.

As this case illustrates, when the decision is between a potentially treatable disorder and dementia, every reasonable treatment should be tried before concluding that nothing can be done. When the results of an assessment are ambiguous or conflicting, a conservative decision rule should be used to prevent overdiagnosis of dementia.

In many cases, the clinician cannot make a definitive statement at the end of the evaluation. A person may have mild memory problems and one or two other soft signs of cognitive difficulties but no deficits in testing or in everyday activities that clearly suggest dementia. At the same time, depression, anxiety, or low levels of prior ability may be strong, competing hypotheses for the cause of the memory problems. In this type of ambiguous or uncertain situation, having the client come back in a year for repeated testing is the appropriate step. After a year, there should either be obvious evidence of decline, or functioning will have remained stable or improved. During the interval, treatment of associated problems such as depression could be undertaken. Testing could be repeated after another interval, should suspicions remain.

The possibility has been raised that early symptoms of Alzheimer's disease may appear many years before they are severe enough to warrant a diagnosis. While a long prodromal syndrome is conceivable, more empirical evidence from longitudinal studies is needed before a reliable diagnosis can be made based on minimal symptoms. Current research suggests that some people with very mild cognitive deficits go on to develop dementia, but others do not (Johansson & Zarit, 1997). In any case, the consequences of a false positive diagnosis are more severe than those of a false negative.

(As noted in Chapter 3, two medications have now been approved for the treatment of Alzheimer's disease, but the benefits are not robust or long-lasting. We do not believe that the availability of these drugs changes the argument presented here for making Alzheimer's disease the diagnosis of last resort.)

Finally, although we emphasize distinguishing one disorder from another, clinicians need to recognize that problems can coexist. A dementia patient may become depressed or develop a delirium. Similarly, someone who is depressed can develop a delirium or dementia. These co-morbidities are important to recognize, because they have different implications for treatment.

Steps in Differential Assessment

Six steps are involved in a differential assessment. The first three, which are discussed in this chapter, are (1) identifying presenting symptoms and problems, (2) obtaining a history of current symptoms and problems, and (3) mental status testing. The remaining steps are discussed in Chapter 6: (4) psychological and neuropsychological testing, (5) coordination with a medical evaluation, and (6), when dementia is present, identifying the probable or likely cause.

In the following sections, we contrast the main disorders of later life—dementia, delirium, and depression—focusing on how they differ from each other and from normal aging. We also point out differences in other problems frequently mistaken for dementia, such as nonprogressive brain injuries and chronic mental health problems.

Identifying Presenting Symptoms and Problems

A careful description of presenting symptoms and problems, including specific examples, how often they occur, in what situations they occur and possible triggering (antecedent) or reinforcing (consequent) events form the foundation of an assessment. Information should be sought both from the older person, and, when possible, from an informant.

The use of an informant is one of the ways that assessment of older people differs from other adults. When an older client has difficulty providing specific details about symptoms or history, an informant can be a valuable source of information. Reports by family informants are usually reliable (e.g., Teri & Truax, 1994). But clinicians should assess each case carefully for the possibility that the informant is presenting a biased or even factually inaccurate version of events. Clinicians should also take steps to protect the client's confidentiality.

The task for the clinician is to compare presenting symptoms with the typical features of syndromes, such as dementia or delirium, to determine whether they match descriptions of the syndrome and meet criteria for a DSM-IV diagnosis. We will elaborate on three presenting symptoms that are especially important in differential diagnosis: perceptions of memory and other intellectual problems, delusions and hallucinations, and affect.

Memory Complaints and Performance. A good starting point in an interview is to ask about perceived memory problems. Questions such as "Are you having any problems with your memory?" are generally non-threatening and provide valuable information about how clients (and informants) view the situation.

As shown in Table 5.1, memory complaints have a paradoxical relation to objective memory problems. People with fewer objective problems tend to complain more about failing memory, while people with significant memory loss often complain little or not at all (Kaszniak, 1987). With dementia, patients are sometimes aware of their deficits in the early stages of their illness. As dementia progresses, they are less likely to be aware of their problems. By the time the disease has become more pronounced, they have little or no recognition that they are having problems. When asked if they are having difficulties with memory, they are likely to respond "No" or to be unable to note any particular problem. They may be applying an inherent adaptive tendency to deny problems in the face of massive brain dysfunction, or they may simply forget episodes of forgetting.

In contrast to this pattern with dementia, older depressed people often create a convincing picture of failing memory, even when no objective evidence of problems can be found (Kaszniak, 1987; Niederehe & Yoder, 1989). When asked about their memory, they often say it is terrible, and they may even worry that they are becoming senile. These complaints are part of the exaggerated negative evaluations typical of depression. An older person who is both depressed and has dementia is especially likely to complain of failing memory (e.g., Johansson, Allen-Burge, & Zarit, 1997; Kahn, Zarit, Hilbert, & Niederehe, 1975).

Normal older people often complain about failing memory, though complaints are less frequent and less severe than found in depressives. Complaints may be present or absent in delirium, though the delirious patient tends to deny any problems. Finally, patients with nonprogressive brain trauma may or may not complain about failing memory, depending on the site and severity of their injury.

Clearly, then, many of the older people who complain about failing memory do not have dementia. What, then, is the basis for their com-

TABLE 5.1. Differential Diagnosis in the Elderly: Reports of Memory Problems

	Dementia	Delirium	Depression	Nonprogressive brain injury	Normal aging
Reported by patient	May report problems, especially in early and mild cases. Some patients recognize that memory is poor but can provide no specific details. Awareness of problems may be greater in vascular dementia	Usually denies problems, may confabulate	Usually complains of memory problems; may fear becoming senile	Depends on the location of the injury; if the damage is not too severe, the patient is usually aware of deficits	May complain that memory is not as good as it used to be; forgets common things (e.g., forgetting to buy an item at the store), but problems do not interfere with everyday activities
Reported by family	Pronounced problems that interfere with carrying out everyday activities	Profound disruption of usual activities	Some absent-mindedness and preoccupation	Depends on location of injury	May report occasional forgetting that does not interfere with everyday activities

plaints? Do complaints reflect normal and expected changes in memory with aging or are they early signs of decline and dementia?

One reason otherwise healthy older people may complain of failing memory is incorrect attributions. Reflecting the common expectation that memory declines with age, they may attribute everyday episodes of forgetfulness, such as forgetting a name or forgetting where they put something, to an age-related irreversible decline. They may have been experiencing the same problem for many years, but now that they are older, they believe it is a sign of aging or senility. This tendency to focus on negative events is heightened with depression.

Another possible explanation is that people complaining of failing memory may be noticing subtle changes that are not yet apparent on test results. To what extent, then, do complaints point to the onset of dementia? Only a few studies have actually followed people over time to evaluate whether memory complaints predict subsequent decline. These studies have found that some people who complain of failing memory but otherwise have no other indications of dementia do go on to develop dementia, but many other people do not (Flicker, Ferris, & Reisberg, 1993; Johansson et al., 1997).

One reason that memory complaints may not be a reliable indicator of decline is that when asked to evaluate their memory, older people inevitably compare their present ability to past performance, while testing evaluates current functioning. A person may indeed have experienced some mild decline in memory compared to 40 years earlier but may function relatively well in the present compared with other people of the same age. For that reason, correlations of memory complaint and performance are low.

In sum, then, when an older person complains about failing memory but assessment reveals no memory problems, the complaints are probably related to other factors (depression, incorrect attributions). On some occasions, however, complaints are an early sign of dementia, even before other indicators are detected.

While complaints of failing memory do not by themselves indicate dementia or depression, clinicians can clarify the situation somewhat by asking for specific examples. This type of questioning can bring out qualitative differences between normal, age-related forgetfulness and the memory problems associated with organic pathology. With experience, clinicians develop a feel for this difference. The more details clients provide about incidents, the better their memory is functioning. Healthy older adults frequently say that they are having memory problems and give many different specific examples of everyday lapses of memory, such as forgetting a name or forgetting to pick up an item at the store. These commonplace incidents of forgetting can occur at any age and do not by themselves indicate anything pathological. These incidents also do not interfere in any significant way with normal functioning.

By contrast, dementia involves memory lapses that go beyond typical forgetting and interfere with everyday functioning. As an example of this type of forgetting, a stockbroker who had always awakened and gone to work early to be in time for the opening of the markets was now going to work at 6:00 in the evening, rather than 6:00 in the morning. This is clearly forgetting of a different magnitude than misplacing one's glasses.

Recurrence of problems is another significant indicator. Forgetting where you parked a car or put your keys is not usually a sign that something is wrong, but doing these things repeatedly suggests that you may have a problem. A high frequency of misplacing objects in a short time frame, being unable to find these objects, and putting them in unusual places all point toward a more significant memory deficit.

An exception is the person who always functioned in an absent-minded way. This person already has a high baseline of everyday forgetting. A careful evaluation can usually determine whether the frequency and type of absent-minded errors has changed. During our training, one of us was involved in an evaluation of a Nobel laureate, who was then in his late 70s and was complaining about failing memory. He was specifically concerned that he could not find what he was looking for in his office. There was, however, nothing new or age-related about the problem. Through his whole career, he had been the prototypical absent-minded professor, always having difficulty finding where he put things in his cluttered and disorganized office. That is not to say that there are never cases of dementia among people who previously had been forgetful or did not pay attention to details of everyday life. Rather, part of the differentiation needs to take into account whether current functioning differs from how that person typically functioned in the past.

The following example illustrates how examining memory complaints can provide useful information about diagnosis. We assessed a client in his early 60s who reported that his memory was failing. He said he could not remember anything anymore and believed he was becoming senile. He had recently been forced to retire because of health problems that interfered with his job, and he reported having no other interests than his work. His wife still worked, and he was at home alone during the day. When asked for specific examples of forgetting, he said he watched daytime television and could not remember what he had just been watching. When asked if he was paying attention, he said no. Besides his concern with memory, he reported feeling very depressed. His cognitive test scores were in normal ranges and did not suggest dementia.

This case demonstrates how depression can lead to memory complaints. Depressed patients are preoccupied with their own thoughts and do not attend to the events around them. When forced to do so, as in a structured testing situation, they can process information adequately, except in cases of severe depression. In this case, treatment of depression was initiated. As the client improved, his complaints of failing memory decreased. Studies of treatment of depression have found a similar decrease in memory complaints with improvement in mood (Popkin, Gallagher, Thompson, & Moore, 1982).

Informants can provide information that can clarify the type and severity of memory problems. Again, the clinician should ask informants to provide specific examples. When informants describe memory lapses that do not interfere with the client's everyday life, that suggests normal memory functioning. On the other hand, serious and recurrent problems are more likely to indicate a disturbance in memory.

Although informants are usually reliable, some are poor observers or do not have sufficient contact with the client to provide adequate information. One situation to be aware of is the "out-of-town sibling" syndrome. In this situation, one child has assumed the bulk of care for an aging parent and sees the parent frequently. This child usually can give a reliable history, perhaps of gradual, steady decline. Then an out-of-town brother or sister swoops in for a visit, is horrified at the "sudden" changes in the parent, and may even blame the local sibling for this condition. Old sibling rivalries, guilt over being so far away, and other family dynamics must be considered in evaluating the reliability of an informant.

In rare instances, the clinician encounters cases that dramatically illustrate how complaints about memory and objective memory functioning can diverge. Knight (1992) reports a case in which a husband was concerned about what he believed was his own failing memory and the onset of dementia. He described his wife as physically frail but mentally alert. Tests did not reveal any evidence of dementia for the man. He was primarily depressed over a move to a new community and the loss of his social support. When his wife subsequently went into treatment, however, it was found that she had a moderately severe dementia.

Both the client and the informant can be asked about other kinds of cognitive problems, such as word-finding difficulties, problems finding one's way around, not remembering how to do familiar tasks or carry out a sequence of tasks, and failing to recognize familiar objects. These problems are more specific to brain disorders, including dementia, and less likely to occur with any frequency in depression or normal aging.

When dementia is suspected, we also find it useful to have the family members complete the Memory and Behavior Problems Checklist (S. Zarit, Orr, & Zarit, 1985) (Appendix 5.1). This instrument is designed to identify common problems associated with dementia as well as which behaviors the family finds particularly troublesome or stressful. Families can complete this instrument in the waiting room while the patient is being interviewed. This instrument allows family members to identify and quantify specific memory and behavior problems, and most take the opportunity to write down concerns they do not want to bring up in front of the patient. An extended revised version of the Memory and Behavior Problems Checklist has been developed by Teri and her associates (1992).

Hallucinations and Delusions. While memory complaints are fairly common and generally nonspecific, hallucinations and delusions occur with a low frequency but indicate a significant disturbance. When there is evidence of hallucinations and/or delusions, clinicians need first to consider the possibility of a delirium (especially when the onset is recent, as indicated in the following sections on history). Lipowski (1990) describes delirium as involving a global distortion in perceptions, in which people cannot grasp or understand what they see. They may experience illusions, that is, mistaking one object for another. As an example, the changing light and shadows from a television screen might be perceived as a small animal running across the room. Hallucinations, or actual false perceptions, are quite common in delirium and are usually visual or visual and auditory. Full-blown delusional systems, in which clients believe in plots and conspiracies against them, can also occur.

We recently evaluated a 103-year-old former nurse who had been moved to an assisted living community 6 days earlier. She had lived independently until she was in her mid-90s and then lived with her one surviving daughter until she required more care and attention than her daughter could provide. After moving into the facility, she began telling her daughter that doctors and nurses were coming into her room in the middle of the night to give her rough gynecological examinations. Staff confirmed going into her room to change a wet adult diaper. In her disorientation, however, the patient had confabulated a more distressing explanation. On another occasion, she identified the assisted-living facility as a resort that she and her husband used to vacation at, and she said she had been to visit the gardens the previous spring. She had not, however, ever been to the facility prior to moving there. These are classic responses typical of a delirium. In this patient's case, the delirium was probably due to her recent relocation, the presence of a hearing impairment, and perhaps mild cognitive impairment. As she settled into the routines at the facility, these experiences diminished.

Hallucinations, illusions, and delusions can also occur in dementia but are less common or may arise as part of a delirium superimposed on an existing dementia, for example, as a reaction to medications or an acute illness. Cummings et al. (1987) report that hallucinations are found in 5% to 20% of dementia patients, while delusions are present in 13% to 33% of cases.

The content of paranoid delusions in dementia often suggests that the patient is filling in information that cannot be recalled due to memory failure. Clients may complain that someone is stealing money or other valuables when they cannot remember where they placed them. These delusions are often intermittent, but in some cases, the older person can become preoccupied with suspicions and accusations. When paranoid delusions become a prominent feature of dementia, it can be very disturbing to the family and other involved persons. As dementia progresses to its later stages, these types of delusions gradually lessen. By contrast, illusory experiences, such as seeing imaginary intruders, become more common, perhaps because of the patient's increasing difficulties perceiving and recognizing objects.

These kinds of disordered perceptions are relatively rare in depression. Other disorders should be considered, however, when hallucinations or delusions are identified. One possibility is that the client is suffering from a lifelong, recurrent problem, such as schizophrenia, or a paranoid personality disorder. Another alternative is a late-life paranoid disorder (see Chapter 4). The distinction between paranoid delusions in dementia and in a late-life paranoid disorder is made on the basis of whether or not there is an accompanying disorder of memory.

Mood Disturbances.   The major mood symptoms, anxiety and depression, can occur in all three disorders: dementia, delirium, and depression. Depressed mood, of course, is the defining characteristic of depressive syndromes and may be accompanied by considerable anxiety. On rare occasions, depressed mood may be muted or absent but the person will have pronounced depressive thoughts—hopelessness, helplessness, worthlessness. This type of pattern is sometimes referred to as a "masked depression."

Depression can be a prominent feature in dementia. Symptoms of depression in Alzheimer's patients can be sufficiently pronounced to warrant a diagnosis of major depression (Reifler, Larson, Teri, & Poulsen, 1986; Teri & Wagner, 1992). The dementia patient's depression often has a realistic component: awareness of one's own decline and disability. As the dementia worsens, depressive symptoms may lessen. In later stages of dementia, depressive symptoms may still occur, though now they are indicated by a sad appearance or crying.

Anxiety is a common component of a delirium, although depressed mood can be a prodromal symptom or can occur in quieter phases. Depressed mood, of course, can be a common part of many other disorders.

We have focused in this section on elaborating how three main symptoms—memory complaints and problems, disordered perceptions, and mood—present in depression, dementia, and delirium, as well as in normal aging. Clinicians, of course, should obtain a complete picture of all presenting symptoms and behavior. The result may well point to other disorders or raise questions that can be addressed during the next steps in assessment.

Assessing the History of a Disorder

An accurate and thorough history probably contributes more than any other factor to correct assessment and diagnosis of an older person. Clinicians should gather information on the onset, course, and duration of symptoms, as well as any fluctuations. Another important piece of information is the occurrence of similar episodes in the past. Clients, family informants, and medical records are all important sources of information about history.

The history of dementia, delirium, and depression usually are distinct from one another and differ from the course of normal aging (Table 5.2). The two main forms of dementia, Alzheimer's disease and vascular dementia, usually have distinct onset and course. Alzheimer's has an insidious onset, a term that captures the terrible nature of this disease. The patient experiences ordinary sorts of forgetting, which gradually increase in frequency. These incidents are at last noticed by other people and begin to interfere with everyday activities. Progression is typically almost imperceptibly gradual. Families may not realize that something serious is going on until a major problem occurs, such as the patient getting lost while driving or walking or forgetting how to do a familiar activity. When the family is interviewed carefully, however, they can often identify other incidents that show a pattern of gradual onset and worsening.

By the time someone is referred for an evaluation, problems may have been going on for anywhere from a few months to several years. This difference in when families seek an evaluation is due partly to when they recognize that the person's forgetting has become a problem and/or when forgetting begins to interfere with performance of everyday activities. The rate of progression can also vary. Some people decline relatively rapidly and others gradually (the more typical course).

The following example illustrates a typical history of onset and progression of symptoms in Alzheimer's disease. A 71-year-old woman was referred to us by a neurologist for evaluation of her memory problems. She was accompanied to the assessment meeting by her husband. When asked if she had memory problems, she said yes but deferred to her husband to provide specific information. When asked how long the problems had been going on, he first said a few months. As we talked, he realized that he had first noticed his wife's problems 5 years earlier. At that time, she was performing in a play in a community theater and uncharacteristically forgot her lines. Everyone regarded the incident as stage fright, but in retrospect, it was the first notable change in her behavior. The changes had been occurring so gradually over the 5-year period, however, that her husband could not pinpoint the onset readily. With some gentle prompting, he was able to give a more complete picture of gradual onset and progression. During this period he had gradually assumed responsibility for more and more household tasks. She no longer could cook, do the laundry, or clean the house. As

TABLE 5.2. Differential Diagnosis in the Elderly: Features of Clinical History

	Dementia		Delirium	Depression	Nonprogressive brain injury	Normal aging
	Alzheimer's	Vascular				
Onset	Insidious	Sometimes sudden	Sudden	Coincides with life changes	Dates to injury	Gradual changes
Duration of problems	Months to years	Months to years	A few days or weeks	Weeks to months	Dates to injury	Minimal changes over long periods of time
Progression of symptoms	Gradual	Stepwise for many vascular dementias	Severe within a few days	Not progressive	Not progressive	Minimal changes over long periods of time
Fluctuations in symptoms	Some daily	More pronounced daily fluctuations with occasional steps down in functioning	Extreme fluctuations from hour to hour	Worse in the morning	Little	Mild situational fluctuations

in many Alzheimer's cases, onset was insidious, progression was gradual, and the duration of symptoms spanned several years.

Patients can fluctuate in behavior from day to day and even from one part of the day to another. Early in the disease families sometimes interpret the "good days" as a sign that nothing is really wrong with their relative and then are surprised or disappointed when the patient relapses the next day. Despite these fluctuations, the course is clearly downward, and good days become fewer and fewer.

Vascular dementia includes several distinct disorders that vary somewhat in onset and progression. The most common pattern, which involves small infarcts or strokes, can have a relatively abrupt onset, occurring in conjunction with a new infarction. Strokelike symptoms, such as mild paralysis, may be observable for short periods of time, although more often symptoms are not observable. Subsequently, there is a pattern of stepwise deterioration, that is, plateaus of stability followed by a sudden drop, which probably corresponds to a new stroke. As with Alzheimer's, the rate of decline can vary. Daily fluctuations can be a little more pronounced in vascular dementia than in Alzheimer's.

The following case illustrates onset and progression of a multi-infarct type of vascular dementia. A 75-year-old woman denied having memory problems. Her family, however, noted that the onset of symptoms occurred quite suddenly 3 years earlier. At that time, she was evaluated by a neurologist, who found evidence of small strokes on a CT scan, a finding that points to vascular dementia. Since then, her family described her as stabilizing for a period of time and then experiencing sudden drops. The most recent drop brought the family in for a consultation. The woman had begun to call up her son every night at dinner time, asking when he was coming home for dinner. She no longer remembered that he was married and lived with his own family. She also did not remember that her husband was dead. The original symptoms, then, had developed suddenly, as opposed to the more gradual deterioration typical of Alzheimer's disease. The progression of symptoms was subsequently stepwise, with the duration covering a period of three years from the time the family knew something was wrong to the point they sought additional help.

There are exceptions to these patterns. Alzheimer's and vascular dementia can coexist in some cases, so onset and course may have features of both disorders. As noted previously, some vascular dementias follow a gradual rather than stepwise pattern of decline. Another apparent exception is when families provide a history of abrupt onset of symptoms associated with a stressful life event in cases that otherwise appear to be Alzheimer's. Triggering events include surgery with a general anesthesia, death of a spouse, and moving to a new location. A typical scenario involving surgery is for the family to report that the patient functioned with no apparent difficulty prior to a surgery. Immediately following the surgery, a delirium occurred with considerable cognitive impairment. The patient improved somewhat as the delirium cleared but never regained prior levels of functioning. Subsequently, a gradual decline occurred. The possibility that a stressful event contributes in some way to the onset of Alzheimer's cannot be ruled out. In fact, there has long been speculation on the possible role of general anesthesia as a trigger for Alzheimer's disease. An alternative explanation, however, is that the stressful event uncovered a degenerative process that the family had not noticed previously. Surgery can sometimes result in brain damage, such as when an anoxia or other problem occurs (e.g., Roach et al., 1996). When the onset of symptoms occurred during surgery, a key distinction is whether there has been subsequent progression. If so, that points toward a dementia; if not, then the cognitive loss can be attributed to a problem that occurred during surgery.

In cases where the triggering event was the death of the spouse, we have usually discovered that the spouse who died was covering up for the other person's cognitive lapses and gradually taking on care. The children did not become aware of the problem until the death, when they were confronted by their surviving parent's behavior.

In contrast to dementia, a delirium typically has a recent and sudden onset and is characterized by dramatic fluctuations. It develops relatively rapidly, over a period of a few hours or days. Functioning changes suddenly and dramatically. The course is also fluctuating: patients can be extremely agitated and restless one hour and nearly comatose the next.

The following example illustrates a typical onset of delirium. The client was a woman in her mid-40s who was suffering from multiple sclerosis. A treatment that is used to slow down the progression of the disease is the hormone prednisone. Prednisone, however, can lead to a delirium. Within a day or two of starting the medication, this client would become agitated, disoriented, and suicidal. Upon stopping treatment, she rapidly returned to her prior level of functioning. As in many deliriums, onset was sudden and was associated with a specific physiological imbalance that in this case was caused by the medication. There was also a rapid resolution of symptoms when the medication was stopped.

A frequent type of fluctuation is for a delirium to become more pronounced in the evening. The term "sundowner's syndrome" refers to a common pattern of mild delirium that occurs only in the evening (Evans, 1987). This pattern is frequently encountered in hospitals and nursing homes. Someone suffering from dementia is especially prone to sundowning, but older people with normal functioning can develop this late-afternoon delirium in response to the multiple stresses associated with hospitalization, such as being in an unfamiliar setting, disruptions of sleep, discomfort, the effects of medications, and anxiety. Exposure to sunlight during the daytime and increased activity has been found clinically to reduce sundowning in institutional settings.

The duration of a delirium is relatively brief. Resolution usually occurs within a few days to a few weeks, ending either in death or in recovery if its cause can be treated. Failure to treat the cause of the delirium may also result in permanent brain damage. Untreated malnutrition would be an example of that pattern.

Most episodes of depression develop over a period of a few weeks. They are typically associated with stressful life events. Duration of a depressive episode is usually several months, but it can be chronic. We have worked with some older people who have had symptoms of a major depression for a few years or longer. These chronic depressions can be differentiated from dementia by the fact that cognitive problems do not get worse over time. Depressed patients can also fluctuate in performance, typically functioning worse in the mornings than later in the day.

The following example illustrates the onset of depression. The client was a 65-year-old woman who had no prior history of mental health problems. She had managed to raise 10 children successfully. When her last child left the home 6 months earlier, the woman's mood plummeted. She became severely depressed and suicidal. It emerged from the history that her symptoms coincided with her child's leaving home. As was the case for this client, it is almost always possible to date the onset of symptoms of depression by specific events.

Clinicians should note any history of prior psychiatric problems that can help formulate hypotheses about current diagnosis. Problems like depression are frequently recurrent. It is important, however, not to be bound by prior episodes of mental health problems when thinking about diagnosis. A person could have had previous instances of depression but now be developing Alzheimer's disease. On the other hand, if there is a history of past problems of a certain type, a recurrence needs to be ruled out before making a new diagnosis.

The following example illustrates how identifying a history of past disorders can be useful in sorting out the probable causes of current problems. A neuropsychological evaluation was requested for a 67-year-old man who was in the stabilization unit of a psychiatric hospital. The psychiatrist wondered whether he might have Alzheimer's disease and asked us to conduct an assessment. In reviewing the medical record, we noticed immediately that the patient had been diagnosed as schizophrenic while in his 20s and had functioned on neuroleptics (major tranquilizers) for the past 40 years, while working as a manual laborer. About 5 years earlier he had retired on disability. The patient was tested and was found to be hypomanic and to have pressured and tangential speech. There were no memory impairments per se. However, in further questioning, it became apparent that the patient would run out of money at the end of each month, fail to take his medication, and become delusional. His family was accustomed to this pattern, but when his behavior had come to the attention of local authorities, he was hospitalized. The chronicity of his schizophrenia had made him a poor historian. He also had performed poorly on a standard mental status examination, primarily because he was so caught up in his own thoughts that he did not pay attention to current events or to the specifics of his surroundings. Thus, the psychiatrist mistook his chronic lack of interest in the world around him for a memory impairment. Once the diagnosis was clarified, treatment was coordinated with the local mental health clinic. They were familiar with the patient and agreed to redouble their efforts to ensure a consistent supply of medication.

In contrast to dementia, cognitive deficits due to a nonprogressive head injury date to the time of the injury. Although these types of injury are relatively rare in an older population, they should be ruled out when conducting a history. We have on occasion encountered cases of older people with nonprogressive brain injuries who were mistakenly diagnosed as demented. Presenting with memory and other cognitive complaints, they were diagnosed as demented solely on the basis of their age.

When there has been a brain injury, an important distinction is whether or not symptoms worsen over time. As was noted in Chapter 3, head trauma may be a risk factor for Alzheimer's disease. We have seen cases where the first symptoms of dementia immediately followed a head injury. Whether the injury was, in fact, a trigger for dementia, or the damage caused by the injury served to uncover a dementia that was already in its beginning stages, cannot be determined. Most people who suffer a serious head injury have deficits that are stable or that improve somewhat over time.

As noted earlier, surgery can result also in nonprogressive brain damage. The following case illustrates the onset of cognitive symptoms following surgery. The client was an 82-year-old man who had been functioning very well. He developed heart problems and was determined to be a good candidate for bypass surgery. During the surgery, he experienced anoxia when oxygen was briefly cut off to the brain. When he awoke after the surgery, he was not himself. The changes were initially believed to be a delirium related to the anesthesia, but they did not clear up. On testing, he was found to have deficits in memory and other cognitive functions that were not evident before the surgery. These deficits were stable over time. The differences from dementia, then, were that symptoms dated from the time of the surgery and did not progress.

Another important consideration is history of alcoholism. Excessive use of alcohol can result in dementia-like symptoms in an older person or even in gradual deterioration (Cummings & Benson, 1992). Older people who were regular, controlled drinkers all their lives may no longer be able to tolerate a similar amount of alcohol, resulting in cognitive difficulties (see Chapter 4). This is often very difficult to uncover as a contributing problem, due to the patient's denial or the norm of having a "cocktail or two" before dinner.

The history of these disorders can be contrasted to changes found in normal aging. A typical history of a healthy older person is one of very gradual changes in memory and cognition that span a long period of time. People may describe themselves as not being able to remember as much as they previously did, but their point of comparison may be 30 or 40 years earlier. Often, people compare their current functioning to a time of life when they were busier and more involved in activities and had more things that were important to remember. Fluctuations in functioning can also occur with normal aging. People report more cognitive problems and other difficulties around stressful events or in association with depressed mood.

Mental Status Testing

The third step in assessment is mental status testing. These tests can address two questions: Is there evidence of an obvious cognitive impairment? What type of impairment is it?

Brief mental status tests are widely used in medical settings and are given by physicians, nurses, psychologists, or other health professionals. Mental status tests are quick and noninvasive and can be used to get an immediate impression of functioning. Although these tests have limitations, clinicians can use them effectively if they understand their shortcomings as well as what they can do.

Mental status tests typically assess recall of overlearned and basic information that people with normal brain functioning rarely forget. A core part of these tests is orientation questions, such as where the person currently is, the address, and the date. Personal information such as one's age and birth date are typically included. General informational questions, such as names of the current and past presidents, and simple cognitive tasks such as recalling three words or serial subtraction may also be assessed.

Mental status tests were developed from items typically asked in clinical examinations to assess altered states of consciousness that are found in delirium and acute psychotic disorders such as schizophrenia. The first systematic compilation of mental status items into a test was the 10-item Mental Status Questionnaire (MSQ) (Kahn, Goldfarb, Pollack, & Peck, 1960; Kahn, Pollack, & Goldfarb, 1961). Designed to be used in conjunction with the Face–Hand Test (described later), the MSQ gave a systematic and quantifiable assessment of functioning. Several other instruments have appeared since that time, usually with an expanded set of questions. Some of these tests are the Extended Mental Status Questionnaire (Whelihan, Lesher, Kleban, & Granick, 1984), the Short Portable Mental Status Questionnaire (SPMSQ) (Pfeiffer, 1975), the Jacobs Mental Status Questionnaire (Jacobs,

Bernhard, Delgado, & Strain, 1977), and the Blessed Information–Concentration–Attention test (Blessed, Tomlinson, & Roth, 1968), which has been adapted for use in the United States by Fuld (1978).

Probably the most widely used test is the Mini-Mental State Examination (MMSE) (Folstein, Folstein, & McHugh, 1975). Somewhat longer than the other standardized mental status examinations, the MMSE supplements questions on orientation with other cognitive tasks, including language, recall, writing, and spatial orientation.

Each mental status test presents cutoffs below which cognitive impairment should be strongly suspected. Because the test items are easy for most people, someone who makes more than a minimal number of errors is likely to have a significant problem. On the MMSE, for example, scores of 23 or below (out of a possible 30 points) are considered to indicate significant cognitive impairment.

Impairment on a mental status test usually indicates dementia or delirium, but it may, on occasions, reflect cognitive deficits associated with other neurological or psychiatric disorders. Severely depressed people, for example, may occasionally fall below the cutoff on mental status tests (Rabins, Merchant, & Nestadt, 1984). Education can affect test results as well. Poorly educated people are more likely to have false positive results, while a well-educated person may be able to answer questions on mental status exams correctly despite obvious evidence of dementia on other tests.

Which mental status test should a clinician use? Obviously, clinicians would prefer the test that yields the most accurate results, but the available data provide little empirical evidence for choosing one test over another. There are, however, practical advantages to using the MMSE. The MMSE has been used in many different studies, including the Epidemiologic Catchment Area studies of the prevalence of mental disorders (see Chapter 3), so considerable normative data are available. Additionally, the MMSE is the instrument most likely to be known and used by physicians, who may even administer it themselves.

The MMSE also has significant drawbacks. It is particularly subject to false positive findings (i.e., identifying someone as cognitively impaired who is not) among poorly educated people (Anthony, LeResche, Niaz, Von Korff, & Folstein, 1982; Folstein, Anthony, Parhad, Duffy, & Gruenberg, 1985; Murden, McRae, Kaner, & Bucknam, 1991; see Tombaugh & McIntyre, 1992, for a review). Murden and associates (1991) suggest using a cutoff for impairment of 17, rather than 23, for people with fewer than 9 years of schooling. Uhlmann and Larson (1991) report 90% accuracy in classifying people with dementia or normal functioning using education-adjusted cutoffs. The education-adjusted lower limits for normal functioning they used were 21 for middle school, 23 for high school, and 24 for college. They also suggested that race, socioeconomic status, and other factors need to be taken into account when examining MMSE results. Crum, Anthony, Bassett, and Folstein (1993) present extensive normative data for the MMSE based on age and education.

Clinicians should be aware of the potential for false negative findings, especially among well-educated individuals. In general, more extensive memory testing must be done to rule out dementia in highly educated patients.

Another problem with the MMSE is that the original version treats two attention tasks as equivalent: serial subtraction of 7's (starting from 100) and spelling "world" backwards. If someone cannot perform serial subtractions, he is then asked to spell "world" backwards. These tasks are not equivalent, however, and probably assess somewhat different underlying neuropsychological functions. Serial subtraction of 7's is a relatively difficult task missed by many people with normal brain functioning. By comparison, spelling "world" backwards is an easier task that can be done even by some people with mild dementia. Because this task is worth 5 out of the total 30 points for the scale, it is given disproportionate weight, despite the lack of equivalence between the two items.

There have been several suggestions for improving and extending the MMSE. The Alzheimer Disease Research Centers, which have been established by the National Institute on Aging, include a standard assessment that incorporates items from the MSQ, the American version of the Blessed scale, and the MMSE (Morris, Mohs, Rogers, Fillenbaum & Heyman, 1988). A common recommendation is that serial subtraction and spelling "world" backwards should be treated as separate items (Tombaugh & McIntyre, 1992). Molloy, Alemayehu, and Roberts (1991) have developed a standardized protocol for the MMSE. Another expanded version of the MMSE has been developed by Teng and Chui (1987).

We have also developed a modified version of the MMSE for use in clinical practice (see Appendix 5.2). First, we administer both attention tasks, serial subtraction of 7's and spelling "world" backwards. Second, we add items from other mental status tests that are useful in identifying obvious cognitive difficulties, specifically asking the client's birth date and age and the names of the current president and the president before him. We also add a series of questions that probe for types of responses that are typically found in a delirium.

When using the MMSE or other mental status tests, it is important to consider both the quantitative score and qualitative information. We report the standard 30-item MMSE score, but we consider carefully performance on the additional items that were administered. When errors have been made, we consider which items were missed and how severe the errors were. Some items are missed fairly often by people with good functioning, such as serial subtractions of 7's. It is also common for people with good functioning to fail to remember one of the three words in the delayed recall task. The additional item, the name of previous president, has varied in its degree of difficulty since it was originally included in the MSQ. When used in the 1950s and 1960s, errors in naming the previous president were relatively rare. Then during the Carter administration, many people with otherwise good functioning either could not name Gerald Ford as the previous president or answered "Nixon." A similar phenomenon occurred during the Clinton administration, with many people naming Reagan as the previous president, rather than Bush. Again, this response should be scored as an error, but it has less qualitative significance than a response of "Roosevelt" or "Truman."

The additional items for identifying delirium shown in Appendix 5.2 are an important part of the examination. Errors in responding to these questions can be classified as denotative or connotative (Kahn & Miller, 1978). Denotative responses keep the same frame of reference as the question. Asked "Where are you?" a patient replies, "In the hospital," but does not know the name of the hospital. This type of response is factually incorrect, but it represents an effort to respond to the explicit content of the question. A typical pattern with dementia is to not know or be unable to recall this information at all. Depressed patients can also make denotative errors on these items. Responses by severely depressed persons are typically characterized by a lack of effort. These patients appear too preoccupied with their own thoughts to respond. Incorrect responses by a person who has pronounced depressed mood and appears distracted or preoccupied during the testing suggests potentially reversible cognitive impairment due to depression.

In contrast, a patient giving a connotative answer is responding in a personal or idiosyncratic way; "it is as though he were responding in a different symbolic system, or that he is answering a different question than the one asked. Thus, if a person is asked where he is his response may actually answer the question of where he would like to be" (Kahn & Miller, 1978, p. 55). These kinds of errors are more likely to indicate a delirium or other acute, rapidly developing condition. These responses are common, for example, among people who recently suffered a stroke or a severe blow to the head.

Some typical connotative responses involve misnaming or displacement. A hospital is identified with a more benign term, such as "country club" or "hotel." It may be displaced spatially, usually by being located near the person's home. The location may also be displaced temporally, for example, if the person identifies a hospital where he or she was treated successfully in the past. This type of response differs from a memory problem. The person may be able to give the address of this other hospital or location. When shown bed sheets or other items that have the current hospital's name, the patient can read the name correctly but may insist that the item is there by mistake. Patients may also claim that they are in a different institution than the one they are in that has the same name. They may ascribe a benign quality to this other institution, such as being the place where people recover or go for minor problems. Other connotative responses include identifying the interviewer or his or her job as unconnected with the hospital or medical care (e.g., calling the clinician "an insurance salesman") and reporting an imagined journey the night before. These kinds of responses are usually accompanied by denial that anything is wrong (Kahn & Miller, 1978; Weinstein & Kahn, 1955).

The following example illustrates these kinds of connotative responses in patients with a delirium. A 55-year-old man who suffered a sudden heart attack a couple of days earlier was transferred from a medical floor to the psychiatric unit of a hospital because he could not be managed in the medical unit. He would alternatively try to escape or climb into bed with a woman patient. When first examined in the psychiatric ward, he responded to the question "Where are you?" by saying he was in the county jail and then giving the correct address for the county jail. Subsequently, he identified himself as being at work and gave his work address. He denied having any problems and tried repeatedly to leave the unit, insisting that he had to go to work. After a few days, during which the delirium resolved, he was able to correctly identify the hospital and its address.

This case illustrates the difference between recall of factual information and connotative responses in a delirium. The patient could provide factual information about the address of his work place and the county jail. The issue was not memory per se but the metaphorical way reality can be transformed during a delirium.

Some patients with a delirium may score above the cut-offs on mental status tests (Tune & Folstein, 1986). The presence of noncognitive symptoms (e.g., inattention, fluctuations, altered level of consciousness) or of connotative responses is a better indication of the presence of a delirium than the total score.

The following case contains many elements typical of delirium, including sudden onset, the interaction of several risk factors, and the possibility for full recovery. This client had some changes in orientation, but the primary symptom suggesting a delirium was her insistence that her recently deceased husband was alive. The patient was a woman who had surgery for breast cancer and went to a rehabilitation hospital for help in the recovery. While at the rehabilitation hospital, she fell and broke her hip. After the fracture was repaired, she was moved to a nursing home. Soon after she arrived in the nursing home, her husband died. During the funeral, the woman showed no grief, and afterwards, she talked about her husband as if he were still alive. An assessment was done and it was discovered that she neither know where she was nor the time or date. Two factors were probably contributing to the delirium. First was the trauma of having suffered a hip fracture and then learning that her husband had died. Second, the pain medication the woman was receiving may have played a role in her delirium. As the fracture healed and she required less pain medication, the delirium gradually cleared, and she was able to move back to her own home. Follow-up evaluation indicated no lingering cognitive deficits, and the woman was fully aware that her husband had died.

New instruments have been developed specifically designed for the detection of a delirium (e.g., Inouye et al., 1990; Rockwood, Goodman Flynn, & Stolee, 1996; Trzepacz & Dew, 1995). One of the most promising, the Delirium Symptom Interview (Levkoff et al., 1991), combines typical mental status items with questions and observations designed to match DSM-IV criteria for delirium. Items for this questionnaire are shown in Appendix 5.3. The scale can detect the presence of delirium symptoms with about 90% accuracy, while not leading to high rates of false positive identifications. Interrater reliabilities are also very good.

The mental status test, then, represents a reasonable screening procedure, but it should never be the only source of information on which a decision about diagnosis is made. The mental status test should be the first screening measure rather than the sole measure used. When used in conjunction with other information about the individual, including education and performance on other psychological tests, it can provide valuable information about the likely presence of cognitive impairments. In the end, the decision about which test to use is probably less important than to administer the same test systematically over a large series of patients who are characterized and followed adequately. In that manner, the clinician can learn how to interpret test results effectively by learning to identify qualitatively different responses on a mental status test, which can reduce the occurrence of false positives and negatives and improve the accuracy of differential diagnosis.

Before leaving the topic of mental status tests, we want to talk about two other procedures, the Face–Hand Test and the Dementia Rating Scale. Developed originally by Bender (1952), the Face–Hand Test evaluates the ability to report two simultaneous stimuli applied to the cheek and back of the hand. Developed serendipitously and without a theoretical foundation, the Face–Hand Test is sensitive to effects of global disturbances of brain function such as those found in dementia and delirium. Its nonverbal content makes false positives among depressed elderly or people with other psychiatric disorders relatively rare (Kahn et al., 1960; Kahn & Miller, 1978; S. Zarit, Miller, & Kahn, 1978).

The Face–Hand Test is shown in Appendix 5.4. Subjects are asked to close their eyes and point to the place where the examiner has touched them. Four blocks of trials are administered, each block consisting of four probes. Errors on the first block are common and do not have any significance. The most common error is to fail to report the hand stimulus. Other errors include displacing the hand stimulus to the cheek or shoulder or out into space. Following the first block, subjects are touched first on both cheeks and then both hands. Each of those probes serve as a learning trial, alerting patients to the fact that they are being touched in two places. Following the learning trials, the pattern of touching cheek and hand simultaneously is repeated. Bilateral errors after the learning trials usually indicate a significant brain problem.

After completing the trials with eyes closed, the clinician can continue testing with eyes open. This step is not necessary if the patient has responded correctly to the previous block of trials. Many patients with cognitive dysfunction continue making errors with eyes open, even though they watch the examiner touch them. Continuing to make errors with eyes open is associated with more severe cognitive impairment (S. Zarit et al., 1978).

One caution in administering the Face–Hand Test is that patients who have long-standing diabetes may have peripheral neuropathy, which impairs tactile sensation in their hands. If a patient is known to have diabetes, trials should be made to determine how hard a touch is necessary for the stimulation of the hands to be felt. It should also be noted that people who have suffered unilateral sensory loss such as following a stroke may make errors only on their affected side. This type of error reflects their sensory loss, not the cognitive problems associated with bilateral errors.

The Face–Hand Test is not widely used anymore, probably because it has no foundation in current neuropsychological theories. It is, however, a relatively brief and nonthreatening test. The information provided, used in conjunction with other tests and information, can add to the overall picture of functioning. Because it is nonverbal, this test may be particularly useful in differentiating pseudodementia from actual cases of dementia. In our experience, a positive indication of brain impairment on the Face–Hand Test, even if other evidence is ambiguous, is often a telling sign of a serious problem.

The Dementia Rating Scale (DRS), developed by Mattis (1976, 1989), provides a comprehensive assessment of functioning in five domains: attention, initiation/perseveration, construction, conceptualization, and memory. Like mental status tests, the DRS can identify obvious cases of cognitive impairment, but because items are relatively easy, it does not usually help in differentiation of early, mild dementia, especially for a well-educated person. It has, however, two major strengths over briefer mental status tests. First, the clinician can obtain a profile of the extent of impairment in different functions. As an example, the DRS may indicate that a patient has poor verbal memory, but visual spatial functioning is relatively spared. This type of observation is useful in planning interventions that build on the patient's remaining abilities, in this case using visual rather than just verbal cues to guide behavior. The second strength of the DRS is for following the longitudinal course of symptoms in mild and moderately impaired cases (Salmon, Thal, Butters, & Heindel, 1990). Recent reports provide additional information on the psychometric properties of this instrument (Smith et al., 1994).

CONCLUSIONS

In this chapter, we have begun an examination of the assessment process. The starting point is how to structure an assessment of an older person to assure that results are not due to lack of rapport, fatigue, sensory loss, conditions in the testing environment, or other factors that might lead to an incorrect estimate of abilities. To answer questions of differential diagnosis, the clinician gathers information from the patient and from family or other reliable informants, including a clear picture of current problems and symptoms and their history. Mental status testing is an important tool that contributes quantitative and qualitative information about current functioning and the likely etiology of symptoms. Clinicians need to be aware of the limitations of mental status testing and to use these tests as part of a comprehensive assessment.

We continue our discussion of differential diagnosis in Chapter 6, focusing on psychological testing and how medical and psychological data are used to differentiate among types of dementing illnesses. We conclude that chapter with a discussion of a different type of assessment issue, evaluation of competency.

APPENDIX 5.1. MEMORY AND BEHAVIOR PROBLEMS CHECKLIST

INSTRUCTIONS TO INTERVIEWER

This checklist has two parts. Part A measures the frequency with which problems occur. Part B determines to what degree the behavior upsets the caregiver. Begin by asking if a problem has occurred and, if so, how often. When you find it has occurred, then go immediately to Part B and determine the caregiver's reaction to that problem *when it occurs*. (In other words, do not go through the whole list for frequency and then come back to get the caregiver's reaction.)

INSTRUCTIONS TO CAREGIVER

Part A. "I am going to read you a list of common problems. Tell me if any of these problems have occurred during the past week. If so how often have they occurred? If not, has this problem ever occurred?" Hand the subject the card on which the frequency and reaction ratings are printed.

Part B. "How much does this problem bother or upset you at the time it happens?" The subject indicates his or her typical reaction on the card on which the frequency and reaction ratings are printed. Reaction is how the person reacts when the problem occurs. When the caregiver's response to frequency is "7," determine reaction by asking: "How much does it bother or upset you when you have to supervise to prevent that?"

Note. From S. Zarit, Orr, and Zarit (1985). Copyright 1985 by the authors. Reprinted by permission.

FREQUENCY RATINGS: How often has the behavior happened?

REACTION RATINGS: How much does this behavior bother or upset you when it happens?

0 = never occurred
1 = has occurred but not in past week
2 = has occurred 1 or 2 times in past week
3 = has occurred 3 to 6 times in past week
4 = occurs daily or more often
7 = would occur if not supervised by caregiver (e.g., wandering except door is locked)
8 = patient never performed this activity

0 = not at all
1 = a little
2 = moderately
3 = very much
4 = extremely

BEHAVIORS	FREQUENCY	REACTION
1. Wandering or getting lost	0 1 2 3 4 7	0 1 2 3 4
2. Asking the same question over and over again	0 1 2 3 4	0 1 2 3 4
3. Hiding things (money, jewelry, etc.)	0 1 2 3 4	0 1 2 3 4
4. Being suspicious or accusative	0 1 2 3 4	0 1 2 3 4
5. Losing or misplacing things	0 1 2 3 4	0 1 2 3 4
6. Not recognizing familiar people	0 1 2 3 4	0 1 2 3 4
7. Forgetting what day it is	0 1 2 3 4	0 1 2 3 4
8. Starting but not finishing things	0 1 2 3 4	0 1 2 3 4
9. Destroying property	0 1 2 3 4	0 1 2 3 4
10. Doing embarrassing things	0 1 2 3 4	0 1 2 3 4
11. Waking you up at night	0 1 2 3 4	0 1 2 3 4
12. Being constantly restless	0 1 2 3 4	0 1 2 3 4
13. Being constantly talkative	0 1 2 3 4	0 1 2 3 4
14. Talking little or not at all	0 1 2 3 4	0 1 2 3 4
15. Engaging in behavior that is potentially dangerous to others or self	0 1 2 3 4 7	0 1 2 3 4
16. Reliving situations from the past	0 1 2 3 4	0 1 2 3 4
17. Seeing or hearing things that are not there (hallucinations or illusions)	0 1 2 3 4	0 1 2 3 4
18. Unable or unwilling to dress self (either partly or totally) or dressing inappropriately compared to previous standards	0 1 2 3 4 7	0 1 2 3 4
19. Unable or unwilling to feed self	0 1 2 3 4 7	0 1 2 3 4

20. Unable or unwilling to bathe or shower by self	0 1 2 3 4 7	0 1 2 3 4
21. Unable to put on make-up or shave self	0 1 2 3 4 7	0 1 2 3 4
22. Incontinent of bowel or bladder	0 1 2 3 4 7	0 1 2 3 4
23. Unable to prepare meals	0 1 2 3 4 7 8	0 1 2 3 4
24. Unable to use phone	0 1 2 3 4 7	0 1 2 3 4
25. Unable to handle money (complete a transaction in a store; does not include managing finances)	0 1 2 3 4 7	0 1 2 3 4
26. Unable to clean the house	0 1 2 3 4 7 8	0 1 2 3 4
27. Unable to shop (to pick our adequate or appropriate foods)	0 1 2 3 4 7 8	0 1 2 3 4
28. Unable to do other simple tasks which he or she used to do—specify (e.g., put groceries away, simple repairs)	0 1 2 3 4 7	0 1 2 3 4
29. Unable to stay alone	0 1 2 3 4 7	0 1 2 3 4
30. Are there any other problems you are having? (specify)	0 1 2 3 4 7	0 1 2 3 4

APPENDIX 5.2. THE MENTAL STATUS EXAMINATION

The standard version of the Mini-Mental State Examination is presented below, along with information on administration and scoring. At the end are mental status test items that we use to supplement the MMSE. These items are useful in differentiating between cognitively impaired and intact people and in identifying delirium (see Chapter 5).

MINI-MENTAL STATE EXAMINATION

Score

1 0		1. What building or place are we in?
1 0		2. What floor are we on?
1 0		3. What city (town) are we in?
1 0		4. What county are we in?
1 0		5. What state are we in?
1 0		6. What is the date today?

Note. Standard MMSE from Folstein, Folstein, and McHugh (1975). Copyright 1975 by Elsevier Science. Reprinted by permission.

1 0   7. Month? (Only the current month is correct, except on last day of the old month or first day of the new.)

1 0   8. Year? (Only the current year is correct, except in January.)

1 0   9. What day of the week is it? (Only the current day is correct.)

1 0   10. What season is it? (Fall = September–December; Winter = December–March; Spring = March–June; Summer = June–September)

1 0   11. Registration: I would like to test your memory now. I am going to say three words and I want you to repeat them after I am done. (Say "ball," "flag," "tree" clearly and slowly for about 1 second each. After you have said all three one time, ask the person to repeat them and record exact responses. Score is the number of words repeated on Trial 1. IF ALL THREE RESPONSES ARE NOT CORRECT on the first trial, repeat the words until the person is able to recall all three, up to a maximum of six trials. Record answers for each trial.)

5 4 3 2 1 0   12. Attention and calculation: Begin with 100 and count backwards by 7's. (Stop after 5 subtractions. DO NOT DEMONSTRATE THE TASK, BUT YOU MAY REPEAT THE INSTRUCTIONS. Record the exact responses. Do not remind the person of the task or the number they were last on. Also, do not tell the person if the answer was correct.)

           ___ 93 ___86 ___79 ___72 ___65

5 4 3 2 1 0   13. Attention and calculation: Spell the word "world." (Person spells.) Now spell "world" backwards. (The score is the number of letters in correct order in the backwards spelling, e.g., dlrow = 5; dlorw = 3.)

           ___ ___ ___ ___ ___
           D   L   R   O   W

3 2 1 0   14. Recall the three words I previously asked you to remember. (Record exact responses, including "I don't know.")

1 0   15. Language: (Show the person a wrist watch and ask what it is.)

1 0   16. Language: (Show the person a pencil and ask what it is.)

1 0   17. Repetition: Please repeat this sentence: "NO IFS, ANDS, OR BUTS." (Be sure to speak clearly and slowly. You may repeat sentence once.)

     18. Three-stage command: (Give the person a piece of blank paper.) Take the paper in your right hand, fold it in half, and put it on the floor. (DO NOT REPEAT THE INSTRUCTIONS. ALSO NOTE THE HAND THE PERSON TAKES THE PAPER IN, AND RECORD EXACTLY WHAT HE OR SHE DOES.)

1	0	Takes paper in right hand
1	0	Folds paper in half
1	0	Puts paper on floor

1 0   19. Reading: (Show the person paper on which is printed: "Close your eyes" in block letters. Ask him or her to read it and then do what it says. Score correct only if person closes eyes.)

1 0   20. Writing: (Give the person a blank piece of paper and ask him or her to write a sentence. To score correct, sentence must contain a subject and verb. Correct grammar and punctuation are not necessary.)

1 0   21. Copying: (Give the person the figure of intersecting pentagons and ask him or her to copy it exactly as it is. DO NOT SHOW THE PERSON WHERE ON THE PAGE TO PUT THE FIGURE. IF THE PERSON DOES NOT UNDERSTAND THE TASK, POINT TO THE FIGURE AND SAY, "MAKE ONE JUST LIKE THIS ONE.")

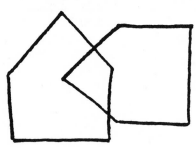

Scoring: 1 point if figures have all 5 sides and intersect at the correct point. Lines must meet at each of the 5 angles.

TOTAL SCORE
    MMSE (extended) _____ (max = 35)
    MMSE _____ (Standard MMSE is computed by taking the highest score for either serial subtraction or spelling backwards; max = 30.)

Scoring (standard version):
    24–30: No impairment
    17–23: Mild impairment
    10–16: Moderate impairment
    0–9:   Severe impairment

ADDITIONAL MENTAL STATUS QUESTIONS

1. Where are you? (Use these probes if necessary: What place is this? What do you call this place? What kind of place is this? If the place is an institution the correct

answer must include both the name and *kind* of place, e.g., hospital, nursing home.) *Note:* This item can substitute for the first item in the MMSE.

2. What is the address of this place? (or What street is this place located on? Generally, the name of any street bordering the block in which the interview takes place is satisfactory.)

3. Have you ever been in another (name of institution, e.g., St. Vincent's Hospital) with the same name? (If yes, Where was that?)

4. Have you ever seen me before? (If yes, Where was that?)

5. What's my job called?

6. Where were you last night?

7. How old are you? (Score exact age as correct, except if one month before or after birthday.)

8. What is your date of birth? Month?

9. Year?

10. Who is President of the United States?

11. Who was the President before him?

APPENDIX 5.3. QUESTIONS FROM THE DELIRIUM SYMPTOM INTERVIEW ACCORDING TO SYMPTOM DOMAIN

Disorientation

Have we ever met before today?
Can you tell me what time of day it is now?
Can you tell me where we are now?
Why are you in the hospital?
During the past day, did you think that you weren't really in the hospital?
Have you felt confused at any time during the past day?

Disturbance of Sleep

Did you have trouble falling asleep last night?
After you fell asleep, did you wake up and have trouble falling back to sleep?
Did you wake up on your own too early this morning?
Were you sleepy during the day?
Did you have nightmares or vivid dreams that were intense or bothersome last night?

Note. From Levkoff, Liptzin, Cleary, Reilly, and Evans (1991). Copyright 1991 by Springer Publishing Company, Inc. Reprinted by permission. This appendix does not include all questions from the Delirium Symptom Interview. For complete interview write to Sue Levkoff, ScD, Harvard Geriatric Education Center, Division on Aging, Harvard Medical School, 643 Huntington Avenue, Boston, MA 02115.

*These are based on observations made of patients.

Perceptual Disturbance

At any time during the past day have you experienced or imagined seeing, hearing, or feeling things that weren't really there?

(Interviewer) During the interview was there evidence of any of the above delusions; for example, did the patient think he/she was at home because things in the room looked like home?

Now I want to ask you about objects that you have seen or sounds that you have heard that you may have misinterpreted; for example, sounds that you have heard were not what they appeared to be.

Did you think that people were trying to harm you, when they weren't?

(Interviewer) During the interview, was there evidence of any of the above misperceptions; for example, did the patient answer the intercom or think a spot on the wall was a surveillance camera?

Now, I'd like to ask you whether things that you recognized correctly looked distorted, or strange. For example, did:

Things look bigger or samller than they really were?

Things move that were not really moving?

Things seem as if they were moving in slow motion?

Your body size, shape, or weight look different from what it is?

(Interviewer) During the interview, was there evidence of any of the above misperceptions; for example, did the patient think a light was swirling that wasn't?

Disturbance of Consciousness*

Did the patient stare into space and appear unaware of his/her environment?

Did the patient talk about something else; for example, did he/she change the subject suddenly (e.g., non sequitur) or tell a story unrelated to the interview?

Did the patient appear inappropriately distracted by environmental stimuli; for example, did he/she respond to questions asked of a roommate (distractible)?

Did the patient show excessive absorption with ordinary objects in the environment; for example, did he/she repetitively fold sheets or examine the IV tube over and over (hypervigilant)?

Did the patient have a recurring thought that prevented him/her from responding appropriately to the environment; for example, did he/she continuously look for shoes that weren't there (persistent thought)?

Did the patient have trouble keeping track of what was being said during the interview; for example, did he/she fail to follow instructions or answer questions one at a time?

Did the patient appear inappropriately startled by stimuli in the environment?

Was the patient awake; sleepy; stuporous; comatose?

Incoherent Speech*

Was the patient's speech:

Unusually limited or sparse?

Unusually slow or halting?

Unusually slurred?

Unusually fast or pressured?
Unusually loud?
Unusually repetitive (e.g., repeating a phrase over and over)?
Characterized by speech sounds in the wrong place?
Characterized by words or phrases that were disjointed or inappropriate?

Psychomotor Activity*

Was there evidence of:
Restlessness (e.g., patient getting in an out of bed)?
Tremors?
Grasping/picking?
Increased speed of motor response (e.g., grabbing for a drinking glass suddenly)?
Wandering?
Lethargy and sluggishness?
Slowness of motor response?
Staring into space?

Fluctuating Behavior*

Did the patient's level of consciousness fluctuate during the interview; for example, did he/she start to respond appropriately and then drift off?
(If present) Did the patient's speech fluctuate during the interview; for example, did the patient speak normally for a while, then speed up?
(If present) Did the psychomotor activity fluctuate during the interview; for example, was the patient at first sluggish, and then moving very quickly?
Did the patient show emotional lability?

APPENDIX 5.4. FACE–HAND TEST

INSTRUCTIONS

1. With eyes closed: "Please close your eyes. I am going to touch you and I want you to show me where I touched you." (On trials 1–4, if person makes an omission, ask: "Anywhere else?")
2. With eyes open: "Now open your eyes. I am going to touch you again. Pay close attention and show me where I touched you." Test is terminated after trial 4, 8, 12, or 16, if the patient has completed the preceding four trials correctly.

Circle omissions; indicate displacements with "D."

Note. From Kahn, Goldfarb, Pollack, and Peck (1960). Copyright 1960 by the American Psychiatric Association. Reprinted by permission.

Eyes Closed

1. Right cheek–left hand
2. Left cheek–right hand
3. Right cheek–right hand
4. Left cheek–left hand
   Right cheek–left cheek
   Right hand–left hand
5. Right cheek–left hand
6. Left cheek–right hand
7. Right cheek–right hand
8. Left cheek–left hand

Eyes Open

9. Right cheek–left hand
10. Left cheek–right hand
11. Right cheek–right hand
12. Left cheek–left hand
    Right cheek–left cheek
    Right hand–left hand
13. Right cheek–left hand
14. Left cheek–right hand
15. Right cheek–right hand
16. Left cheek–left hand

SCORING

Results suggest brain damage if the patient continues to make errors on the fifth trial or after. Severity of damage is related to the number of errors. Errors before the fifth trial have no clinical significance.

6

Psychological Testing for Differential Diagnosis and Competence Evaluations

In this chapter we continue describing the assessment process. Chapter 5 presented the first three steps in differential diagnosis: identifying presenting symptoms and problems, obtaining a history of current symptoms and problems, and mental status testing. We now turn to the next three steps: psychological and neuropsychological testing, coordination with a medical evaluation, and, when dementia is present, identifying the probable or likely cause. We end the section on differential diagnosis with three case examples and a discussion of additional issues in assessment. The second half of the chapter addresses competence evaluations and how psychological evaluations contribute to the determination of competence.

PSYCHOLOGICAL AND NEUROPSYCHOLOGICAL ASSESSMENT

Psychological testing is a systematic way of assessing current performance under standardized conditions, yielding findings that can be compared against normative data. These objective results help clarify the more impressionistic findings from clinical examinations. Test performance can also be assessed over time, which is especially important when initial findings are ambiguous. Results from psychological tests have been found to be as accurate as medical evaluations in differentiating dementia from normal aging and other disorders of later life (Tuokko, Kristjansson, & Miller, 1995). Of course, tests should not be used alone in a dementia workup. Just as a medical evaluation is often incomplete without neuropsychological testing, test results also tell only part of the story. Patients are served best when testing is part of a comprehensive evaluation that includes medical and other relevant assessments.

A full neuropsychological evaluation is expensive and time-consuming, but it need not be conducted in every case. In cases of obvious cognitive deficits, brief testing can confirm the pattern and severity of deficits. To do more would often just be frustrating for the patient without clarifying the situation further. A thorough evaluation is warranted when the initial findings from medical and neuropsychological data are unclear or ambiguous, when a baseline assessment is needed to follow people over time, when definitive proof is needed, such as to clarify the situation for a family that is arguing over diagnosis, or if legal issues are involved. We discuss these situations in detail.

A thorough psychological or neuropsychological assessment serves a number of purposes in differential assessment. The most frequent question raised in clinical practice is whether there is evidence of dementia or other significant cognitive impairment. To address this question, test findings should be evaluated in light of age norms for the test (when available), the client's education, and any other noncognitive factors that might affect performance, such as hearing or vision loss, fatigue, or distractions during the testing session (see Chapter 5). If there is evidence of impairment, the next consideration is which abilities are affected and what types of errors are made. The pattern of test results provides evidence for differentiation of dementia from other causes of brain damage and from depression. Findings may also suggest what type of dementing illness is present. Dementia is generally characterized by global impairment, that is, memory, abstract reasoning, judgment, language, and other abilities are affected. In frontal dementias and subcortical dementias, however, some abilities are spared until later in the disease. Traumatic head injury is usually characterized by specific neuropsychological deficits that correspond to the damaged region of the brain. Patients with a focal injury have problems in one or two areas but stable and relatively intact performance on other abilities. With depression, patients perform within normal limits or have minor memory deficits. Compared to dementia patients, however, people with depression and other psychiatric disorders improve in memory performance with successive learning trials and have little or no deficits in delayed recall or in recognition memory (Butters, Salmon, & Butters, 1994).

The use of a test battery makes it possible to detect early and mild cases of dementia that would not be identified through mental status testing or other clinical procedures. Many people with high intelligence and education get a perfect score on a mental status test or miss only one or two items, even though they are having obvious difficulties in cognitive functioning. The mental status test items represent overlearned and familiar information that well-educated people can answer easily. Neuropsychological tests include items with a range of difficulty. The more difficult or challenging tasks can identify mild deficits in someone with a high education. If findings remain ambiguous, however, the results from testing can be used as a baseline and performance then tracked over time. A comprehensive evaluation can also identify specific strengths and weaknesses in cognitive abilities, which is important in planning interventions with the patient, family, or other caregivers.

An extensive literature on neuropsychological abilities, aging, and dementia has developed in recent years (see, e.g., Albert & Moss, 1988; Flicker, 1988; Kaszniak, 1990, 1996; Lezak, 1995; Storandt & VandenBos, 1994). The debate over which test or test battery is best can be contentious. Rather than taking the position that there is one best test for a particular ability or one battery that represents the gold standard, we believe that any approach has strengths and limitations. The most important step is to gain a lot of experience with a set of tests that meet the criteria discussed. In that way, clinicians learn to recognize the patterns of scores associated with different disorders. It is also important to know the limitations of a test battery, and to supplement it with other tests, as the situation requires. Perhaps the primary advantage of employing a standard set of tests is that it is easier to learn how to use the information that does not go into test scores. What clients say about their performance and how they answer questions or solve problems is often as important as whether a response is right or wrong. By using the same set of tests, clinicians can develop an understanding of the significance of this part of testing. (See Lezak, 1995, for a thorough discussion of qualitative responses.)

Five main considerations should be taken into account when choosing a test battery. First, the degree of difficulty of the tests should be considered. Tests can be thought of as having floors and ceilings. A test with a high ceiling has a lot of difficult items and can test people's limits. A test like that is useful for identifying subtle or mild problems, especially in someone who is well educated. A test with a high ceiling would be used when evaluating someone for possible early dementia. In contrast, some tests have a low floor, that is, they contain many easy items, some of which can be solved by people suffering from dementia or other cognitive disorders.

A second consideration is that tests have age norms so that actual performance can be compared against expected levels of functioning. As will be discussed, several tests now have adequate norms into very late life.

A third consideration is that the test battery evaluate several functions. A person may have problems in only one or two domains but not across all neuropsychological abilities. The pattern of errors is important for diagnosis. A discrete problem may suggest focal brain damage or some other cause of symptoms besides dementia. By comparison, a pattern of mild deficits across several abilities might suggest early dementia. In cases of dementia, identification of functions that are relatively spared can be useful in planning treatment.

Albert (1988) proposes that an assessment of an older patient should evaluate five functions: attention, memory, language, visuospatial, and conceptualization. The clinician can accomplish this goal by choosing comprehensive test batteries such as the Wechsler Adult Intelligence Scale (WAIS-III) (Wechsler, 1997a), the Halstead–Reitan Battery (Reitan, 1969), or the Luria Nebraska Neuropsychological Battery (Golden et al., 1982), which include tests for measuring most or all of these functions. Another approach is to select specific tests for each function. Whatever the choice, the main goal is to obtain a broad-based evaluation of cognitive performance.

The fourth consideration is to evaluate the risks associated with different kinds of errors in assessment. Some tests are more likely to yield false positive findings, suggesting dementia when it is not present, while other tests do not reliably identify early, mild cases. In general, the more challenging the test, the more likely that false positive results will occur. Conversely, relatively easy tests such as mental status tests yield fewer false positive findings but more false negatives. As discussed previously, a false positive diagnosis of dementia carries with it more negative consequences than a false negative outcome. As a result, there must be a preponderance of evidence that is clear and unequivocal before assessing someone as having a dementing illness. By contrast, failure to detect delirium and depression can have serious or even catastrophic consequences. It is better, then, to err on the side of diagnosing these disorders and to initiate appropriate treatment.

Fifth, it is important to obtain follow up information on clients, including repeated testing when that is appropriate. Many difficult diagnostic questions are clarified over time. If dementia is suspected but the evidence is not really clear, conducting follow-up assessments one year later will provide conclusive evidence of whether or not there has been progression of symptoms. During that period, the client could receive treatment for any potentially treatable component, such as depression symptoms. Follow-up evaluations are especially valuable in cases that had atypical findings at the initial testing or that have a rare diagnosis (e.g., Pick's disease). We include examples later in the chapter that illustrate the use of repeated assessments.

Tests and Test Batteries

This section describes several tests and test batteries that are useful in the assessment process. Sources for these tests, including information on ordering them, are found in Appendix 6.1. Lezak (1995) provides a comprehensive listing of tests and valuable information on their clinical application and interpretation. The Geropsychology Assessment Resource Guide (VA National Center for Cost Containment, 1993) is another useful resource that provides primary sources for tests, how to obtain them, and the availability of age norms. (Copies can be ordered for $30 from the National Technical Information Service, U.S. Department of Commerce, 5285 Fort Royal Road, Springfield, VA 22161, order number PB 93-213684.)

General Intelligence

The WAIS remains a popular test, due in no small measure to the extensive literature and adequate age norms on it (Ryan, Paolo, & Brungardt, 1990; Ivnik et al., 1992b). Although the normative work was largely done with the previous edition (WAIS-R), the newest version (WAIS-III) (Wechsler, 1997a) contains all the scales from the earlier version, and so the available norms can be applied.

The WAIS-III comprises six verbal tests and eight performance tests (Table 6.1). Dementia is suggested if the verbal, performance, and total scores are lower than would be expected for a person of a given age and educational background. Performance scores decline with normal aging (about 12 points by age 65 and 20 points by age 80; see Ryan et al., 1990). This decline occurs in part because many of the performance tests are speeded. They also include more challenging and unfamiliar tasks than the verbal subtests. Low performance but not verbal scores can reflect normal aging or a disease process that disrupts response speed or visual spatial functioning (see Kaszniak, 1996, for a review). By contrast, verbal performance is relatively stable until very late life. A lower than expected verbal score can be a very important indicator of cognitive problems.

TABLE 6.1. WAIS-III Subscales and the Abilities They Measure

Verbal tests	Abilities
Information	General knowledge, verbal recall
Comprehension	Reasoning, social judgment
Vocabulary	General mental ability; verbal recall, language fluency
Similarities	Concept formation, abstract reasoning
Arithmetic	Computational skill, short-term memory, concentration
Letter–number sequencing	Working memory, attention

Performance tests	Abilities
Digit span	Attention, concentration, short-term (working) memory
Digit symbol coding	Attention, psychomotor performance, response speed
Block design	Visuospatial organization and construction, conceptualization
Object assembly	Visuospatial organization
Picture arrangement	Visuospatial ability, social judgment, reasoning
Picture completion	Visual reasoning, visual search, recall
Matrix reasoning	Visual information processing, abstract reasoning
Symbol search	Visuospatial ability

The WAIS-III can be used in its entirety or subscales selected to measure specific abilities, as discussed in the following sections.

Attention

Attention is assessed directly and through observation. Two commonly used tests are digits forward from the digit span task of the WAIS-III and a letter cancellation task (Lezak, 1995), in which subjects are instructed to cross out particular letters (e.g., all the E's and C's) from a long series. Cancellation tasks can also use geometric figures or pictures. Observations of how the patient focuses on other tasks can also provide good evidence of attention problems (Albert, 1988).

Attention tasks are generally performed well by healthy older people. Impairment in attention is a central feature of delirium. People with early, mild symptoms of dementia do not show attentional deficits, but difficulties develop as the dementia progresses. Patients who are depressed or have other psychiatric disorders may be preoccupied with their own thoughts and show poor attention. Poor attention scores by themselves do not indicate a disorder, but they must be considered in combination with other tests and the overall clinical picture.

Memory

As the most central feature of dementia, memory plays a critical role in an evaluation when dementia is suspected. Memory is not a single function but comprises several different and interrelated processes. Identifying which aspects of memory are impaired is an important part of an assessment. Among the distinctions that testing should make are the following:

Differentiating initial acquisition from subsequent recall
Identifying rates of acquisition and retention of new information
Distinguishing immediate and delayed recall
Assessing both verbal (semantic) and nonverbal recall
Assessing both recall and recognition

Memory for old, well-learned information, such as prominent historical events during the person's lifetime, can also be assessed (e.g., Butters, Salmon, & Butters, 1994).

A well-constructed battery assesses these different types of memory. Tests of short-term memory that involve several learning trials and both immediate and delayed recall are particularly useful in differentiating early dementia from normal aging. In dementia, the rate of learning and retention of new material is poor (e.g., Butters, Salmon, & Butters, 1994; Delis et al., 1991; Johansson & Zarit, 1997; Morris et al., 1991; Welsh, Butters, Hughes,

Mohs, & Heyman, 1991). People with dementia have lower than expected performance on initial trials and show little or no improvement with repeated presentation of the stimuli. Some healthy older people also have poor initial recall but show improvement over repeated trials. Delayed recall also helps in differentiating between dementia and normal aging (Welsh et al., 1991). Dementia patients have a greater drop-off in delayed recall than normal older people. More intrusions during recall as well as poorer overall delayed recall can differentiate Alzheimer's disease from other dementias, particularly subcortical disorders such as Huntington's disease (Delis et al., 1991). Intrusions have been found for verbal as well as nonverbal stimuli, for example, recall of geometric designs (Jacobs, Troster, Butters, Salmon, & Cermak, 1990).

Depressed patients can be differentiated from those with dementia on many of these indicators. People who are depressed may have lower recall than normal elderly on initial trials of a memory test, but in contrast to dementia patients, they improve with repeated presentations of stimuli. Delayed recall and recognition are also good, compared to dementia patients (Blau & Ober, 1988; Butters, Salmon, & Butters, 1994; Kaszniak, 1986). Depressed patients also do not typically have intrusions. Of course, some individuals may have both dementia and depression, complicating the process of differential diagnosis.

The revised Wechsler Memory Scale (WMS-R) (Wechsler, 1987) provides a comprehensive assessment of different memory functions. The test has five index scores: general memory, verbal memory, visual memory, attention/concentration, and delayed recall. Normative data suggest functioning declines with age and dementia, particularly in delayed recall. This test gives a comprehensive measure of paired recall, both visual and verbal, and includes delayed recall of most of the tasks. There is normative data up to age 97 (Ivnik et al., 1992b; Ivnek, Smith, Malec, Kokmen, & Tangalos, 1994). The scale has spawned countless research studies comparing different populations of patients with neurological disorders (such as amyotrophic lateral sclerosis, Huntington's chorea, and Korsakoff's psychosis) (e.g., Butters et al., 1988).

In 1997, the WMS-III (Wechsler, 1997b), an updated and expanded version of the WMS-R, was released. This version retains all the former tests except visual paired associates. The items in the subtests have been changed and the tasks expanded to eliminate early ceiling effects. New subtests have been added: faces, family pictures, word lists (similar to the Auditory Verbal Learning Test, described later), and letter–number sequencing. Since the WMS-III has only recently been released, little research is available on it and little is known about how it compares to the WMS-R. The entire WMS-III takes about 2 hours to administer, compared to 1 hour for the WMS-R. The WMS-R and WMS-III may be experienced as frustrating by someone with significant memory impairment. These tests are also fairly challenging for people with low education and occupational attainment. Given the length of both tests, but particularly the WMS-III, clinicians may want to select only those subtests most pertinent to the referral question.

As an alternative to the WMS-R or WMS-III, clinicians can put together their own battery from the many tests available in the literature. We describe several tests on which good data on older people are available.

The Auditory Verbal Learning Test (AVLT) (Lezak, 1995) comprises 15 unrelated words that are presented over five trials. Immediate and delayed recall and recognition are scored. Extended age norms have been reported (Ivnik et al., 1992a). Dementia is associated with lower immediate and delayed recall and also with a higher rate of intrusions of words that were not on the original list (Bigler et al., 1989).

Some clinicians prefer the California Verbal Learning Test (CVLT) (Delis, Kramer, Kaplan, & Ober, 1987; Butters, Salmon, and Butters, 1994) because the stimulus words can be organized into semantic categories— types of food that make up a shopping list. The CVLT has been found to identify very early, mild changes in people with a family history of Alzheimer's disease who subsequently developed the illness (Bondi et al., 1994). Measures of response bias can be computed from the CVLT, which can be useful in differentiating dementia from depression (Massman, Delis, Butters, Dupont, & Gillin, 1992). Depressed patients have a more conservative response style, refusing to guess even though they might know the answer, while dementia patients give more incorrect answers.

The Fuld Object Memory Test (Fuld, 1978) has been used extensively in research on dementia. This test provides the opportunity to assess rates of learning and recall by selectively reminding patients which items they missed after each trial. Other advantages of this test are its use of familiar objects and the opportunity for the patient to use multiple sensory modalities in learning. Patients are presented with a bag that contains 10 common objects. They are asked first if they can identify the objects by touch in the bag. If they are not successful, then they are asked to name the objects by sight. Following identification of the objects, there is a short distraction (60 seconds). Then patients are asked to recall the objects. Following this trial, patients are reminded of any item they missed, distracted for 60 seconds, and then tested again for recall. There are a total of five trials of recall, followed by a multiple-choice recognition test. A delayed recall (15 minutes) is also administered.

Dementia patients are able to recall fewer items over the five trials than are normal elderly or those who are depressed. Delayed recall is also likely to be significantly lower. Norms are included with the test kit. The Object Memory Evaluation has been found to successfully differentiate between depression and dementia (La Rue, D'Elia, Clark, Spar, & Jarvik, 1986).

A related procedure, the Selective Reminding Test (Buschke & Fuld, 1974), has also been found to differentiate normal from demented elderly

(Masur et al., 1989). In contrast to the Object Memory Test, patients are presented with a series of 12 words. Alternate forms of the test are available.

Finally, we want to note that recall of past information is typically impaired in dementia, though not in normal aging or depression. Some tests of well-known historical events are available (e.g., Butters, Salmon, & Butters, 1994; Wilson, Kaszniak, Bacon, Fox, & Kelly, 1982; Squire, 1974; Flicker, 1988). One caution about tests of past information is that it is difficult to separate initial exposure and learning from subsequent forgetting. An alternative is to ask people about personal information, such as when they got married, or about children and grandchildren. Errors in remembering names of children or grandchildren are highly significant and usually indicate a serious cognitive problem. People who are healthy or who are depressed rarely forget this information. Occasionally, someone with a large number of grandchildren may have a bit of trouble recalling all their names and ages but will have no other memory problems. A severely depressed person may refuse to answer or avoid answering, which should be distinguished from being unable to recall the information.

Language

Language deficits in dementia can be subtle and not noticeable to the untrained observer. Because syntax, grammar, and phonology can be preserved until late in the disease (Flicker, 1988), speech can seem superficially normal. In Alzheimer's disease, a particular kind of language deficit, namely, empty language or an overall impoverishment of speech, is often an early symptom. Instead of saying, "Oh, look at the girl," a patient will say, "Oh, look at, um, her." Patients use pronouns instead of nouns and gradually stop using adjectives. Eventually, they use no nouns or adjectives at all. Patients also use a restricted vocabulary and may begin to paraphrase when they cannot recall a word, use an inappropriate word, or misname objects or combine words. Patients may be able to engage in the social process of speech, but the richness of their language declines. As the disease progresses, their speech has little content and frequent repetitions.

The vocabulary subscale of the WAIS-III provides information about language functioning. Patients with dementia have increasing difficulty recalling words. Their attempts to define words may be characterized by circumlocutions; they talk around the definition but are not able to produce the specific words needed for an adequate response.

A useful procedure for differentiating normal functioning from dementia is the Boston Naming Test (BNT) (Kaplan, Goodglass, & Weintraub, 1983). The BNT is a confrontation naming test in which patients are shown a series of pictures and asked to give the names. The test starts with a series of easily recognized objects and moves on to harder ones. If the patient does not respond after 20 seconds, the tester gives a phonemic cue, the beginning sound of the word. Not identifying the picture even with a cue is a more serious type of error.

Patients with mild dementia have tip-of-the-tongue experiences; that is, they say that they know the word but are not able to recall it. They usually are helped by the phonemic cues. Inability to identify items and misnamings are common with dementia but are relatively rare in normal aging. Norms are reported by Van Gorp, Staz, Kiersh, and Henry (1986). Equivalent short forms can be extracted from the full test (Flicker, Ferris, Crook, Bartus, & Reisberg, 1986).

Another common pattern of language deficit in dementia is in word fluency. Word fluency can be assessed by having patients recall items from categories. The Controlled Oral Word Association Test (Benton & Hamsher, 1976) asks patients to recall words starting with the letters F, A, and S. Norms are also provided for two other sets of letters: CFL and PRW. One letter in each set has a high frequency in the language, one has a medium frequency, and one a low frequency. There is a time limit (60 or 90 seconds) and the items recalled within each 15-second segment are noted. Other fluency tests involve recalling items from semantic categories, such as naming animals, fruits, or items from a supermarket. Dementia patients who sometimes cannot perform when the stimulus is a letter can respond to categories of animals (Morris et al., 1989).

Alzheimer patients recall fewer items from both letter and semantic categories than normal controls (Ober, Dronkers, Koss, Delis, & Friedland, 1986). In addition, Alzheimer patients make more incorrect responses to the category and have more perseverations as severity of dementia increases. Tests using semantic categories may be more sensitive to problems of early dementia (Butters, Granholm, Salmon, Grant, & Wolfe, 1987). People who are depressed may be slowed in their responses but usually perform at adequate levels without intrusions. Fluency tests can be used as the distractors between trials of various memory tasks.

Visuospatial Abilities

Visuospatial ability can be assessed with figure copying, such as with the Benton Visual Retention Test (Benton, 1974). Norms up to age 89 have been reported (D'Elia, Boone, & Mitrushina, 1995; Spreen & Strauss, 1991).

Drawing tasks can also reveal deficits. Clients are asked to draw a familiar object such as a house, tree, bicycle, or person (see Lezak, 1995, for a review) or to draw a clock, setting the hands to specific times (Johansson, Zarit, & Berg, 1992; Tuokko, Hadjistavropoulos, Miller, & Beattie, 1992; Watson, Arfken, & Birge, 1993). Errors on the clock test are particularly significant because performance does not decline with normal aging (Albert, Wolfe, & Lafleche, 1990). When drawing a clock, some dementia patients cannot maintain the shape of the clock face, while others are unable to put the numbers in the shape or to set the time. A step-down procedure is to give patients predrawn clocks, asking them to set the hands to specific times.

The Bender–Gestalt test, although widely used with other age groups, does not adequately differentiate mild dementia from normal aging (Storandt, 1990). The WAIS block design test provides a good evaluation of visuospatial ability, but it is often too frustrating for patients, even early in the dementia process.

The Rey–Osterrieth Complex Figure Test (Osterrieth, 1944; Lezak, 1995) has the advantage of assessing drawing a figure with the copy present and from recall. Clients are presented a complex figure and asked to copy it. After a delay, they are asked to reproduce the figure from memory. Both immediate (after 3 minutes) and delayed (approximately 30 minutes) recall are tested. Obvious spatial deficits are apparent in the copying task, while the recall task identifies more subtle problems. Rapid decay of the visual icon is typically associated with dementia. Patients with primarily right or left hemispheric damage make characteristic errors. Left-sided lesions are more typically associated with slow organization of the complex details while performance improves with recall. In contrast, right-sided lesions are associated with difficulty in both copying and recall of the figure. Age norms have been reported for this test (D'Elia, Boone, & Mitrushina, 1995; Spreen & Strauss, 1991).

Conceptualization

Concept formation can be assessed in several ways. The similarities subtest of the WAIS-III provides a well-documented approach to concept formation. The comprehension subtest also assesses conceptual abilities in making social judgments. Block design assesses concept formation in a nonverbal task. Other tests of conceptualization include the Proverbs Test (Gorham, 1956) and the Trail Making Test (Reitan, 1958), which involves drawing paths between a sequence of letters and numbers. Age norms for the Proverbs Test are reported by Albert, Duffy, and Naeser (1987). Sorting tasks, such as the Wisconsin Card Sorting Test, are lengthy and do not adequately differentiate dementia from normal aging (Flicker, 1988). A short version of this test, such as that developed by Nelson (1976), may be more useful.

Two Composite Batteries: UCLA Screening Battery and Mayo Clinic Battery

As an alternative to selecting from individual tests, two test batteries are now available that have been developed specifically for use with older adults, the UCLA Screening Battery (Drebing, Van Gorp, Stuck, Mitrushina, & Beck, 1994) and the Mayo Clinic Battery (Smith et al., 1992; 1994). The main advantages of these batteries are their extensive norms and cutoff scores. The tests within each battery are shown in Table 6.2.

The UCLA Screening Battery takes under an hour to complete, even by a demented patient. The battery can be administered to someone who is moderately demented, yet it is sensitive enough to be given to someone in the earliest stages to help make the differential diagnosis. Cutoff scores are provided that indicate probable cognitive impairment. It can be readministered in 6 months or 1 year to determine if there has been change.

The scoring system with the UCLA battery, when used in conjunction with other information, leads to clear clinical decisions about diagnosis. Based on our experience with a large number of patients, however, the bias of this battery is toward overdiagnosing dementia. That may in part be due to reliance on timed tests. Digit symbol is a challenging, time-oriented test in which clients have 90 seconds to fill in numbers that match each symbol as shown in a key. Trail Making is also timed. This weighting toward speeded tests means that people who are depressed or slowed down for other reasons (e.g., Parkinson's disease) do more poorly on the test.

The Mayo Clinic Battery (Table 6.2) is much more extensive, incorporating the complete WAIS-R and WMS-R. This battery requires 4 to 6 hours of testing, in addition to the time for scoring and interpreting the findings. When a patient's status is questionable and the clinician is not sure what is going on, or when there is some other reason to pull out all the stops in doing an assessment, such as for a court case, the Mayo Clinic Battery is a good choice. A big advantage of this battery is that by spending a lot of time with the patient, the psychologist gets a lot of useful clinical information in addition to test scores.

Age norms are available up to age 97. Factor structure of the core battery and a short form have also been reported (Smith et al., 1992; Smith, Ivnik, Malec, Petersen, et al., 1994). Software for scoring is available through

TABLE 6.2. UCLA Screening Battery and Mayo Clinic Battery

UCLA Screening Battery[a]	Mayo Clinic Battery[b]
WAIS Digit Symbol Subscale	WAIS-R
Trail Making Test, Forms A and B	Wechsler Memory Scale—Revised
Auditory Verbal Learning Test	Auditory Verbal Learning Test
Rey–Osterrieth Complex Figure Test (copy and delayed recall)	
Mini-Mental State Examination	

[a]Drebing et al. (1994).
[b]Ivnik et al. (1994).

The Psychological Corporation.

Although both of these batteries are comprehensive, there is no direct assessment of language. For that reason, we supplement these batteries with language tests, usually the Controlled Oral Word Association Test and the Boston Naming Test. When there are additional questions about spatial functioning, we add the Rey–Osterrieth Complex Figure Test to the Mayo tests.

We want to emphasize again that this discussion of tests is not meant to be exhaustive. Many other tests and batteries have been reported for use with older clients and in the differentiation of dementia from other disorders (e.g., Kaszniak, 1996; Parks, Zec, & Wilson, 1993; Tuokko, Kristjansson, & Miller, 1995). The important issue in testing involves selecting a sensible battery that will address the particular question to be assessed. That can be accomplished in different ways. It is also critical to know the limitations of the tests that are used.

Qualitative Test Results

Interpretation of test findings depends both on objective scores and on qualitative information about how patients responded to tasks or the types of errors they made. Although there is less research that validates these more qualitative aspects of testing, experienced clinicians make use of the nuances and subtle differences in performance. Qualitative features can be of particular help in differentiating depression from dementia. Among the qualitative differences that have been noted: depressed patients often are reluctant to guess, while dementia patients make more frequent incorrect answers or intrusions during recall trials; depressed people generally have more variable performance, compared to dementia patients who score consistently low on tests except in the earliest stages of their illness; depressed patients can improve with prompts or other cues, while dementia patients show little or no improvement; depressed patients are often aware of or exaggerate their deficits, while dementia patients typically have less insight into their deficits (Kaszniak & DiTraglia Christenson, 1994).

Early Diagnosis of Alzheimer's Disease and Other Dementias

A major challenge for neuropsychological assessment is to differentiate early, mild dementia from normal aging with low rates of false negative and false positive results. This is a difficult task, because cognitive performance can vary for many different reasons besides mild dementia. Norms and cutoff scores represent population averages. An individual who is depressed, has another psychiatric illness, or has a poor educational background may perform below those levels and not have an early dementia. Estimation of likely premorbid performance can reduce but not eliminate these problems.

Another problem in early diagnosis is that there may be heterogeneity in the earliest symptoms of dementia. That is certainly the case with Alzheimer's disease and vascular dementia. Early symptoms in vascular dementia depend on the location of infarcts or other damage, so they can be quite varied. With Alzheimer's, there is some evidence that early symptoms primarily affect visuospatial functioning in some patients and language and verbal memory in others (Becker, Huff, Nebes, Holland, & Boller, 1988).

One of the most thorough investigations of early diagnosis has been conducted by Storandt and her colleagues (Storandt, Botwinick, Danziger, Berg, & Hughes, 1984; Storandt & Hill, 1989). In the first study, four tests were identified as differentiating mild dementia patients from age- and sex-matched controls. These tests were the logical memory and mental control subtests of the WMS, Form A of the Trail Making Test, and word fluency for the letters S and P. A subsequent evaluation used the same battery of tests to differentiate very mild cases of dementia from normal aging. The questionable group overlapped considerably in test performance with both normal people and mild dementia patients.

These findings suggest that very early detection remains problematic. In cases that cannot be classified clearly as dementia or normal, the best approach remains to treat any treatable problem and adopt a wait-and-see attitude. Retesting after an appropriate interval (usually a year) clarifies the initial findings. Decline in performance confirms the presence of dementia, while stable or improved performance indicates some other cause of the person's cognitive difficulties.

ROLE OF THE MEDICAL EXAMINATION IN ASSESSMENT

A medical examination is a critical part of an overall assessment. It has two primary goals. First, it should be used to rule out treatable components of the presenting problems. Particularly when dementia is suspected, it is important to rule out the many potentially treatable causes of cognitive symptoms. Disorders such as depression and anxiety can also be caused by various illnesses and/or medications. Second, when dementia is diagnosed, a medical evaluation can contribute to identifying the specific type of disorder.

An evaluation should include assessment of all main systems and current medications. A recommended evaluation is shown in Table 6.3. Laboratory tests can uncover infections and endocrine, metabolic, and electrolyte disturbances. Nutritional deficits also need to be considered, since they can contribute to cognitive problems and delirium. Older people living alone are prone to not eating properly. Another element that should be evaluated

TABLE 6.3. Recommended Medical Tests in the Assessment of Possible Dementia

1. Complete blood count
2. Chem 21 panel, including electrolytes, kidney function, calcium, albumin, liver function and glucose
3. Thyroid function tests
4. Vitamin B12 and folate levels
5. Tests for syphilis and, depending on history, human immunodeficiency antibodies
6. Urinalysis
7. Electrocardiogram
8. Chest X-ray

Note. From National Institutes of Health (1987).

is pain. Patients sometimes do not report pain, so the possibility of an undetected fracture, fecal impaction, or similar disorder should be explored.

It is especially important to review medications for possible adverse effects. Medications are a common cause of reversible cognitive impairment and delirium. They can also lead to symptoms of depression and anxiety and other mood changes. Both prescription and over-the-counter medications should be considered by the physician. Commonly used over-the-counter drugs, such as antacids, can have cognitive effects, especially when used in combination with other medications. Alcohol use, which can potentiate the effects of many medications, should also be evaluated. Caffeine can play a role in anxiety and sleep problems. Even vitamins and other dietary supplements can become toxic under certain conditions or can interact adversely with a prescription medication.

A brain scan is recommended as part of an initial assessment when dementia is suspected. Scans generally can be used in ruling out other possible causes of symptoms, such as a brain tumor, but they do not provide definitive information for a diagnosis. Diagnosis of a dementing illness should never be based on results of a scan alone, in the absence of evidence of cognitive decline.

The type of scan done, CT, MRI, or other, often depends on local availability. Enlargement of the ventricles on CT scans is usually consistent with Alzheimer's disease. Longitudinal analysis indicates that increases in ventricle size and neuropsychological decline are highly associated (Luxenberg, Haxby, Creasey, Sundaram, & Rapoport, 1987). Some enlargement, however, is found among otherwise apparently healthy older people. Enlargement alone without other evidence of dementia should not be used to make a diagnosis. Both CTs and MRIs can identify multiple large-vessel strokes associated with multi-infarct dementia (Román et al., 1993). MRIs can also identify white matter lesions. As discussed in Chapter 3, white matter hyperintensities have an uncertain relation to dementia and to cognitive performance. Unless there is clinical evidence of dementia, white matter hyperintensities alone are not sufficient to make a diagnosis or a prediction that the person will become demented in the future.

The following case illustrates the importance of a careful medical examination in differentiating delirium from other conditions. It also demonstrates how a change in medications can have catastrophic effects. The client in this example is a 76-year-old woman who lived alone. She suffered from diabetes, high blood pressure, and emphysema but was otherwise was in good health. Her physician had gone on vacation, and she went in to see one of the physician's partners for a minor complaint. Unrelated to her complaint, the partner decided to change the woman's antihypertensive medication. The patient had not been having any trouble with the antihypertensive she had been taking, but the physician thought the new drug would work better.

A few days later the woman was found in her apartment by her niece. She was aphasic and had a right-sided weakness. She was taken to the emergency room, where she was treated as if she had had a stroke. Findings from an MRI, however, indicated no evidence of a recent stroke. She was very difficult to manage in the emergency room and struggled with staff. She was disoriented, delusional, and also incontinent.

The neurologist who was called in on the case continued exploring other hypotheses besides a stroke. Her blood work indicated severe sodium depletion (hyponatremia), which had apparently been caused by the new antihypertensive medication. She had been monitoring salt in her diet very carefully, and the result of the new medication was to reduce salt levels too low. The emergency room treated her for the sodium depletion by giving her salt water and changing her medication. Within two days the delirium had cleared. She has no remaining cognitive deficits, except for having no memory of the events in the emergency room.

In this case, the onset and pattern of symptoms were consistent with a stroke. Changes in mental status and behavior suggested a delirium, but that could have been the aftermath of a stroke. When neuroradiological findings did not provide confirmation of a stroke, however, the neurologist looked for other causes and found the change in antihypertensive medication. As in many cases of delirium, the woman recovered fully.

DIFFERENTIATING ALZHEIMER'S DISEASE
FROM OTHER DEMENTIAS

At the completion of a comprehensive assessment, there should be sufficient information to identify the likely type of dementia. Guidelines have been developed for diagnosis of Alzheimer's disease (McKhann et al., 1984) and vascular dementia (Román et al., 1993). These criteria, which are shown in Appendices 6.2 and 6.3, complement DSM-IV. The main distinction between these disorders is that there are positive diagnostic indicators for vascular dementia, such as focal neurological signs, evidence of infarcts on CT or MRI scans, and evidence of an abrupt onset and stepwise course. Alzheimer's disease, by contrast, is diagnosed by exclusion, that is, when there is no evidence for other causes of the symptoms.

Frontal dementias can be differentiated from other dementias based on the more frequent occurrence of characteristic symptoms, such as disinhibition, poor judgment, apathy, and indifference. There can, however, be some overlap in these symptoms with other dementias. Two brief screening instruments, the Executive Interview (Royall, Mahurin, & Gray, 1992), and the Qualitative Evaluation of Dementia (Royall, Mahurin, Cornell, & Gray, 1993) can be used for identifying frontal dementias.

Neuropsychological tests aid in differentiating among the dementing illnesses. In Alzheimer's disease, memory and language deficits are prominent. By comparison, there are some retrieval difficulties in subcortical disorders and little or no aphasia (Butters, Salmon, & Butters, 1994). Differences in test performance between Alzheimer's disease and vascular dementias are less clear-cut, because site of the damage in vascular dementia can vary so widely from case to case. It has been suggested that vascular dementia is characterized by greater variability in test scores than Alzheimer's, rather than any specific pattern of deficit (Erker, Searight, & Peterson, 1995).

Often the history of the appearance of deficits is more revealing than the pattern of tests. The differentiation between frontal dementia and Alzheimer's usually can be made based on initial presentation of symptoms. Initial symptoms of frontal dementias involve changes in attention, personality, and possibly language (in Pick's disease), with memory impairment developing later. As symptoms progress, it may no longer be possible to differentiate frontal from Alzheimer's cases based on test performance. Similarly, history can differentiate Alzheimer's and vascular dementia, especially when patients show the classic patterns typical of these disorders— gradual onset and progression in Alzheimer's and sudden onset and stepwise progression with many cases of vascular dementia.

In the end, however, it may not be possible to be certain about diagnosis, because many symptoms overlap and a significant number of people have mixed pathologies, for example, brain pathology typical of both Alzheimer's and vascular dementia. Improved diagnosis will come when there are definitive markers for the various dementing illnesses and will be important when there are effective treatments to control or reverse the degenerative process.

CASE EXAMPLES

The following cases illustrate the use of a test battery as part of an overall evaluation and the decision making process in clinical assessment.

Case 1. Determining the Etiology of Mild, Atypical Cognitive Symptoms

The patient, Ellen, was an accomplished 67-year-old woman. She was college educated, had a successful career, and had raised four adopted children. She was in many ways an ideal client. She had a pleasant personality, always showed up for appointments on time, and was always perfectly groomed.

Ellen was referred because of findings of white matter hyperintensities on an MRI. She hadn't been feeling quite herself, and she went to her doctor complaining of fatigue and memory problems. He referred her to a neurologist who did an evaluation including the MRI. He then asked for psychological testing to determine if this was a case of vascular dementia.

In the clinical assessment, Ellen was able to tell us about all the specific types of memory problems she was having. Diagnostically, that type of memory complaint with specific recall of incidents points to depression, not dementia. She had a score of 29 out of 30 on the MMSE. Her one error was that she was able to recall only two of the three words after interference. One error, particularly on recall, does not indicate any problem.

Another important piece of information was that Ellen's mother had Alzheimer's disease before she died. As a result, Ellen was worried about developing Alzheimer's disease. When she forgot something, she worried that it might be a sign of Alzheimer's. Her worries increased when the neurologist told her about the MRI findings.

A complete test battery was administered including the WAIS, WMS, and language tests. The WAIS indicated that she had high to very high overall intelligence. Scores on the WMS revealed an interesting pattern. Her general memory was above average, but verbal memory was not as good as visual memory. This pattern is unusual, especially in someone with high education and good verbal skills. Typically, verbal memory is higher than visual memory. The lowest scores were in attention and delayed recall. That is a pattern often seen in dementia. Because dementia is a disorder of short-term memory, tests of delayed recall are particularly sensitive to its effects. The language tests were normal.

At this point the test findings confirmed that Ellen was a very bright woman who was generally performing at a level we would expect for someone with her background and history, but there were a few areas of weakness. Tests of attention and delayed recall showed some questionable performance but were not clearly out of line with her overall functioning. We had, then, evidence of high performance on most tests, a few areas of difficulty, and findings of white matter hyperintensities on the MRI. What should be done next?

We told her that her test performance did not currently indicate Alzheimer's disease or similar problems and that her memory problems could be explained by depression. We discussed with her that depression might be affecting attention so that she was not taking information in efficiently, leading to test scores in that area that were lower than expected. We also clarified with her that white matter hyperintensities have an undetermined significance and prognosis; that is, we do not always know what they mean for functioning, but they did not indicate Alzheimer's disease. We proposed testing her at a later time.

Retesting was done a year later. Ellen's WAIS scores were the same as before. The WMS was also almost identical, but delayed recall was improved. Clinical examination indicated that her mood was also improved. These findings suggest that whatever the white matter hyperintensities might have meant, they were related neither to obvious cognitive problems nor to progressive impairment. Ellen's stability in performance was good evidence for ruling out Alzheimer's disease.

This case had a very positive outcome. In some instances, very mild findings of impairment in attention and delayed recall can very well be the first manifestation of a dementing illness. But very mild deficits can have multiple causes. Because it is often not possible to separate out the effects of depression as well as other sources of individual differences in test performance, we find it better to wait until there is evidence on the course of symptoms before making a diagnosis. Repeated testing is not necessary when symptoms of dementia are obvious during the first assessment, but it is an essential step in cases with unclear or ambiguous findings.

Another feature of this case is the family history. A history of Alzheimer's disease in a parent or other close relatives increases the risk of developing the disease. Relatives can also become fearful of developing Alzheimer's and become more vigilant of even minor problems in their memory, as happened in this case. Testing can be a powerful tool for providing reassurance and clarifying the significance of minor problems.

Case 2. Alzheimer's Disease Exacerbated by Alcohol

History provides valuable information for the clarification of diagnosis. In this case, a 66-year-old retired business executive, Robert, was referred for a neuropsychological assessment by a neurologist. The referring physician said he found signs of dementia in his neurological examination, but that the MRI was normal.

Robert gave a loose and unreliable history, so much of the information came from his wife. Robert had been very successful in business, rising to an executive level in a midsize company. He retired 14 years earlier because of hypertension but subsequently took some part-time jobs teaching business classes. He was not asked to return to his last job. Since 1981, he had two surgeries on his spine and became addicted to painkillers. Throughout his life he had been a heavy social drinker, though his wife reported some decrease in alcohol consumption in the past 4 months. His use of pain medication also decreased. His only other current medication was for hypertension. He had no friends or activities, apart from swimming 5 days a week. He spent his days at home alone.

There was a family history of Alzheimer's disease. His mother died 10 years earlier after a long course of Alzheimer's disease, and a sister with Down's syndrome was showing Alzheimer's symptoms. Robert was very fearful of having Alzheimer's.

Current symptoms included significant word-finding and short-term memory problems. His wife reported that he had problems remembering and following recipes (he did the cooking), but that he was able to cook and shop competently. She was concerned about his driving, however, particularly his ability to judge the speed of oncoming traffic. For the past 4 months, she stopped serving wine with dinner, telling him that it was giving her headaches. This step cut down his alcohol consumption considerably.

Robert was cooperative during the testing, though at times he did not seem to put his whole effort into it. His responses were often impulsive. He frequently had to be redirected to tasks or to have the instructions repeated. He was frequently frustrated with his performance.

Testing revealed significant problems with memory. Robert scored in the mildly impaired range on the MMSE, mainly because of difficulty recalling the three words and repeating the phrase "No ifs, ands, or buts." On the WMS, he scored about two standard deviations below normal on most tests of visual and verbal memory, as well as on attention and concentration. Delayed recall was somewhat better. On the WAIS, his scores were in the average range, with little difference between verbal and performance scores. There was, however, considerable interscale variability, particularly on the verbal scales. Comprehension was relatively high (scale score = 14), possibly indicating high premorbid reasoning ability. But other scores indicated considerable decline, given his prior occupational functioning. Digit span and arithmetic, which are measures of attention and concentration as well as higher executive function, were among the lowest scores (scale scores of 5). His score on the Boston Naming Test was within normal limits, but he had 11 literal paraphasias, for example, saying "wrath" for "wreath" and "date" for "dart." Word fluency as measured by the Controlled Oral Word Association Test was in the high normal range. Scores on Trail Making A and B and on the Rey-Osterrieth Complex Figure Test were low. Recall on the Rey Auditory Verbal Learning Test also was consistent with considerable memory impairment.

Although the overall pattern of impairment was consistent with dementia, the history and some features of the test results suggested the possibility that the problems were related to chronic alcoholism, perhaps in combination with painkilling medications. In particular, the scatter of scores on WAIS subscales, with sparing of some abilities and somewhat better performance on delayed compared to immediate recall on the WMS, suggested the possible effects of chronic alcoholism. It is, of course, possible that both processes were at work, that is, that symptoms were due to a combination of dementia and alcohol use.

To differentiate between these possibilities, we recommended eliminating all alcohol and painkillers to determine if there would be a stabilization or improvement in functioning. To reduce his anxiety over Alzheimer's disease, Robert was told that his memory problems were due to high blood pressure and his use of alcohol and painkillers. Although there was a family history of Alzheimer's, we were reluctant to make that diagnosis until the alternatives were ruled out.

Unfortunately, the decrease in drinking did not slow the progression of symptoms. As it became apparent that Robert had a progressive dementia, his wife decided she did not want to try to control his alcohol intake. Rather, she felt it would be better that their last years together were not filled with conflict.

One year later, a comprehensive medical and neuropsychological examination was done, and it revealed evidence of continued decline and confirmed a diagnosis of probable Alzheimer's disease, though with alcoholism as a secondary cause. A factor pointing toward Alzheimer's was Robert's MRI, which in contrast to previous tests now showed evidence of brain atrophy. While an initial finding of atrophy is nonspecific in the absence of pronounced cognitive deficits, longitudinal evidence of changes point toward Alzheimer's disease.

In retrospect, Robert's alcoholism probably hastened his decline, but his wife made a decision that preserved his autonomy and, in a way, their relationship. Pressing the issue about his drinking could have had some positive benefits, but his wife's decision to let him live out his life as he preferred had to be respected.

Case 3. Early-Onset Dementia Complicated by Medications

Following is a case of early-onset dementia, with symptoms exacerbated by medications. The client, Donna, was accompanied to the appointment by her husband, Fred, who provided much of the detail about background and history, as Donna had difficulty giving accurate information. Donna was a 50-year-old schoolteacher with a master's degree in education. She had a successful career in elementary education that spanned the past 28 years. She had had a number of health problems, including severe hypertension and headaches. For over 2 years, she had been having increasing difficulties with memory and functioning in the classroom. When the problems started two years earlier, she had been referred by her primary care physician to a neurologist for an evaluation of her memory problems and headaches. An MRI revealed tiny zones of increased signal intensity in the midbrain and left periventricular white matter changes, suggesting the possibility of vascular disease, but the MRI was otherwise considered normal. The results of a brief cognitive screening were also in the normal range (her MMSE score was 28). Over the next 2 years, her problems in functioning increased, but both her primary care physician and the neurologist still felt there was nothing wrong. Finally, her husband became exasperated by the discrepancy between the doctors' lack of concern and his observation of continuing decline, and he asked for a referral for a neuropsychological evaluation.

Donna was very anxious during an initial testing session but was more comfortable during a second visit. She wanted to perform well and put forth a lot of effort. Her MMSE score was 28, as it had been two years earlier. Other tests, however, showed significant impairments. On the WMS-R, her general memory score of 72 was three standard deviations below normal. Verbal memory was much lower than visual memory. Her performance on two learning tests, the Rey Auditory Verbal Learning Test (RAVLT) and the California Verbal Learning Tests (CVLT), showed much lower rates of learning and retention (delayed recall) than would be expected. On the RAVLT, for example, she recalled 1, 3, 5, 7, and 9 words (out of 15) over the five trials, and then only 3 on delayed recall. The Boston Naming Test was within normal limits (54 out of 60 spontaneously named), but Donna made semantic errors, literal paraphasias, and circumlocutions. These types of errors indicated a problem with language, though she was able to compensate for the most part at this time. The UCLA Screening Battery was consistent with a moderate degree of impairment.

An immediate problem was whether Donna should continue teaching. She had been functioning in the classroom only with the help of two assistants. We encouraged her to take a leave of absence and to reevaluate the situation in the summer. Reports were sent to the neurologist and primary care physician. Although they acknowledged the findings, both of them continued to show unconcern about her memory problems, at least according to her husband.

In cases such as this one, where there is some controversy over the diagnosis and where the implications are significant (in this case, whether Donna could return to work), we like to refer the client for another opinion. Six months after our initial evaluation (a minimum period for seeing changes in functioning in cases of dementia), we referred Donna and her husband to a memory disorders clinic at a medical center in another town. She was seen there by a neuropsychologist and a geriatrician.

The neuropsychologist repeated most of the same tests. Donna now scored only 23 on the MMSE, a drop of 5 points in 6 months. As in the previous testing, she had a great deal of difficulty learning and retaining new information. This problem was more pronounced on verbal tests but was also found on nonverbal tasks. Other tests were stable or showed a mild decline from the previous testing. Given her functioning, the finding was similar to ours, that she was no longer capable of continuing in her old job.

A diagnosis was given of vascular dementia or possibly mixed vascular and Alzheimer's disease. The medical findings, a history of hypertension and the MRI abnormalities, pointed toward a vascular dementia. Alzheimer's disease, however, could not be ruled out from the test performance. In fact, all three clinicians involved, the two psychologists and the geriatrician, felt that Donna seemed in behavior, appearance, and test performance more like an Alzheimer's patient, a clinical sense based on having evaluated many dementia patients.

The geriatrician who saw Donna recommended several changes in medications. She suggested changing the two antihypertensives Donna was taking because they have more cognitive side effects than other available drugs, discontinuing two common over-the-counter antacids that can affect cognition, and discontinuing a pain medication (Ultram) that also has cognitive side effects. After making these changes, her husband reported an immediate improvement in her functioning. Donna's memory was a bit better, and she asked fewer repetitive questions. She generally seemed more alert. Although it was clear that she still had dementia, the medications had obviously been contributing to her problems.

This case shows how dementia can affect someone relatively early in life. Early-onset cases are often difficult for everyone involved, because the illness seems premature. Whereas someone who is over 65 has a number of safety nets, such as Medicare and Social Security, a person under 65 must deal with early retirement and disability. The financial consequences can be catastrophic if the person does not have sufficient resources. Patients often encounter obstacles trying to qualify for disability and Medicare. It takes a lot of determination and usually an appeal to get on disability, so unless the patient has a family member who is an effective advocate, the patient's resources can easily be depleted.

The other noteworthy feature of this case is that the patient's cognitive functioning and behavior improved following changes in medication. This improvement illustrates that there can be treatable components in cases of dementia, a fact that is often overlooked because of the pessimism associated with the diagnosis.

OTHER ISSUES IN ASSESSMENT

Our discussion of assessment emphasizes the differentiation of dementia from other problems. Assessment does not end at that point. After determining diagnosis, clinicians need to identify the most pressing problems that need to be addressed in treatment, as well as gathering information such as the following that will help in planning treatment.

1. *Resources:* What psychological or social resources or strengths does the patient have that can be brought to bear in treatment? A depressed client, for example, may have had good planning skills in his or her job. These skills could be used in developing and implementing a treatment plan.

2. *Deficits:* Besides the main presenting problem, what other deficits are present? A person who is disorganized and a poor planner, for example, may have trouble with some features of highly structured therapy approaches.

3. *Social network:* Who are the people to whom the client can turn for support and help, and are there problematic relationships?

4. *Substance abuse:* Along with evaluation of prescription medications, it is important to find out if an older client may be abusing alcohol or other medications.

5. *Suicidal and homicidal thoughts:* Clinicians need to determine if an older client is thinking about suicide. In couples where one person is disabled, the possibility of a double suicide or a homicide–suicide should also be evaluated.

6. *Sleep and appetite disturbance:* How well is the person eating or sleeping? Appetite and sleep problems are both indicators of the severity of psychiatric disorders and can contribute to making problems worse. We often find that part of the treatment involves restoring good sleep habits or addressing eating problems. In contrast to younger clients, overeating is a more frequent issue than not eating enough. Another issue is that medications can be affected by when and what the person eats.

7. *Prior treatment history:* What prior treatment experience did the client have? Treatments that helped with similar problems in the past should be noted because they are likely to be effective again. Clients with no prior history of psychological treatment may require more explanations about how treatment works and how they can benefit from it.

We expand on these issues and discuss treatment planning in detail in subsequent chapters.

COMPETENCE

Clinicians who practice with older people are increasingly called on to make complex judgments about competence. Questions about competence address three main areas: Can an older person (1) live alone, (2) manage his or her finances, or (3) refuse medical treatments. These situations are complex and can literally have life-and-death implications. To evaluate competence, clinicians must be able to conduct sophisticated and objective assessments that carefully weigh the evidence from several sources. It is also necessary to understand state law and legal practices that pertain to competence proceedings. Competence evaluations pose many intellectually challenging puzzles for clinicians. The well-trained geriatric specialist can provide an informed opinion to resolve in an optimal way an often tangled or difficult situation.

Psychological testing forms a central part of a competence evaluation because it provides an objective assessment of a person's ability to process information and to make decisions. Interviews with the person and other involved individuals and direct observations of behavior are also important parts of the evaluation.

Defining Competence

Competence and incompetence are legal terms and their determination is the outcome of a defined legal process. Competence, of course, is used in everyday speech, and the various professions (e.g., medicine, psychology) have their own definitions. But the decision of whether someone is or is not competent depends on legal statutes and procedures. Because the laws governing competence in the United States are a state issue, the definitions and procedures for determining competence vary somewhat from one state to another. There are, in effect, 50 definitions, so clinicians must familiarize themselves with the laws in their own state.

Though the definition of competence differs from state to state, there are some common features. Legal statutes address in varying degrees three key issues. First, competence is now generally regarded as applying to specific domains of functioning. In the past, incompetence was a global term and a competence evaluation involved an all-or-none decision. Now, a person can be judged not competent to make decisions in one area but competent to carry out other activities. The finding that someone is incapable of managing money, for example, does not presume an inability to take care of personal needs or make decisions about where to live. Sabatino (1996) notes the increasing use of the term "incapacity" rather than incompetence, which connotes a more specific disability.

Second, current legal definitions usually include both medical and functional components. At one time, courts used sweeping, global terms for determining incompetence, such as finding a person to be "insane" or "senile." In some state statutes, "old age" was a sufficient condition for determination of incompetence (Willis, 1996). In the 1960s, a gradual reform of state laws incorporated medical diagnosis into definitions of competence. Using medical criteria, a determination of incompetence could be made based on the presence of a specific illness or disabling condition, such as dementia or mental retardation. In the ensuing years, most states added a functional component to this definition; that is, the person must have an illness or disabling condition that has led to being unable to carry out activities or make decisions in a competent manner. Under this type of law, someone diagnosed with Alzheimer's disease would not be considered incapacitated without evidence of functional deficits in decision making and behavior. A few states, such as California, no longer include a medical component in their definition (see Sabatino, 1996, for a review of the development of state statutes).

Definitions of functional competence vary from state to state, particularly in the degree to which cognition and behavior are emphasized. Cognitive competence involves the capacity to make reasoned decisions, for example, to be able to evaluate information and make plans. Behavioral definitions concern the ability to carry out plans and activities in an adequate or competent manner. Some states (such as California, again) place emphasis on behavior and others stress cognition (Sabatino, 1996). Despite these differences, we recommend that clinicians should attend to both cognition and behavior: Does the person have the cognitive ability to make decisions and understand the implications of those decisions, and is the person able to carry out intended actions in an effective way (see also Kapp, 1996)?

A third component of legal statutes is that a person is considered competent until court procedures determine otherwise. Determination of incompetence involves due process, that is, a court proceeding in which the "defendant" has the right to representation and to contest the proceeding. Some states now require the person to be present during the proceedings. Historically, absence of due process in competence evaluations led to occasional misuse. A person with a history of mental illness or who was old could be ruled incompetent without any presentation of evidence or without being able to challenge the proceeding. Family members or other individuals sometimes tried to get control of an older person's assets this way. Legal safeguards are now in place in most states that assure that determination of incapacity can occur only when there is appropriate evidence and due process.

When someone is found to be incapacitated, the court assigns a guardian who is given specific responsibilities, for example, managing the person's finances and/or care. The legal procedure to obtain guardianship is often expensive and can be avoided in many situations. One alternative is for families to obtain power of attorney. Power of attorney can be given for the purpose of managing financial affairs and/or for making health care decisions. This procedure gives the designated individual the ability to make decisions if the older person becomes incapacitated. Power of attorney provides a smooth transition as long as there is no conflict in the family that leads to questioning the decisions of the person or persons holding power of attorney.

A drawback is that the person giving power of attorney must be legally competent to do so. Increasingly, older people are aware of the usefulness of power of attorney and arrange for it when they make a will, in advance of any disability. But it is still common to encounter people who have become incapacitated without arranging for formal power of attorney. State laws allow families to make decisions about health care if the elder cannot do so. But the family cannot legally make other important decisions, such as where the older person should live or how the person's financial assets should be used.

When caught unprepared, some families obtain power of attorney even though the person is no longer able to give consent. The proper approach at this point is to seek guardianship, but as we noted, that is often expensive and can be perceived by families to be humiliating to the older person, especially if a court appearance is required. Power of attorney obtained under questionable circumstances is usually not challenged unless there is conflict in the family or some indication of abuse. Lawyers are often willing to help the family with power of attorney in these circumstances, especially if they know the family. Sometimes dementia patients have better-functioning days when they can understand the implications of giving power of attorney to a family member, so legally can do so.

Compared to guardianship, power of attorney does not include safeguards against abuse. A guardian for a person's financial affairs must submit records to the court on a regular schedule. In contrast, decisions made by someone with power of attorney are not reviewed. Fortunately, most families act in the patient's best interest and do not abuse their power of attorney.

Questions of competence of terminally ill patients to refuse treatment can be complex. Sometimes a family member or the physician doubts the patient's competence to refuse treatment. More typically, the issue is how to assure that the patient's preferences are honored. Two prior legal steps are helpful. First, there should be an advance medical directive telling the family or other involved caretakers what the patient's preferences are. Second, the family should have power of attorney for health care. We discuss these situations in more detail in Chapter 14.

As with competence issues, power of attorney and advance directive statutes vary from state to state, so clinicians should be familiar with the laws in their home state. For decisions about their legal options, older people and their families should consult attorneys who have familiarity with this part of the law.

Competence Evaluation

State laws vary in their definitions of competence, and experts in the field disagree on what constitutes competence. As a result, there is no standard prescription for which tests and other procedures should be included as part of a competence assessment (e.g., Grisso, 1994; Kapp, 1996; Willis, 1996). Most experts agree, however, that competence evaluations should include three components: (1) psychological or neuropsychological tests, (2) functional assessment, and (3) interviews with the person and with family or other individuals who can provide relevant information. Kapp (1996), for example, recommends that an evaluation include the following areas: (1) orientation; (2) recent and remote memory; (3) intellectual capacity, including ability to understand abstract ideas and reasoning; (4) affect, including suicidal ideation; (5) the occurrence of delusions, hallucinations, or illusions; (6) overt behavior; and (7) a history of prior episodes of psychiatric problems that affected competence.

A specific competence evaluation should be constructed around the type of question being asked, for example, ability to make financial decisions, ability to make medical decisions, or ability to make life decisions (i.e., to live at home or go to an institution). Rather than having one approach to assessment of competence, clinicians need to tailor their assessment to evaluate abilities and decision-making processes that are related to the reason for the evaluation.

Psychological Tests

Psychological testing provides evidence on the capacity to make competent decisions and judgments. Testing has the advantage of providing objective information obtained in a structured and systematic way, with results that can be compared against population norms.

In conducting an evaluation of competence, we select tests from the batteries discussed earlier in this and the preceding chapter. We usually begin with the Mini-Mental State Examination (MMSE) (Folstein, Folstein, & McHugh, 1975). The MMSE provides a gross estimate of the degree of impairment. If testing reveals severe dementia, it does not usually make sense to put the person through a whole battery of tests. In that case, we do fewer tests, so as not to frustrate the patient or the tester.

In considering other tests, we try to select a battery that assesses the abilities that are most directly related to competence. We want to know if a person can attend to, process, and retain information in an adequate way. For that reason, we include a test of attention (usually the digit span subtest from the WAIS) and tests of verbal memory and language. We are also interested in judgment and reasoning and use the comprehension and similarities subtests of the WAIS. If there is a question about ability to manage finances, we use the arithmetic subscale of the WAIS, which assesses ability to do simple computations involving spending money and making change.

These tests constitute a minimum battery, provided the person is not severely demented. The amount of additional testing depends to some extent on the person and the question that is being asked. We do not believe it necessary or desirable to have everyone complete a long and comprehensive test battery. Many tests do not bear directly on the question of competence. How, for example, would the block design or picture completion subtests of the WAIS relate to a decision about competence? These tests would provide information on general capacity but would not necessarily help us with an evaluation of a specific domain of competent functioning. A comprehensive battery of tests (e.g., a complete WAIS and WMS) is useful, however, when the competence issues are complex, when results from a short battery of tests reveal ambiguous findings, or when the case is highly contested.

In addition to focusing on test scores, clinicians need to examine the quality of reasoning and judgment the person reveals in responding to test items (Kapp, 1996). Often we ask the person to explain answers or to discuss the reasoning used in giving a response.

As with testing for differential diagnosis, the clinician needs to keep in mind that factors such as fatigue and sensory impairment can interfere with test performance. Testing should be conducted under optimal conditions, but the clinician should also note the role that fatigue or sensory loss might play in performance of everyday activities.

Evaluation of Functioning

Questions of competence focus on the ability to understand and make judgments about information and carry out decisions or plans in the performance of everyday activities. Psychological tests examine decision-making capacity, while functional assessments address people's ability to carry out their intentions in everyday situations. In this section, we discuss some of the assessment instruments available in evaluation of functioning. Much of the pertinent information about performance of everyday activities, however, comes from interviews with the person and informants.

TABLE 6.4. Activities of Daily Living

Activities of Daily Living (ADL)	Instrumental Activities of Daily Living (IADL)
Feeding oneself	Taking medications
Bathing	Doing housework
Using the toilet	Preparing meals
Dressing	Shopping
Grooming (shaving for men, applying make-up for women, hair care)	Managing money
	Using the telephone
Transferring from bed to chair or from chair to standing	Using transportation
Walking for short distances or up and down stairs	

The typical assessment of functioning involves activities of daily living (ADL). There are two levels of ADL, basic or personal activities such as dressing, bathing, and using the toilet and instrumental activities, including using public transportation, using the telephone, or managing finances (see, e.g., Fillenbaum, 1987a, 1987b; Katz, Ford, Moskowitz, Jackson, & Jaffee, 1963; Lawton & Brody, 1969). A list of ADL activities is shown in Table 6.4. The sources of information about performance of these activities are usually the person being evaluated and/or a relative or other informant. People with dementia and forms of head injury are likely to deny problems in carrying out everyday activities. Informants, on the other hand, may not have accurate information, may not be good observers, or may have their own agenda that leads them to give misleading reports. For that reason, the information provided by these instruments may be of limited value in a competency evaluation.

Several performance-based measures have been developed to overcome difficulties in self-reports of functional abilities. Among the measures are the Community Competence Scale (Loeb, 1983), the Direct Assessment of Functional Status Scale (Lowenstein et al., 1989), the Structured Assessment of Independent Living Skills (Mahurin, DeBettignies, & Pirozzolo, 1991) and the Everyday Problems Test (Marsiske & Willis, 1995; Willis & Marsiske, 1993). These tests use specific tasks to assess functional abilities, for example, telling time or being able to understand the information on a prescription drug label. Table 6.5 gives examples of sample tasks. These performance tests provide a more direct assessment of competence, but they may not necessarily bear on the specific question being asked. For example, a person might not be capable of making decisions about different Medigap plans but may still be able to handle daily expenses. There is no agreement as yet on what critical tasks might assess domains such as financial management or being able to live independently (see Willis, 1996, for a review of these issues).

Furthermore, as with traditional psychological tests, people with low

TABLE 6.5. Examples of Tasks That Assess Instrumental Activities of Daily Living

Domain	Exemplar task
Managing medications	Determining how many doses of cough medicine can be taken in a 24-hour period
	Completing a patient medical history form
Shopping for necessities	Ordering merchandise from a catalog
	Comparison of brands of a product
Managing finances	Comparison of Medigap insurance plans
	Completing income tax return form
Using transportation	Computing taxi rates
	Interpreting driver's right-of-way laws
Maintaining household	Following instructions for operating a household appliance
Meal preparation and nutrition	Evaluating nutritional information on food label

Note. From Willis (1996). Copyright 1996 by Springer Publishing Company, Inc. Reprinted by permission.

education may appear incompetent on these measures. Willis (1996) notes that many older people with low education are marginally competent in everyday life even without Alzheimer's disease or other disorders that impair cognition and functioning. When they have dementia, their performance may look very poor, even though it has not changed much compared to premorbid levels. As a consequence, it is important to take into account how someone functioned in the past and how much of a change the current situation represents.

Performance measures, then, represent an advance in our ability to assess competency, but they also have limitations. Both ordinary and performance-based functional measures can be a useful part of an overall competence evaluation, but as with psychological testing, they must be complemented with as much specific information as possible about the person's judgment and performance in a specific domain, whether it is management of finances, ability to care for one's self, or ability to make health care decisions.

Interviews with the Patient, Family, and Friends

Assessment of competence should include a focused interview with the person being evaluated and when appropriate and possible, interviews with other people who can provide information about the person's daily functioning. Questions should be specific and should reveal both decision-making capacity and the ability to carry out plans effectively. When financial management is the focus, the older person should be asked about where his or her money is and about managing it. If the competence evaluation concerns whether the person can remain at home, questions can probe judgment in making adequate decisions in key situations and the ability to provide for self-care and safety.

Kapp (1996) suggests examination of five specific and two general factors that reflect competency. The specific factors follow.

1. Can the individual make or express choices about life situations?
2. Can the person offer reasons for these choices?
3. Is the reasoning process that underlies these choices rational, that is, based on facts rather than delusions?
4. Can the person understand the implications of these choices?
5. Are the choices consistent with the person's values and preferences or do they represent a departure that might be due to illness or excessive influence by another person?

Two general factors to consider reflect the capacity for making decisions:

1. Can the person take in factual information?
2. Can the person understand his own situation as it relates to the facts?

Interviews with family members, neighbors or other pertinent people can provide observations of the person's behavior in key situations. Of course, clinicians need to take into account the possibility of bias in these reports.

A home visit can be a very important part of a competence evaluation when the question has to do with the person's ability to continue living at home. Home visits are recommended by the American Bar Association as part of competence evaluations whenever possible (Kapp, 1996). In a home visit, it is possible to observe the person's performance directly and to get a firsthand look at possible safety hazards. Many older people function better at home than in an unfamiliar situation, as illustrated by the following example.

We were asked by the court to evaluate a 96-year-old woman who lived alone in a house in the country. There was a dispute between her daughters concerning her ability to live safely at home. One daughter felt that she should be placed in a nursing home because she was no longer safe at home. The other daughter believed that her mother was better off remaining at home and that it was safe for her to do so. Psychological testing revealed a significant deficit in short-term memory, but no other obvious cognitive deficits. The woman's memory problems may have been an early manifestation of dementia, but in the absence of other obvious cognitive problems, it was not sufficient for diagnosis of dementia. Her memory deficits may have been due to advanced age (or age-associated memory impairment, see Chapter 3) or to a problem other than dementia.

The main question posed in the evaluation was her safety at home, so we visited her there. The home was small, but neat and clean. We talked about food preparation and had her show us how she went about preparing her meals. We also questioned her about what she might do in an emergency situation, such as a fall. She told us she had a neighbor who checked in on her regularly. The neighbor made sure she was safe and also gave her reminders, for example, that it was time to prepare dinner. With her permission, we talked to her neighbor who confirmed that she checked on the woman regularly and indicated that she was willing to continue doing so. From the information we obtained, we concluded that the woman was competent to remain in her home.

Evaluation of Driving

Clinicians are increasingly asked to give an opinion concerning whether an older person should continue driving. This question comes up in cases of Alzheimer's disease or other dementia but can also be raised about people suffering from vision loss or various other health problems and people taking medications that interfere with attention and reaction time. Dementia patients who continue to drive are a common concern to families. Families are often reluctant to take the car away from the patient themselves or may be unable to do so because the patient objects. Although many patients voluntarily give up driving, a minority (mostly men) continue to drive long past the point the family considers them to be unsafe (Kaszniak, Keyl & Albert, 1991).

Studies of driving and dementia indicate that patients are at greater risk of having accidents and getting lost while driving (Kaszniak et al., 1991; Tuokko et al., 1995). Cognitive deficits are strongly related to ratings of driving performance on a test course and in traffic (Odenheimer, Beaudet, Jette, et al., 1994). For one of the most informative studies, trained driving instructors evaluated actual driving performance in a road test (Hunt, Morris, Edwards, & Wilson, 1993). Older people without dementia and those with very mild dementia were judged to be competent drivers, but 40% of people with mild Alzheimer's were rated as unsafe. Participants in the study also completed a variety of psychological tests, virtually all of which were found to be correlated with unsafe performance. The highest correlations, however, were between driving performance and two specific predriving screening measures, traffic sign recognition and an attention-switching task in which subjects had to circle only numbers or only letters until instructed by the tester to switch. These results suggest that significant proportions of Alzheimer's patients are no longer safe drivers fairly early in the disease process and that cognitive deficits are associated with increasing risk.

Some states require that people with Alzheimer's disease or other disorders be prohibited from driving or be required to have their licenses reviewed. Evaluation of competency for driving is a relatively new area, and there are few guidelines about how to conduct an assessment or what tests have the best validity. Carr and associates (1991) recommend assessing both the person and the driving environment and vehicle. A person who drives in daylight in a familiar and low-traffic area is at less risk than someone driving at night or on high-volume roads. Evidence of actual or near accidents is important, but in the absence of clear findings, it is very difficult to evaluate the degree of risk. Recommendations should be consistent with state law. We believe, however, that it is prudent to err on the side of being overrestrictive in cases of dementia, because the risk increases over time and patients sometimes do not have the ability to recognize the danger themselves.

Examples of Competence Evaluations

The following case illustrates constructing the competence assessment around the type of competence that is being questioned.

An older man became depressed when his wife discovered he had been having a long-standing affair. He took a gun and shot himself through the head. The bullet entered and exited through the frontal region of the brain but did not kill him. His wife subsequently divorced him and he was living on his own. He was in charge of his own finances.

The man had two daughters, and he gave power of attorney to one of them. This daughter promptly spent about $60,000 of his money on herself and her family. The other daughter went to an attorney to protect the father's assets. Her concern was that he would run out of money and be left with nothing to live on if her sister continued spending his assets. The attorney referred the patient for an evaluation of his ability to make decisions about his finances.

Testing in this case proved to be a challenge. The man had frontal lobe damage and was hard to manage. In the middle of testing, he would lose track of what he was doing. For example, he would suddenly stand up during the testing and start to walk around or get ready to leave. These interruptions did not reflect resistance or hostility; he was simply forgetting what he was doing.

We performed a thorough evaluation that included the WAIS, the WMS, and language testing. Because the main question was his competence to make decisions about finances, we focused particularly on tests of comprehension and ability to abstract. Could he think logically and develop and implement a plan?

Based on the test findings and discussions with him, it became apparent that he was highly suggestible. If someone presented a scheme to him, he would turn over some money. But the situation was complicated because he was also capable of making logical plans. Testing revealed that comprehension and reasoning were adequate. When we asked him specifically what he wanted to do with his money, he could give a logical answer.

The assessment, then, indicated that he was capable of logical decisions but had difficulty implementing them. Because he was very distractible, it was possible to confuse him and take his money from him. Based on these findings, the judge put safeguards in place to prevent his daughter from continuing to spend his assets on her own needs.

A very important competence question concerns situations in which the patient wants one thing and the family another. In this example, a woman was living in a nursing home but wanted to move back to her own home. She had been placed in the nursing home by her sister, who felt that she was not making good decisions about her care at home. On a couple of occasions, the woman had returned home on a trial basis but would not take her medications properly. As a result, she would become sicker, and her family would put her back in the nursing home. The patient would then get very depressed and say she did not want to go on living.

The patient's attorney requested an evaluation to determine whether she was competent to decide to go home, even if it might compromise her care. The key to the evaluation was talking with her in depth to determine if she really understood what the implications of going home would be. We asked her specifically if she understood that if she went home, the likelihood was that she would die sooner. She replied, "I know I am sick and am going to die soon, and I'd rather die at home." Given that that was her wish and that she was cognitively able to make that decision, the judge ordered that she be permitted to go home. She went home and lived there for about three months before she died.

This case illustrates that people can competently make decisions that put them in potential danger. This woman understood the implications of going home and therefore was competent to make that decision. In contrast, the man in the previous example was not competent because of his suggestibility and therefore needed protection from one of his daughters.

One other important type of competence evaluation concerns decisions about medical treatment, especially refusal of treatment with terminal conditions. We give examples of those evaluations in Chapter 14.

CONCLUSIONS

In this chapter, we have discussed the uses of psychological testing in differential diagnosis and in evaluations of competence. Testing provides a structured evaluation that yields data that can be compared to age norms, thereby helping to clarify the significance of presenting symptoms. When there is a question of possible dementia but initial assessments do not provide conclusive evidence, subsequent evaluation can confirm the presence of a degenerative process or symptoms due to something other than a progressive dementia. Just as dementia is the focal point for differential diagnosis of older adults, so is cognitive functioning the central issue in evaluations of competence. Competence evaluations require integration of interview and testing data with an understanding of individual and family issues out of which questions about competence arose. The issues that are typically addressed, such as driving, making decisions about medical care or place of residence, and handling finances lie at the heart of a dialectic between respecting individual rights and providing protection when someone's judgment is impaired. With the continued growth of the older population, we expect these questions to become even more common and more complicated.

APPENDIX 6.1. SOURCES AND REFERENCES FOR COMMON TESTS

Wechsler Memory Scale—III; Wechsler Adult Intelligence Scale—III;
Boston Naming Test; Auditory Verbal Learning Test
  The Psychological Corporation
  Order Service Center
  P.O. Box 839954
  San Antonio, TX 78283-3954
  (800) 211-8378
  FAX (800) 232-1223

Clock Drawing: A Neuropsychological Analysis
  WPS
  12031 Wilshire Blvd.
  Los Angeles, CA 90025-1251
  (800) 648-8857
  FAX (310) 478-7838

Clock Test
  MHS
  908 Niagara Falls Blvd.
  North Tonawanda, NY 14120-2060

Rey–Osterrieth Complex Figure Test (CFT)
  PAR
  P.O. Box 998
  Odessa, FL 33556
  (800) 331-8378
  FAX (800) 727-9329

Trail Making Test
  Reitan (1958); Lezak (1995).

UCLA Screening Battery
  Drebing et al. (1994).

MAYO Clinic Battery
  Ivnik et al. (1994).

APPENDIX 6.2. CRITERIA FOR CLINICAL DIAGNOSIS OF ALZHEIMER'S DISEASE

I. Criteria for the clinical diagnosis of *probable* Alzheimer's disease include the following:
   A. Dementia established by clinical examination and documented by the Mini-Mental State Examination, Blessed Dementia Scale, or some similar examination, and confirmed by neuropsychological tests
   B. Deficits in two or more areas of cognition
   C. Progressive worsening of memory and other cognitive functions
   D. No disturbance of consciousness
   E. Onset between ages 40 and 90, most often after age 65
   F. Absence of systemic disorders or other brain diseases that in and of themselves could account for the progressive deficits in memory and cognition

II. Diagnosis of *probable* Alzheimer's disease is supported by the following:
   A. Progressive deterioration of specific cognitive functions such as language (aphasia), motor skills (apraxia), and perception (agnosia)
   B. Impaired activities of daily living and altered patterns of behavior
   C. Family history of similar disorders, particularly if confirmed neuropathologically
   D. Laboratory results of (1) normal lumbar puncture as evaluated by standard techniques; (2) normal pattern or nonspecific changes in EEG, such as increased slow-wave activity; and (3) evidence of cerebral atrophy on CT with progression documented by serial observation.

III. Other clinical features consistent with the diagnosis of *probable* Alzheimer's disease, after exclusion of causes of dementia other than Alzheimer's disease, include the following:
   A. Plateaus in the course of progression of the illness
   B. Associated symptoms of depression, insomnia, incontinence, delusions, illusions, hallucinations, catastrophic verbal, emotional, or physical outbursts, sexual disorders, and weight loss
   C. Other neurological abnormalities in some patients, especially with more advanced disease and including motor signs such as increased muscle tone, myoclonus, or gait disorder
   D. Seizures in advanced disease
   E. CT normal for age

IV. Features that make the diagnosis of *probable* Alzheimer's disease uncertain or unlikely include the following:
   A. Sudden, apoplectic onset
   B. Focal neurological findings such as hemiparesis, sensory loss, visual field deficits, and incoordination early in the source of the illness
   C. Seizures or gait disturbances at the onset or very early in the course of the illness

Note. Adapted from McKhann et al. (1984). Copyright 1984 by Lippincott–Raven Publishers. Adapted by permission.

V. Clinical diagnosis of *possible* Alzheimer's disease
   A. May be made on the basis of the dementia syndrome, in the absence of other neurologic, psychiatric, or systemic disorders sufficient to cause dementia, and in the presence of variations in the onset, in the presentation, or in the clinical course.
   B. May be made in the presence of a second systemic or brain disorder sufficient to produce dementia, which is not considered to be *the* cause of the dementia.
   C. Should be used in research studies when a single, gradually progressive severe cognitive deficit is identified in the absence of other identifiable cause.

VI. Criteria for diagnosis of *definite* Alzheimer's disease are the following:
   A. Clinical criteria for probable Alzheimer's disease
   B. Histopathological evidence obtained from a biopsy or autopsy

VII. Classification of Alzheimer's disease for research purposes should specify features that may differentiate subtypes of the disorder, such as the following:
   A. Familial occurrence
   B. Onset before age of 65
   C. Presence of trisomy-21
   D. Coexistence of other relevant conditions such as Parkinson's disease.

APPENDIX 6.3. CRITERIA FOR DIAGNOSIS OF VASCULAR DEMENTIA

I. Criteria for the clinical diagnosis of *probable* vascular dementia include *all* of the following:
   A. Dementia (i.e., cognitive decline in memory and two or more other intellectual domains)
   B. Cerebrovascular disease (focal neurological signs; evidence from brain imaging of large vessel infarcts or a strategically placed single infarct, white matter lacunes or extensive periventricular white matter lesions, or combinations of these features)
   C. Onset of dementia within 3 months following a recognized stroke, an abrupt deterioration in cognitive functions, or fluctuating, stepwise progression of cognitive deficits

II. Clinical features consistent with the diagnosis of *probable* vascular dementia include the following:
   A. Early presence of a gait disturbance (small-step gait or march à petit pas, or magnetic, apraxic–ataxic or parkinsonian gait)
   B. History of unsteadiness and frequent, unprovoked falls
   C. Early urinary frequency, urgency, and other urinary symptoms not explained by urological disease
   D. Pseudobulbar palsy
   E. Personality and mood changes, abulia, depression, emotional incontinence, or other subcortical deficits including psychomotor retardation and abnormal executive function.

Note. Adapted from Román et al. (1993). Copyright 1993 by Lippincott–Raven Publishers. Adapted by permission.

7

Basic Issues in Treatment

Our client was a 68-year-old man who had recently retired and was trying to decide what to do with the rest of his life. His initial plan was to leave the town where he had spent his life. He associated the town with his work and he was bitter toward his former employer for not giving him the recognition he believed he deserved, and toward his colleagues, who he believed prevented him from being promoted to senior management. By moving away, he thought he would avoid being reminded of the disappointments he had in his career.

Like many professionals, this man derived much of his sense of identity from his job. His work had been his main interest, and the few friends he had made were colleagues. When he retired, his relationships with them ended. We focused treatment on coming to grips with his bitterness toward his former employer and finding an interest that would be an outlet for his talents. He was able to give up the hope of receiving recognition from his former employer and to explore activities he had always wanted to pursue but had not had the time to do because of work. Instead of ruminating about the past or running away from his problem by moving, he got involved in a new activity, painting watercolors, which provided him with a sense of accomplishment.

This example illustrates how psychotherapy can address issues and problem of later life and help restore people to a fulfilling and productive life. Treatment in this case was fairly typical. It focused on an age-related transition, retirement, as well as the client's long-standing beliefs. Psychotherapy can address many different types of problems and transitions in later life. Timely psychological intervention can improve functioning and may even be cost effective, for example, in reducing unneeded physician visits or improving rehabilitation following an illness or injury. Furthermore, psychotherapy with older people is effective, perhaps as much so as with younger clients (Gallagher-Thompson & Thompson, 1996; Gatz et al., in press; Scogin & McElreath, 1994; Smyer, Zarit, & Qualls, 1990).

This chapter begins with a discussion of planning and initiating treatment. It then focuses on how basic psychotherapy skills are applied in the treatment of older people and the main ways that treatment can differ with older clients. We conclude with case examples that illustrate treatment issues.

Our goal is to provide a framework for treatment of mental health problems in later life. Treatment of older people is sometimes similar to and sometimes different than treatment of younger people. We do not believe in a single or unique type of psychotherapy to be used with every older client. Rather, therapists working with older people modify basic psychotherapy skills as needed to meet the special circumstances and qualities older clients bring into treatment. Treatment also requires specialized knowledge of problems and issues that are different with aging, such as the more frequent interaction of medical and psychological problems and the differences in how older people respond to medications.

Subsequent chapters extend this framework and apply it to common disorders, problems, and settings. We examine treatment of three disorders in detail, depression (Chapter 8), paranoid disorders (Chapter 10), and dementia (Chapter 11). We look at common and often complex issues that arise when working with community-dwelling older adults; how to coordinate mental health treatment with health and social services (Chapter 9) and how to work with family caregivers (Chapter 12). We then present a multilevel approach to treatment in nursing homes and other institutional settings (Chapter 13). We conclude with an examination of ethical issues in treatment of older adults (Chapter 14).

PLANNING AND INITIATING TREATMENT OF OLDER CLIENTS

Starting the treatment process off right depends on careful planning and preparation. During the initial phase of treatment, therapists draws on specialized knowledge and skills for working with older clients. We highlight several issues that are particularly significant in preparing to treat an older client: (1) assessment, (2) treatment setting, (3) preparing the client for treatment, (4) goals, (5) role of the family, (6) medical conditions and medications, and (7) preparing the client for psychotherapy.

Assessment

We want to reiterate the importance of conducting a careful initial evaluation. Sometimes, however, the initial assessment does not answer important questions, and so we continue gathering information to clarify diagnosis. As an example, it is helpful to proceed slowly before reaching a conclusion about diagnosis, especially when there is a possibility of a personality disorder. We gather a lot of information and listen carefully to clients to sort out and make sense of the information. More than with younger clients, we have found that some older clients initially present themselves and their experiences in a disorganized way. Their thinking may initially seem loose and tangential, suggesting a psychotic process or personality disorder. The problem, however, can turn out to be how clients are describing their experiences rather than their underlying thought processes.

As an example, we once saw a client whose initial description of an event sounded bizarre and possibly psychotic but turned out to be more understandable once she provided more details. The client, who was a 70-year-old woman, talked in the first session about an incident that occurred when she was a teenager. She recounted that her high school principal told her that her father had been convicted of a crime and that she then bled all over the principal's office. Her unconnected way of telling the story suggested loose or even psychotic thought processes. Throughout the first session, the woman described other events in similarly unconnected ways. During the second session, the client was more relaxed and less pressured in her speech. She talked about how she had had recurrent nosebleeds when she was a teenager and that her nose would bleed copiously when she was under stress. This information filled gaps in the story she told previously, when she had not mentioned nosebleeds. The client also commented on the fact that she had felt nervous in the previous session. Although some of her stories remained tangential, it was clear once we got to know her better that she did not have a thought disorder.

This case illustrates how important it is not to reach a judgment about diagnosis based on one example. If there is a possibility of a thought disorder, we try to get multiple examples. In this case, we then could ask about other incidents in which her nose bled.

Some older people communicate in ways that can contribute to incorrect initial impressions. If they spend a lot of time alone, their style of interacting with other individuals can become somewhat impoverished. In fact, the woman with the nosebleeds spent nearly all her time with her demented husband and did not interact much with anyone else. When people do not have much everyday social interaction, their initial recounting of stories may reflect thought processes that have become somewhat idiosyncratic. Accustomed to examining experiences only for themselves, they recount events without providing the context or connections for anyone else to make sense out of them.

Another factor that contributes to misunderstandings is differences in conversational patterns. Older people have different patterns of speech and vocabulary than younger people. They may use jargon that was contemporary many years ago but that the therapist does not recognize. They also may relate experiences differently. They often take longer to get to the point, or they go off on digressions. They may think the therapist understands the context of the event they are relating or the connections between events, even though they have not provided the details. This manner of communicating creates the impression of loose and tangential thinking. Whether these patterns are due to generational differences or age cannot be determined. The therapist, however, must patiently sort through the information provided in order to determine if it does, in fact, make sense. This is done by asking questions and also learning to grasp a client's perspective and meaning. After a few sessions, it often emerges that the person's experiences and thought processes are quite normal but that he or she related experiences initially in an unusual way.

Another reason for proceeding more slowly before reaching a conclusion about diagnosis is that older clients have more history to relate than younger clients. Therapists need to be patient when listening to history, learning how to direct and sort through the information that clients provide about their past. Of course, therapists need to hear only the more pertinent parts of the history, not every detail. Some clients are not good at selecting the relevant portions of their story, or they believe they have to relate everything to the therapist for the therapist to understand them. In these cases, the therapist needs to create a balance, listening to enough of the history so as to convey understanding and obtain sufficient clinical information to proceed with treatment, but also moving clients along in a gentle way.

Treatment Setting

Treatment of older people can take place in a variety of settings. The therapist needs to decide at the outset where treatment will take place and what the implications of the location will be.

Most older clients can either drive themselves or arrange for transportation to a therapist's office. In many locales, special transportation is available that can bring older people to an appointment. For people who do not get out often, a trip to the therapist's office can be helpful in itself and contribute to discussions concerning increasing activities outside the home. Information on transportation services is available from local Area Agencies on Aging (see Chapter 9).

There are, however, times when it is important to make home visits, for instance, to establish rapport with a reluctant client or to see a disabled client who cannot get to the therapist's office.

When older clients live in a nursing home or other residential setting, it is often more practical to treat them there, rather than in the office. Residents in those settings, however, have very little privacy. The therapist needs to find a place to conduct therapy that is private and where there will be no interruptions from staff or other residents. Case records also need to be confidential. Since case files in a nursing home can be accessed by anyone on the nursing staff, they are not an appropriate place to keep confidential information about sessions. We return to this issue in Chapter 13.

Preparing the Client for Psychotherapy

Psychotherapy has changed greatly during the lives of our older clients, in terms of how it is practiced and how it is viewed by the general public. When today's older people were young, the predominant treatment was psychoanalysis, and only people who were "crazy" took medications. We think it is useful to find out the client's ideas and expectations for therapy. We also explain to clients how therapy works and how they can benefit from it. Explanations about how the clinician will conduct treatment can clear up misconceptions and also allows clients to be more active in their own treatment. This type of socialization for treatment has been found helpful in many different types of psychotherapy (e.g., Lewinsohn, Muñoz, Youngren, & Zeiss, 1992; Orne & Wender, 1968) and results in improved outcomes.

Therapists should also find out about a client's past treatment experiences. Some older clients have a great deal of knowledge and sophistication about psychotherapy. They may have been in and out of therapy throughout their lives and can recount the whole history of psychotherapy in the United States. Over the years, we have encountered people who were treated by some of the most famous therapists from earlier generations: Rogers, Perls, Minuchin, Ellis. Although clients with a history of prior treatment are more sophisticated about therapy, we still discuss with them how we plan to proceed. In particular, these clients often have been passive in their past treatment, while we work with them in a more collaborative role. While we use contemporary treatment approaches, we do try to build on what may have been helpful in past therapies.

Older clients sometimes have had bad experiences in therapy when they were younger. These incidents were often due to practices that are now outmoded or theories that have been discredited. As an example, we once treated a 68-year-old gay man who had spent his young adulthood in and out of therapy with therapists who tried to "cure" him of homosexuality. Rather than helping the problem, the therapists only made him feel more guilty and confused and provoked a couple of psychiatric hospitalizations. Given this history, it was essential to convey acceptance of his homosexuality at the outset and assure him that we would focus on the problem that

brought him back to treatment; what to do with his life now that he was retired.

Goals of Treatment

Given the diversity of the older population, goals of treatment necessarily
vary depending on clients and their circumstances. Goals should be developed as part of the interaction between client and therapist. What clinicians
believe to be realistic or possible inevitably influences what goals are set. If
a therapist believes that not much can be accomplished, little will be attempted. On the other hand, therapists who hold unrealistically positive expectations will be frustrated when treatment does not yield the good outcomes they hoped for.

How much can older people change? When working with younger
clients, therapists often believe that far-reaching changes in behavior and
personality structure are possible. Some of our colleagues have expressed
wonderment that we would work with older people whose capacity for
change is more limited. In fact, older clients' maturity and experience is often an asset, and they possess knowledge and abilities that can be brought
to bear on their current problems. In the example we used to start the chapter, the retired man embittered about his job, the treatment goal was to decide whether or not he should move, which was related to coming to terms
with retirement. This discussion led the client to uncover interests and abilities he had not pursued when he was employed. By comparison, our col-
lege-age clients often do not have the basic life skills for finding and keeping a job or a relationship. Although the possibilities may be more limited
with older clients, therapists can find strengths to build on.

While the specific goals that emerge depend on the unique features of
every case, two general principles should guide the selection of goals: identifying treatable aspects of the situation and supporting autonomy. Many
older clients have problems that seem at first to be intractable. They may be
suffering from a chronic and degenerative illness. Or they may have long-
standing psychological problems that have not responded to treatment in
the past. In instances such as these, parts of the problem may still be modifiable. For example, the person with Alzheimer's disease can benefit from interventions at different points in the progression of the disease. Early on,
counseling may be useful to help patients come to terms with their illness
and make plans for their future while they are still able to consider the alternatives. Throughout the course of the illness, interventions with family
caregivers can lower the stress they are experiencing, enabling them to take
better care of the patient (see Chapter 12). Even when dealing with a late-
stage patient living in a nursing home, it is often possible to improve quality of life by working with staff or family members. Similar treatable compo-

nents can be found in other chronic physical or mental health problems. Even when a complete recovery is not possible, treatment of some features of the situation may result in significant improvements for the patient or the patient's family.

The second overarching principle in treatment of the elderly is supporting autonomy. Therapists often deal with older clients facing immediate or potential threats to their autonomy. Some clients may be facing a move from home to an institution; for others, family members are trying to take over making decisions for them. These issues can be complex. Older clients may, for example, have chronic health problems that make it difficult for them to continue living independently. Their families may be concerned about their ability to stay alone safely or get needed medical care. Placing older people in a protected setting can reduce these concerns. But the potential gains of relocation have to be weighed against the risks associated with taking away someone's autonomy and independence. Older people often function better in familiar settings, maintaining their mobility and self-care activities longer at home. In general, it is best to support autonomy as long as it is feasible and to take steps that compromise an older person's independence only after other avenues of treatment have been explored.

We believe that treatment of older people should be guided by a general strategy that the pioneering geropsychologist Robert Kahn (1975) called the "principle of minimum intervention." Minimum intervention means treatment that is the least disruptive to clients' usual functioning. While important when working with people of any age, minimum intervention is especially critical for older adults, who maintain a fragile balance between independence and dependence. Minimum intervention supports continued independence whenever possible, because that maximizes the choices of older clients, and assures that they have the opportunity to make decisions about how they live consistent with their own values.

Minimum intervention can be practiced in many different ways. A basic principle of geriatric medicine is that the more one does, the more the potential for adverse or unintended effects. It is better not to make changes when a person is doing all right, for instance, to switch a medication. Fewer medications are usually better than more. Tests or surgeries should be considered carefully, weighing the potential gains against possible losses and complications. As one geriatrician told us, a guiding principle in her practice is "If it isn't broken, don't fix it."

We stress a similar approach in mental health practice. To the extent possible, we try not to upset a client's usual way of doing things or to undermine remaining areas of competency. We also try to support people so that they can live at home as long as possible. We do not do more than clients ask.

There is often a lot of pressure to institutionalize an older person, but trading autonomy for security introduces new problems, for example, inducing dependencies. In Chapter 9, we return to the issue of helping people stay at home and look at the resources and strategies that make it possible.

Role of the Family

One way treatment of older people often differs from that of younger adults (but is similar to interventions with children) is that the family of the client is often involved. Families may initiate contact with the therapist or may contact the therapist during the course of treatment. Friends of an older person or other concerned individuals sometimes become involved. From the clinician's perspective, it is often helpful to contact families of older clients (or friends, if no family are involved) to clarify diagnostic questions or to provide information about key issues. Therapists, of course, should protect the confidentiality of their clients and not talk to children or other interested persons without explicit permission.

A family member sometimes accompanies an older client to a first visit, so the clinician must initially decide who is the client. In some cases, the older person is unwilling or unable to participate in treatment, but the relative who brought the older client may still want help for him- or herself in dealing with the older person. Dementia is the most frequent of these situations. Another such example is children of parents with long-standing personality disorders. As these parents age and develop health-related problems, they may begin making excessive demands on a child's time, such as calling repeatedly in the middle of the night. Their children may initially seek help for the parent, but the parent may not agree to participate in anything more than an assessment and, indeed, may see nothing wrong with his or her own behavior. In this type of situation, the therapist can redefine the problem as the child learning to cope with and set limits with the parent and can help the child examine the care options available for the parent.

In other situations, the therapist's assessment suggests that the older person's problems could best be addressed by couple or family therapy. Involving a child for one or two sessions can help clarify key issues and results faster than seeing the older client alone. These sessions allow us to assess the relationship better and to share important information about the course of treatment—if our client agrees.

Medical Conditions and Medications

One of the biggest differences in treatment of older people is the importance of coordinating psychotherapy with medical care. Older people typically have one or more chronic health problems that may either be the cause of feelings of depression or anxiety or be affected by the person's behavior and emotions. The medications prescribed for medical conditions can influence mood and cognition. Psychiatric medications must be evaluated carefully for possible adverse effects on the patient's medical conditions and for possible interaction with other medications the person may be taking.

An understanding of the interface of health and mental health in later life is very helpful in the practice of psychotherapy with older people. Therapists should become familiar with the common medical illnesses in later life, the medications and other treatments used for them, and their influences on mental health. Morrison (1997) provides a comprehensive summary of psychological symptoms associated with medical disorders.

Typically, the influence of medical problems is indirect, that is, clients react to the discomfort and/or implications of their illness in unique ways. When clients have a chronic illness or disability, clinicians need to be able to identify reasonable opportunities to improve functioning and when the best course is to adjust to current levels of discomfort or disability. Obviously, therapists do not want to encourage dependence when there is a possibility for rehabilitation and recovery. Conversely, they should not foster false hopes that cannot be realized.

It is important to keep abreast of new developments in medical treatment of common diseases of later life. If we encounter a client with an illness we are not familiar with, we read up on it and consult with the client's physician, if our client consents. That way we get a better idea about what might be realistic goals and how psychotherapy can contribute to the situation.

Another important area is familiarity with psychotropic medications and their benefits and risks with older people. There are many situations in which psychotropic medications are an integral part of treatment. Rather than seeing medications and psychotherapy as opposed, we view them as complementary, facilitating improvement at different levels. Newer medications that are more targeted to symptoms and have fewer side effects increasingly are an important part of practice. In subsequent chapters, we discuss the more widely used psychotropic medications.

A fundamental issue is that the use of medications, whether for psychiatric symptoms or medical problems, is more complicated in older people than in younger ones. Physiological changes in the aging body result in differences in how drugs are processed. Generally, medications are absorbed, distributed, metabolized, and eliminated more slowly by older people (Beizer, 1994). As a result, medications reach a therapeutic level more slowly and also have a longer half-life; that is, they remain in the body longer. The result is an increased risk that drugs will build up to toxic levels. Compounding this problem are changes in how medications affect the target tissue or organ, or what is called "pharmacodynamics." Some changes with aging decrease the effectiveness of a medication at its target site, while other changes increase sensitivity (Beizer, 1994). There are, of course, considerable individual differences. These changes can be especially pronounced in some patients; for example, people with reduced kidney function eliminate most medications very slowly.

Identifying a therapeutic window in dosage is a major problem with older people. Often there are no specific guidelines for how much of a medication to give to an older person. With psychotropic medications, geriatric specialists often start with lower levels than for younger patients, but there are wide individual variations in dosages that are effective and tolerated.

Problems can occur when only one drug is involved. Typically, however, older people are taking several medications. When introducing a new medication, physicians need to evaluate carefully how it interacts with the other medications the patient is taking, including any over-the-counter drugs. A medication can also affect chronic health problems. Some antidepressant medications, for example, should be used cautiously in someone with a history of cardiovascular disease. In turn, medications can have a variety of behavioral and cognitive side effects. When toxic levels are reached or there is an adverse interaction between medications, a delirium is often the result. It has been estimated that up to one third of hospital admissions of older people are due to the results of unwanted or unanticipated side effects of medications (Cooper, 1994).

People are increasingly turning to natural substances for treatment of their health problems or for preventive purposes. Often people believe that these substances are not harmful because they are "natural," but that is not the case. Just like other medications, natural substances, including vitamins, can become toxic in high dosages or can produce adverse side effects by themselves or in combination with each other or with prescription medications.

These issues about the interface of health and mental health problems lead us to another facet of geriatric psychology, learning how to consult with physicians and other health care providers to clarify issues about medications and illnesses. In a typical outpatient practice with younger adults, the need to consult with a client's physicians rarely arises. When it does, the discussion usually involves psychotropic medications. With older clients, consultation is a frequent and often a key part of treatment. Consultations can clarify the significance of current somatic complaints and lead to coordination of treatment efforts. They can also address issues such as identifying the therapeutic dosage of common psychotropic medications or changing medications to reduce side effects or improve the therapeutic response.

Physicians are often very busy and may not understand or appreciate the contributions to treatment that can be made by mental health practitioners. We have found, however, that it is possible to build collaborative relationships with physicians through several means. First, it is important that the mental health professional have a familiarity with common illnesses and medications. That is the physician's area of expertise, but it helps in discussions of clients' problems if the mental health professional understands common terms and issues. Second, information should be presented to physicians in a succinct way, free from psychological jargon. (Of course, any release of information should be done only with a client's written consent.) Third, the therapist's own treatment plan should be presented briefly and clearly. When physicians understand that therapists can actually help their patients, they welcome collaboration and, indeed, often become a source of new referrals.

BASIC SKILLS IN TREATMENT OF OLDER PEOPLE

Psychotherapy with older adults involves incorporation of the knowledge and skills of geropsychology with a solid foundation of psychotherapy technique. Many different psychotherapy approaches have been used successfully with older clients. Rather than providing a comprehensive overview of psychotherapy, we have chosen to highlight the strategies that have been the core of our approach over the years. We will look at why these skills are useful and how they may differ with older adults.

We draw on concepts and techniques primarily from four traditions: (1) a Rogerian, client-centered approach; (2) behavior therapy; (3) cognitive-behavioral therapy; and (4) family systems. In the following sections, we discuss at a general level how we use these approaches with older clients. In subsequent chapters, we look at the application of these skills to treatment of specific disorders.

Core Skills: Empathy, Warmth, and Genuineness

Rogers (1951) proposed that certain core skills are necessary for any therapy relationship to be successful. These skills include empathy, warmth, and genuineness. In our clinical work and in the supervision of students, we are repeatedly reminded of the value of empathy. Empathy is a familiar concept. It involves being able to understand the client's feelings and behavior from his or her own perspective and to convey that understanding. Clinicians must try to see the world through their clients' eyes.

Empathy is especially important when there are marked differences in background that separate client and counselor. Since there is usually an age difference and sometimes cultural and social differences between client and therapist, empathy is critical. In these situations, empathy works in two directions. For the clinician, empathy provides a check against accepting biases or stereotypes about clients. By communicating empathy, clinicians push past overt characteristics and social stereotypes to a more individuated view of the client. Older clients feel understood despite being older than the therapist or despite differences in social class, education, or ethnic background. Empathy bridges the differences.

The following example illustrates how empathy can address the age difference between client and therapist. The client was a woman in her early 70s who was depressed and lonely, and her counselor was a student trainee in her mid-20s who looked even younger. During the first session, the client was reviewing her problems but then stopped and said to the counselor, "You haven't been through what I have been. You're not old. You can't possibly understand." The counselor had been trained to use a medical analogy in this situation, that a doctor did not have to have had chicken pox in order to know how to treat it. Instead, she responded spontaneously, "It's true I am not old, but I have been lonely, too." This response identified the client's core feeling of loneliness and conveyed understanding through self-disclosure. This brief exchange was crucial in establishing an effective therapeutic relationship between client and counselor, which subsequently contributed to a successful treatment outcome.

Two other core qualities in the therapeutic relationship are warmth and genuineness. As with other clients, therapists should be warm and accepting toward older clients and not hide behind the role of "expert" or "doctor." A particular issue with older clients is touching. We do not believe that therapists should touch clients routinely because touching can easily lead to misunderstandings. Occasionally, however, touching is appropriate, such as when a client is retelling a very painful story. Therapists need to overcome the culturally induced apprehensions about touching an older person so that they can convey comfort in the same way as with a younger client. In fact, it may be more helpful to touch an older client because some are rarely touched by another person. But while touching has therapeutic potential, it needs to be used on a limited basis. Because of the improprieties taken by some therapists with their clients, companies that provide malpractice insurance now mandate that physical contact be restricted to touching a client's hand.

Older clients may express opinions that upset therapists and make it difficult to convey empathy or warmth. Some older clients hold racist or sexist beliefs that are offensive to the therapist. It is important for therapists to recognize that these attitudes were more socially acceptable in the past and so not overreact to them.

Over the years we have been struck by the way some clients assume that we have the same ethnic background they do, even when it is not the case. By developing an empathic relationship, we have reduced the likelihood that differences in our backgrounds will interfere with treatment.

Behavioral Approaches

Behavioral approaches such as relaxation, desensitization, and shaping new responses have many potential applications when working with the elderly (Zeiss & Steffen, 1996b). Outpatient treatments are effective with insomnia, depression, and anxiety and in helping families manage problem behaviors of an elder with dementia or a chronic mental illness (Bootzin, Engle-Friedman, & Hazelwood, 1983; Burgio & Burgio, 1991; Gallagher et al., 1981; Green, Linsk, & Pinkson, 1986; Lewinsohn, Antonuccio, Steinmetz, & Teri, 1984; Hussian, 1986; Hussian & Davis, 1985; Haley, 1983; Pinkston & Linsk, 1984; Scogin, Rickard, Keith, Wilson, & McElreath, 1992; Wisocki, 1991). Many behavioral interventions have been conducted in institutional settings. The targets of these problems have included increasing social participation, increasing exercise, improving self-care activities, managing incontinence, training social skills, and, particularly, controlling problems such as wandering and agitation (see Carstensen & Fisher, 1991; Hussian & Davis, 1985).

As with Rogerian therapy, behavior therapy is valuable with older clients as much for its basic concepts and approaches as for specific techniques. Behavioral approaches focus on observable, countable problems. They emphasize identifying the specific behaviors, thoughts, or feelings that are problematic, their frequency (or absence, when the problem is a deficiency of behavior), and the circumstances in which they occur. This direct approach to problems appeals to the practical side of older people. The focus on overt behavior also helps therapists and clients alike get beyond age stereotypes and other incorrect attributions about why a problem is occurring and instead look for treatable aspects of the situation. Clients, for example, may mislabel problems (e.g., saying they are anxious when depressive symptoms predominate). They may describe a problem as occurring more or less often than it actually does. Similarly, they may fail to note antecedents and consequences of their problems, that is, the events that trigger and reinforce behaviors or feelings. By obtaining the specific details of what the problem is and when and how it occurs, the clinician gains valuable information for planning interventions.

As an example, a woman who was caring for her mother who had a dementing illness reported that her mother was driving her crazy by asking the same question over and over again; "When will your husband come home?" A behavioral assessment was made in which the woman noted in writing each time her mother asked the question. This behavioral record showed that the mother did not ask the question often. Rather, it greatly annoyed the caregiver when she did ask it because the caregiver interpreted it as a criticism of her marriage—if she were a better wife, her husband would be home already. By getting the specifics of what happened and when, we changed the formulation of this problem from an excessive rate of verbal behavior by a dementia patient to the client's own cognitive appraisal of a verbal statement.

Another feature of behavioral approaches that is especially useful with older clients is the emphasis on implementing new behavior in specific, graduated steps. Rather than instructing a client to carry out a complex set of behaviors, tasks are broken down into steps or components. In many instances, clients agree to carry out new behaviors but delay or put off actually doing anything new. Behavioral approaches address this problem with schedules for specific behaviors and reinforcements for carrying them out. The detailed, concrete steps in planning and scheduling new behaviors are often critical in helping depressed or dependent clients break out of a cycle of passiveness and inaction.

In a broader sense, behavioral approaches encourage clients to take an active role in treatment, which is especially useful for older clients who feel helpless or overwhelmed. The strong educational component helps clients understand why they are having problems and how new behaviors can help them overcome those problems.

Probably the most useful feature of a behavioral orientation is its emphasis on evaluating the outcome of treatment. A great deal of pessimism about the ability of older people to change and improve, whether through psychotherapy or any other method, is held by health care professionals, family members, and older clients themselves. To counter this skepticism about the value of therapy, it is critical to obtain evidence of its efficacy. The detailed assessment that is part of behavioral treatment provides a clear baseline against which outcomes can be evaluated. By obtaining concrete evidence of progress, clinicians can reassure clients who are pessimistic about their capacity to improve or benefit from psychotherapy.

Cognitive-Behavioral Treatment

What older people believe about themselves and their experiences is a major focus of treatment. Cognitive-behavioral approaches (e.g., Beck et al., 1979; Zeiss & Steffen, 1996b; Gallagher-Thompson & Thompson, 1996) provide a systematic framework for identifying and modifying thoughts that lead to maladaptive behaviors and emotions. In a sense, cognitive-behavioral therapy addresses many of the same issues as traditional psychodynamic approaches, but it uses a structured framework to bring these thoughts out in the open more quickly and to treat them in a direct manner. Clients become aware of how they distort or misinterpret the events in their lives and how these distortions relate to negative concepts about themselves.

Several features of cognitive-behavioral therapy make it particularly well suited for work with older people. First, as do behavioral approaches, it emphasizes educating clients about their thought processes and how thinking affects behavior and emotions. Clients learn how to apply cognitive-behavioral techniques to their everyday life. As in behavior therapy, the detailed planning and scheduling of interventions helps break a client's passivity. Another feature that cognitive approaches have in common with behavior therapy is the emphasis on evaluating treatment outcome.

A main part of cognitive therapy is identifying what people think about themselves and their circumstances. There are so many negative stereotypes about the elderly that clients readily incorporate these stereotypical beliefs into their self-concept.

The issues older people raise often have a basis in reality but also have a component of exaggeration. One of the most complex issues for therapists is differentiating realistic implications of losses from exaggerated beliefs. In other words, a portion of a client's negative thoughts may have a factual basis, but there is also usually an exaggerated component. Cognitive-behavioral techniques provide tools for therapists to explore the difference between a reasonable sense of sadness or grief over loss and an overgeneralized and excessive preoccupation. Clients who have experienced losses often believe that life is not worth living or that they cannot be happy anymore because of a particular problem or loss. The cognitive-behavioral therapist can discuss the appropriateness of being sad over a loss while challenging the exaggerated belief that the client will never again be happy. When therapists use cognitive-behavioral approaches with younger clients, they can readily identify which beliefs are excessive or exaggerated. If a college student proclaims that her life is over because her boyfriend has broken up with her, the therapist recognizes the exaggeration right away. He or she knows that the client will have more and probably better relationships in her life, and so feels secure in challenging this negative belief. When an older client makes a similar generalization following the death of a spouse, clinicians may accept it uncritically. The death of a spouse is, of course, more serious than breaking up with a boyfriend or girlfriend, and a period of grieving is normal. But when grief persists long after the spouse's death, it is usually due to exaggerated beliefs that make the loss worse than it needs to be.

Cognitive-behavioral therapy provides the tools for differentiating the realistic and reasonable consequences of loss from exaggerated components. Through a gentle process of questioning and challenging beliefs, the therapist can usually help clients identify overgeneralizations or other distortions and activate more realistic appraisals of themselves and the options available to them, despite their loss.

Family Systems Perspective

As mentioned earlier, family members are frequently involved in treatment of older adults. They may encourage the client to obtain therapy or may seek information from the therapist as treatment proceeds. The content of treatment frequently touches on family issues as well. Therapists must make complex judgments about what actually may be going on within a family and when to bring in other family members for the purpose of gathering information or to be involved in treatment.

Given the central role that families have in the lives of older people, we have found it useful to take a family systems perspective when working with this population (e.g., Herr & Weakland, 1979; Haley, 1976). Several features of a family systems approach are particularly relevant. First, we look at how the family functions. We consider who is influential or powerful within the family, who makes decisions, who is viewed positively by other people and who is seen as weak, needy, or problematic. We also look at how the family members communicate with each other. Building on these observations, we conceptualize problems as caused by interactions rather than the behavior of one person or another. Viewing problems in this way opens up more possibilities for intervention. In many situations—for example, in cases of dementia or chronic psychiatric problems—the "patient" cannot change. Nevertheless, it is possible to change the interactions others have with that person and thereby lessen strain on the family.

Another feature of a family systems perspective is that the therapist does not take sides, assign blame, or support one person against another. Clinicians are often caught up in tense family situations rife with disagreement about what is best for an older client. An issue likely to produce disagreements is whether an older person should move to a institutional setting. We have often seen therapists in this situation reflexively taking sides, advocating relocation without considering the elder's preferences or capability to remain at home or how the roles the family members play have shaped the conflict. In many instances, of course, relocation is in everyone's best interests or is necessary for the older person's safety. But this is an area where clinicians need to tread cautiously rather than assuming that one perspective is correct .

Families are not always involved in treatment nor should they always be involved. But when the older client wants their involvement or is dependent on them, they need to be included at least to some extent. Even when the family is not included in treatment, a systems perspective is useful for understanding an older client's relationships with them.

The following case example illustrates using a family systems perspective. Nadine sought help for her sister, who was the primary caregiver for their mother, Sophie. According to Nadine, Sophie was suffering from dementia, and the family wanted to keep her at home as long as possible. The caregiving sister, Anne, had always lived with her mother. An initial assessment confirmed that the mother indeed had dementia.

Nadine's goal was to enlist the clinician's help in getting her sister to be a better caregiver. She described her sister as always having been slow and inept. Anne had never married and had worked at a series of marginal jobs. She was taking care of her mother now because no one else had the time for it. This view of the caregiver was reinforced by Nadine's sons, who were successful businessmen. Like their mother, they saw Anne as ineffectual and incompetent. In fact, they said she had always been considered incompetent by the family and was the butt of the family's jokes.

In a separate interview, Anne indicated that she was struggling to do everything her mother needed. It appeared that she was managing some tasks fairly well, though she was under a lot of stress.

Anne's one-down position in this family system was a critical factor to take into account in making an intervention. Given how this family functioned, efforts to build Anne up would have to be done in ways that did not activate the long-standing patterns of putting her down and devaluing her efforts. In other words, we felt we could not tell Nadine directly that her sister was doing a good job. Since Anne wanted help with problems she was having caring for her mother, we began working with her individually to build up her skills as a caregiver. The overt purpose was to help her in caregiving, but as her skills improved, that could lead to more positive interactions between her and her sister. At the same time, we agreed with Nadine that many of the tasks Anne was facing were overwhelming and that she needed occasional help with them. We then discussed with her the need to bring some help in so that Anne could get a break and could carry out her responsibilities more effectively. Over time, we were able to provide help with the immediate problem, providing adequate care for Sophie. Nadine was pleased to see her sister become more effective in managing care-related problems, and Anne gained a small measure of approval for her activities.

HOW THE PROCESS OF THERAPY CAN DIFFER WITH OLDER CLIENTS

We now turn to some of the ways that conducting therapy can differ. The challenge for therapists is to use their basic skills but with some subtle and not-so-subtle variations in style that make treatment work better for many older clients. It also involves being comfortable with discussions of issues that do not arise frequently with younger people. We do not mean to imply that it is necessary to make all these adjustments with every older person. In fact, the similarities in treating older people usually outweigh the differences (Miller & Silberman, 1996). Rather, therapists need to be ready to modify their basic approach some of the time in order to improve the effectiveness of treatment.

Being Patient with the Pace of Treatment

The biggest change we have to make when working with older clients is to be patient with the pace of treatment. Older people move at a slower pace and change comes in smaller increments (e.g., Zeiss & Steffen, 1996b). In part, this slower pace is due to differences in communication style. Older clients frequently take longer to get to the point. They may digress, telling anecdotes or recounting events that seem unrelated to the issue we are discussing. Some clients feel they have to tell the therapist everything about an issue or problem or about their lives.

We allow older clients as much time as they need to say what they have to say. Allowing them to take the time they need is helpful in building a therapeutic relationship. There may not be many people in their lives who take the time to listen to them. When few people value or pay attention to what they have to say, they may adopt the strategy of holding onto someone's attention for as long as they can—and then feel that doctors and other professionals are rushing them. A therapist needs to build a different kind of relationship and should not be in a hurry. We often remind ourselves that we may be the only ones who give this older client our undivided attention, and that helps us be more tolerant of the slower pace.

There is always a delicate balance between directing conversations too much and allowing too many digressions. Early in treatment we allow more digressions. Sometimes we learn something important during a digression. As we get to know clients better, we can redirect them when a digression seems to be a distraction.

There is also more repetition when treating older clients, both of things they say to us and what we say to them. We sometimes go over a point several times. Although this process may feel repetitious to the therapist, it does not to the client.

The slow pace and repetitions may partly reflect the learning process for some older clients. Older people generally learn more slowly and thus benefit more from repetitions and a slower pace. They may also make decisions more cautiously, which may contribute to the slower pace (see Chapter 2). Clients who are not sophisticated about how to use therapy also may make slower progress.

A counterforce is sometimes at work: older clients are frequently more goal-oriented in their treatment than younger people. They want to work on some specific problem or issue and then move on with their lives. Of course, older people who are excessively dependent or for whom the therapist is their main social outlet prolong therapy as long as possible. But many older clients are comfortable with time-limited and goal-oriented treatment.

The slower pace of treatment with older people is a concern because of the emphasis on managed care in the United States. As the number of older people joining managed health care programs grows, therapists can expect to run into limits on the number of covered sessions they can offer. Session limits are based on expectations developed with younger clients, and even then they are often too restrictive. In efforts to manage mental health care of older people, carriers need to understand that the pace of treatment is slower. Providing an adequate amount of treatment in the first place saves costs later on.

Addressing the Youthfulness of the Therapist

One of us referred a client to another member of our practice. When we told the client that she would be seeing Dr. Young, the client responded by asking, "Is she?" The answer was "Yes," which was a concern for this client.

Most therapists who work with older adults are younger than their clients. Although age differences are usually not a barrier, they may become an issue in treatment. The geriatric specialist learns to recognize and address problems associated with age differences that might arise during treatment.

In the example, the client was concerned not about the therapist's youth per se but about her experience. In other instances, clients feel that a young person cannot understand what they are going through. We have found that explaining in a nondefensive way our training in geropsychology usually is sufficient. As noted earlier, the development of a therapeutic relationship quickly allays most of these concerns.

We start a relationship with an older person with the assumption that although we are one up on our client in our role as therapist, we are one down in terms of age and experience. We always treat clients with respect. One of the reasons we allow older clients more leeway in getting to the point is that it is not respectful to interrupt. As the relationship evolves, it becomes more collaborative.

Giving Clients Control

An important issue for many older clients is actual or perceived threats to their independence. As part of how we deal with these threats, we allow clients to take control of some therapy issues. As an example, we sometimes allow clients to take control over how frequently they see us. After an initial period of weekly visits, they may decide to come biweekly or just once a month. It is often not clear why they want to reduce the frequency of visits. In some instances, they may not want to overuse their resources. In other cases, we have thought that clients did not want to indulge themselves by coming too frequently.

Irregular clients use their sessions productively. They get clarification of what has been going on in their lives, or they get help sorting out medical or other problems they may have been having.

Accommodating Sensory Problems

Just as sensory loss can affect assessment, it can also be a problem in therapy. When working with older clients, we have trained ourselves to talk louder (though not too loud), slower, and at a lower pitch. If someone hears better in one ear, we make sure we sit on that side. The office in which treatment is conducted should be free from background noise and be well lighted, without excessive glare. Older clients should not be positioned so that they are looking directly toward a window or a bright light.

Using Written Records

Because therapy places a considerable load on a client's short-term memory, some therapists recommend approaches that help older people compensate for deficiencies in memory (e.g., Zeiss & Steffen, 1996b). Using written notes, summaries, reminders, and similar approaches can reduce the load on a client's memory. Forms for recording events, behaviors, or feelings between sessions can also compensate for memory problems.

Frequent Themes in Treatment

Another source of differences is the topics or themes older clients discuss in therapy (Knight, 1986). We highlight four themes that are not typically encountered with younger clients or that take a different form when working with older clients: (1) medical issues; (2) dealing with "what if" questions; (3) death and dying; and (4) relationship issues and sexuality.

Medical Issues

The focus of treatment with older clients is often on medical problems. Just as we take medical issues into account when conducting an assessment and planning treatment, we also spend time understanding and interpreting the ongoing medical problems and experiences clients have.

Emphasis on medical problems takes different forms. Since many of our older clients have medical problems, we frequently work closely with physicians to coordinate medical and psychological treatment. We spend a lot of time gathering information, explaining, and clarifying. Sometimes we help the physician understand the symptoms the client is presenting; sometimes we help the client understand what the physician is recommending. We often play a consulting role with clients, going over with them what the physician has recommended and examining their choices. If a client is confused about what the doctor said, we offer to consult with the physician and get a copy of the medical records so that we can go over them with the client.

Some clients talk excessively about somatic symptoms. We have heard more about digestive problems and bowel movements from older clients than we ever wanted to know in a lifetime. We have learned to listen to these complaints, however, to find out if there is something psychological that leads a client to be so focused on a somatic symptom or if there could be a real medical problem. Interestingly, many somaticizing older clients do not think of themselves as frail or vulnerable. Rather, they are not good at identifying which complaints are important.

Generally, older clients present themselves to physicians in the same way they do to therapists, that is, they have trouble getting to the point and identifying which complaints are important. As a result, physicians sometimes stop paying attention and may fail to identify important new symptoms.

To deal with this problem, we teach clients a set of strategies for communicating with their doctors. We developed this approach based on conversations with physicians about how they evaluate and respond to patients' symptoms. Physicians have been trained to listen for certain kinds of information. When they do not hear that information or get distracted by too many complaints or digressions, they become frustrated and even lose interest. We teach clients how to phrase their complaints so that physicians are likely to pay attention. It could be argued that physicians should be skilled enough at interviewing patients to draw out the information they need, and some certainly are. Nonetheless, it is more practical to instruct patients how to present their problems effectively than to wait for physicians to change how they practice.

The starting point is for clients to plan an agenda for each visit. Their agenda should be limited to one or two problems. Physicians often stop listening when the patient brings a long list of complaints, dismissing the patient in their mind as a hypochondriac or complainer. The problems should be relatively recent, typically originating within the past three months. Physicians tend to lose interest in a problem that has become chronic, believing that there is less they can do to treat it. We work with clients to be as specific as possible when presenting symptoms, for example, stating "I have had a sticking pain in my left shoulder" rather than "I have had lots of pain recently." Even though the doctor may start the conversation by asking, "How are you feeling," he or she is really interested in finding out what the patient's main concern is. Getting to the point and being specific helps the interaction. Patients, however, should let the physician ask the first question, rather than launching into a list of complaints. Another step is working with clients to plan the questions they want to ask the doctor. Some clients may need to work on their listening skills so that they can process what the doctor says. Besides these specific suggestions, we help clients understand the time pressures modern physicians face and that they cannot expect the more leisurely and personalized care they received in the past.

These procedures help people present information to a physician in a clear and organized manner. That creates a favorable impression and also gives doctors the information they need to make a diagnosis and develop a treatment plan. With the immense financial pressures on medical practice, the physician's time is at a premium. The more efficiently patients can present their concerns, the better the process will work.

Medical problems come into play in a direct way in many cases. Clients with whom we work for any length of time invariably experience an unexpected illness, such as a heart attack or stroke. As their therapist, we need to be able to deal with clients' health changes, conveying support during the acute phase of their illness and then helping them maximize their potential for recovery. Therapists working with older people need to be comfortable talking about illness and disability and dealing with problems that sometimes cannot be changed.

When treating older clients with a serious illness or disability, clinicians sometimes focus on how they would feel in that kind of situation. As a result, they may not be able to help clients deal with what they are feeling or explore the practical alternatives for managing their situation. As an example, one of us developed a counseling program that was part of a treatment center for people with vision problems. At the beginning, we found ourselves at a loss for words when clients said that their life was no longer worth living because they could not see. With more experience, however, we became familiar with the many ways people can overcome vision loss and engage in satisfying and meaningful activities. Our role became helping clients explore the full range of options available to them rather than identifying with their feelings of loss.

Dealing with "What Ifs"

Another difference we find with older clients is the amount of time they dwell on possible risks, or "what ifs." Many older people are concerned about what would happen to them if they fell or needed help for other types of emergencies. Probably the biggest "what if" is the fear of going into a nursing home. People who already have lost some functioning are particularly concerned about what will happen to them if they decline further. There are exceptions, of course, but generally people prefer retaining as much independence as possible.

To deal with "what ifs," we help people identify resources that can address their concerns, either right now or in the future. We also help them differentiate between realistic and exaggerated fears. Finally, we help people develop scenarios that they are comfortable with, should they need more help. Finding ways of controlling what might happen reduces feelings of helplessness.

Death and Dying

Older clients are often concerned about their own death or about the loss of significant people in their lives. As Knight (1986) points out, much of the literature on counseling people about death is based on case studies of younger people with illnesses that have predictable trajectories, such as cancer. In contrast, older people's ways of dealing with death are likely to be more varied. Fear and anxiety about death are not common among the elderly but can be significant for some clients. Some people are concerned about controlling the circumstances of their dying, such as not having unwanted medical procedures. Some have unfinished emotional business with their family or issues that they want to resolve before they die. Other people are grieving for the loss of a spouse, child, or other significant people. They may question why they have been left behind or believe they cannot go on with their lives.

Therapists need to be comfortable talking about death and dying and letting clients know they can talk about these issues. Therapists also need to know where they stand on end-of-life issues and not let their own beliefs interfere with clients making their own decisions.

It is possible to be too focused on issues of death and dying. We once supervised a doctoral student who had a great deal of interest in death and dying. When her first client began focusing on these issues, we thought it was a good coincidence that the client's concerns matched the therapist's interests. When her subsequent clients also began dwelling on death and dying instead of their presenting problems, we realized that the therapist was shaping their responses to what she believed was the main issue, rather than letting them define their concerns in their own way. Therapists need to come to terms with their own beliefs and feelings so that they do not distort or misinterpret what clients say or feel.

Therapists also have to be prepared to lose clients. We find ourselves in an ambiguous situation; we are not a family member but we have some of the feelings a family member would have. When appropriate, we attend the funeral, both for ourselves and to respect our client and his or her family.

Relationship Issues and Sexuality

Though old age is often a time of losses, it is also a period in life when important relationships continue and even when new relationships form. Older clients may be concerned about relationship issues, for instance, working out problems in a long-standing relationship and developing new relationships. They may want to address conflict with a spouse or child, or they may seek help with family strains that have emerged as the result of recent stresses or changes.

Sexuality and sexual feelings are not frequently part of treatment, but therapists need to be aware that they can emerge as an important issue. Clinicians can be helpful in a number of ways. They need to convey acceptance of a discussion of sexual feelings. Because of stereotypes about sexuality and aging, some older people believe that they should not have these feelings or should not talk about them. Several years ago, one of us conducted an initial assessment with an older woman who was concerned that she might have a sexually transmitted disease. She had been to her doctor, who told her that that was impossible for someone her age. Yet she had recently had unprotected sex with someone she did not know well, and there was a foundation for her concern. While this example is extreme, it underscores the importance of recognizing sexuality and helping clients feel comfortable talking about sexual issues and feelings. Therapists also need to be aware of generational differences in sexual beliefs and practices and the degree of comfort different people have in talking about their sexuality.

When an older client has a sexual problem, the therapist should be able to assess and treat it. As with other problems of aging, sexual difficulties may have their origins in illnesses and/or medications. A careful assessment to determine the extent to which illness and medication may contribution to sexual difficulties is necessary. When physiological factors do not play a major role in sexual difficulties, sex therapy techniques that have proven effective with younger clients can be used with older people (Whitlatch & Zarit, 1988). These techniques include the use of specific procedures and exercises to improve functioning, as well as helping clients recognize and adjust to changes that occur with aging, such as more time needed to become aroused.

Issues for Clinicians

We also want to highlight three professional issues for therapists working with older clients: (1) the client–therapist relationship; (2) the duration of treatment; and (3) the use of empirically validated treatment.

Client–Therapist Relationship

Many of the issues we have presented in preceding sections have to do with not letting one's own biases enter the therapy situation. When working with older people such issues as illness and death and dying, as well as age and generational factors, can touch on a therapist's prejudices.

Therapists also need to monitor their feelings and reactions toward clients to avoid bringing into the relationship issues or conflicts they have or have had in their personal lives. When undetected, such responses interfere with treatment. Therapists who develop strong positive feelings toward a client may overlook or minimize important problems or deficits in the client's behavior. Sometimes new or inexperienced counselors see their role as overcoming the negative bias and stereotypes about old age through their relationships with clients. But as with any other group, the elderly include people who are not likable or who engage in self-defeating or otherwise aggravating patterns of behavior. An overly positive counselor will fail to detect these behaviors, which may, in fact, be contributing to the client's adjustment difficulties. Conversely, we often experience negative reactions to clients. These feelings can help identify ways in which the client is having trouble in other relationships. But it is important to be able to differentiate between reactions to the client's behavior and reactions because the client in some way reminds the therapist of someone in his or her life. Therapists are obligated to work the latter issues out on their own or through consultation or supervision.

Clients, of course, can have a distorted view of the therapist. Therapists must learn to monitor how clients are responding to them and how to recognize and use distortions in treatment. Sometimes distortions reveal how clients approach other relationship in their lives. Rather than pointing out distortions to clients, which would not do any good, we develop strategies for using them. When clients view us in an exaggeratedly positive way, we build on that to encourage new behaviors. It is also possible to use negative reactions creatively. As an example, an older woman who is angry with her children may regard a therapist who is the same age as her children as taking their side or failing to understand her needs. Empathizing with this client, that is, agreeing that the therapist cannot really know or understand what the woman has gone through, can paradoxically provide understanding and build the basis of a therapeutic alliance.

Duration of Treatment

Most therapy with older clients is relatively brief, lasting 4 to 6 months. We see a small number of older clients on a long-term basis. These clients often have chronic physical and mental health problems and either have no family at all or relatives who live at some distance. Therapy serves as a sounding board for relatively isolated individuals. It helps them address problems and concerns and probably reduces inappropriate use of medical services for their psychological complaints. We often see these clients monthly, or as needed when problems develop.

The role these long-term clients often place us in is that of the valued child who is supportive and accessible. We can accept this role while keeping in place appropriate boundaries on our time and involvement.

Developing Empirically Based Treatments for Older Adults

There is a growing movement toward using treatments that have at least some empirical support for their effectiveness. Toward that goal, the Division of Clinical Psychology of the American Psychological Association has developed criteria for empirically validated treatments (Chambless et al., 1996). Using these criteria, Gatz and her colleagues (in press) reviewed the literature on treatment of older people. Although there have been far fewer controlled outcome studies of older adults than younger adults, many approaches met the standard for effective treatment (see also Gallagher-Thompson & Thompson, 1995; Scogin & McElreath, 1994).

We support this effort to develop a more rational, research-based body of knowledge for making treatment decisions. Much still has to be learned, however, about treatment of older people, and it is likely that other treatments that have positive outcomes will emerge in time. Thus, while it is useful to identify which treatments have been empirically validated, it would be premature to limit practice to only those treatments. That type of approach would stunt development of clinical practice by preventing therapists from taking new and creative directions in their work. It would also greatly limit older people who could receive treatment to those who fall within the diagnostic categories investigated to date. Standards of practice are necessary, and clinicians should use empirically validated approaches when possible. For the majority of people seeking help, however, no such empirically based guidelines are available. In these situations, clinicians are obliged to evaluate the success of their treatment by carefully monitoring progress. Clinicians need to know when treatment is not helping so that they can discontinue it and try something else. With the growth of managed care and the ongoing cost pressures on Medicare, we expect that there will be efforts to restrict psychotherapy of older adults. By practicing responsibly, therapists can contribute valuable clinical findings on the uses of psychotherapy with older adults that justify the cost and point to the benefits that their clients receive.

CASE EXAMPLES

The following examples illustrate some of the unique features of working with older clients. The first case examines the role medical problems play in treatment and how therapists can help their clients clarify and make decisions about their medical care. The client, previously presented in Chapter 5, had suffered a delirium when a physician changed a blood pressure medication she had been taking. She was referred for treatment to get help in her recovery from the delirium and to deal with the consequences of her health problems.

The client was a 75-year-old retired nurse with multiple health problems. In her 60s she had developed emphysema. More recently, she had had heart bypass surgery. She suffered from hypertension and diabetes and diabetic retinopathy was affecting her vision. Despite her health problems, she was completely independent, living in her own apartment in the community. (People with multiple health problems whom we might expect would have a great deal of difficulty functioning independently are often able to continue an active lifestyle with little or no modifications. Of course, sometimes the opposite is true, that a person with relatively circumscribed health problems does not feel able to carry out his or her usual activities.) One factor contributing to her good functioning was that, as a retired nurse, she kept exact records of her health. In a notebook, she wrote down her vital signs, when she took each medication, and every calorie she ate. As a result, her diabetes was in very good control.

The initial plan was for short-term treatment to get her back on an even keel. After making gradual progress over the course of several sessions, she took control of the frequency of visits, setting appointments about one month apart. We could insist that a younger client come every week. But we believed the ex-nurse needed to feel in control of her life, so we let her set the frequency.

The focus of sessions was initially her anxiety that the delirium would return. The feeling of being out of control during the delirium greatly unnerved this woman. Despite her understanding of her medical problems, it took her a year to feel competent again and not embarrassed over what she had said and done during the delirium.

Gradually, the focus of treatment shifted to consultation on her medical problems. During the year we were treating her, all her medical doctors changed. Her therapist was the one constant for her during this time. Changing physicians is another frequent issue older clients face, when their physicians retire or, as in this case, move out of the area. The readjustment to new physicians is often associated with anxiety, especially for someone whose medical condition is fragile.

We helped this client understand the plans developed by her new doctors. For example, she went for the first time to see an optometrist about the vision problems caused by her diabetic retinopathy. After that visit, we had the optometrist send over a copy of her records so that we could review them with her. We played a similar role with her other doctors. Although her problems were mainly medical, there was a component of anxiety that potentially could have made her condition worse. The monthly therapy visits, however, had a calming effect.

Other concerns arose as well. Winter driving worried her. She did not want to drive in icy or snowy conditions but feared being completely cut off, unable to shop or get to the doctor. To deal with this concern, we introduced her to a geriatric case manager, who could arrange help if she needed it. The winter turned out to be relatively mild, and she did not need a driver, but it relieved her anxiety to know she had someone to call.

This case illustrates several typical features about treatment of an older person. First and foremost was the focus on the client's medical problems and our role in clarifying and helping her interpret what her doctors were doing, thereby lowering her overall anxiety. This case also illustrates an older person taking control of the frequency of visits. Last, we linked her to a community service, in this case, to a care manager who could arrange for a driver.

The next case involves a woman in her late 60s who had become progressively anxious and depressed, though there was no clear precipitating event. Seeking treatment for the symptoms, the family took her to a psychiatrist, who wrote a prescription and then went on vacation. When the patient worsened on the medication and could not get hold of the psychiatrist, the family had her hospitalized. After a brief examination by a hospital psychiatrist, she was given a major tranquilizer and a drug for a bipolar disorder. (There was no apparent history of manic depression, and the reason for prescribing these medications was not clear.) Her condition worsened on these medications and she gradually withdrew and became inactive. Discharged from the hospital, she came under the care of a third psychiatrist, who changed the medications once again, this time to an antidepressant, a tranquilizer, and a sleeping pill. At this point, the daughter contacted us for an assessment and treatment.

The initial session was conducted in the client's home. The client lived with her husband. Both of them had been very active in community organizations until her depression. At this time, she was very depressed, but there was no indication of cognitive impairment. She was spending most of her time in bed and was not engaging in self-care activities. Her husband was continuing his activities while providing assistance to his wife.

The treatment plan was psychotherapy for depression. We consulted with the most recent psychiatrist, who decided to continue the current medications for awhile (the change had been made quite recently) to determine if they were having any effect. The patient was advised, however, to wean herself off the sleeping pill, as sleeping medications are most effective for short-term treatment of insomnia and could now be making her situation worse.

Treatment involved building an empathic relationship and utilizing behavioral and cognitive-behavioral strategies to reduce depression. A major goal of these approaches was to encourage the patient to resume activities that she had previously enjoyed and valued and to address negative beliefs that prevented her from increasing her level of activity. Because her husband was involved in helping her with self-care activities and in trying to get her to resume some of her former activities, it was decided to have one session a week with both of them and one session with the patient alone. In this manner, the husband could work with her in encouraging specific activities or in supporting the steps she was taking in treatment. Leaving him out would have left open the possibility that he would work at cross-purposes with us or that the client would resist his encouragement to become more active and therefore also resist our efforts. By holding a joint session, we could pursue a strategic approach that enlisted both husband and wife in agreed-on assignments. The client showed gradual but steady improvement and was able to resume her normal activities.

This case incorporated several common features of therapy with older clients. A critical first step was coordinating psychotherapy with the use of psychotropic medications. A basic approach to psychotherapy for depression was initiated that incorporated a family approach as well as individual treatment. The complexity in this case is by no means typical, but it does indicate the types of knowledge and skill therapists must draw on when working with older clients.

CONCLUSIONS

In this chapter, we have presented basic issues in psychological treatment of older people. Is psychotherapy with older people different from treatment with younger age groups? In many instances, treatment proceeds in similar ways and is equally effective. But there are subtle and not-so-subtle differences. The psychotherapist needs to draw on a wider range of skills when working with older clients. Medical comorbidities are likely to be of far greater importance with older clients, as is an understanding of the client's family system. Goals may be more focused and limited and treatment may proceed more slowly than with younger clients. More needs to be learned about the efficacy of various treatments and the conditions under which treatment response can be maximized. Nonetheless, a growing body of clinical studies and controlled research is emerging that indicates that psychotherapy is an effective treatment with older people. In subsequent chapters, we explore how psychotherapy approaches have been adapted for treatment of specific problems.

8

Treatment of Depression

Depression affects more older people than any other mental health problem. Fortunately, a growing body of evidence suggests that treatment of older depressed people is very effective, whether with medications, psychotherapy, or a combination of the two. Despite these optimistic findings, older people frequently do not receive optimal treatment or any treatment at all. In this chapter we examine treatment for depression, with particular attention to features of treatment that are unique or different when working with older people. Case studies demonstrate how treatment principles are implemented.

We focus extensively on depression because of its prevalence and as a model of key treatment issues with older people. An extensive literature on treatment of depression has developed, including outcome studies that document the effectiveness of different approaches. No other area of geropsychology has as well-developed an empirical foundation for treatment. In addition, treatment of depression illustrates the major problems and issues that clinicians encounter when working with older people. Our discussion highlights these issues, including modification of basic treatment approaches for use with older clients, comorbidity of psychiatric and medical problems, coordination of medications and psychotherapy, and the involvement of the family. While our emphasis is on depression, it will be apparent how the basic treatment framework can be applied to other disorders.

PSYCHOTHERAPY AS A TREATMENT FOR DEPRESSION

Studies with younger clients have established the effectiveness of psychotherapy as a treatment for depression. In a review of 58 studies, Robinson, Berman, and Niemeyer (1990) found that psychotherapy is associated with consistent and significant improvements in mood, compared to control conditions, that the benefits are long lasting, and that the amount of improvement is comparable to treatment with antidepressant medications. Although the literature on treatment of depression among older people is more limited, Scogin and McElreath (1994) drew similar conclusions. Reviewing 17 studies that used a control group, they found that psychotherapy was reliably associated with decreases in depression. In fact, the effect size (a statistical estimate of the amount of improvement, expressed in standard deviation units) was somewhat greater in the studies of older clients than that reported for younger clients. Older clients receiving psychotherapy improved on average three quarters of a standard deviation on depression measures.

Outcome studies have thus far documented the effectiveness of psychotherapy compared to control conditions but have not identified which psychotherapeutic approaches are most likely to be effective. Many treatment studies, however, have focused on three structured psychotherapy approaches that have been developed specifically for use with depression. These approaches are behavioral therapy for depression, particularly the method developed by Peter Lewinsohn and his associates (Lewinsohn et al., 1992); cognitive-behavioral treatment, developed by Aaron Beck and colleagues (1979); and interpersonal psychotherapy (IPT), developed by Gerald Klerman and associates (1984). These therapies were initially developed for younger people, but each has been adapted for use with older clients. In the following sections, we look at the main elements of these three therapies and review evidence of their effectiveness. We also consider the many features that these treatments have in common. Although starting from different theoretical orientations, the three approaches converge in the methods they use, which suggests that some techniques may be essential in treatment of depressed clients. Clinicians may be able to combine elements from each of these approaches in creative ways to develop individualized treatment plans for particular clients.

Behavioral Therapy for Depression

Building on the work of Peter Lewinsohn (Lewinsohn et al., 1992), a behavioral therapy for depression has been developed that has had good outcome results with both younger and older adults (Gallagher-Thompson & Thompson, 1995; Scogin & McElreath, 1994). The starting point for this approach is observation of what depressed people do and don't do. As Lewinsohn and his associates detailed in a series of studies, depressed people engage in fewer behaviors than do nondepressed people, particularly pleasant or reinforcing behaviors, or what they have termed pleasant events (PE). This low rate of output of behaviors that are reinforced or reinforcing leads to a vicious cycle in which mood is lowered, further decreasing the output of behavior, and so on. Given this association between mood and pleasant events, the most parsimonious approach to treatment of depression is to increase the frequency with which clients engage in behaviors they find enjoyable.

As experienced clinicians know, giving direct advice to clients to change their behavior is usually not successful. Lewinsohn and his colleagues (1992) have developed a sophisticated approach that goes beyond simple advice and facilitates change. Seven features of treatment are particularly relevant to treatment of older, depressed patients:

Clients as Active Participants in Treatment

Clients are actively involved in the treatment process. Lewinsohn's model includes a strong psychoeducational component, which instructs clients about their problems and about the process of change. Treatment begins with an explanation of the rationale of the approach, in effect instructing clients how they can use therapy to get better. The therapist explains that the client's mood is related to everyday activities. Engaging in more pleasant or rewarding activities will improve mood, while engaging in fewer of those activities worsens mood. Depression is viewed as the result of a vicious cycle in which a person may feel sad because of events in his life, then decrease pleasant activities, feel worse as a result, and then decrease activities further. Treatment involves breaking out of this vicious cycle.

As treatment proceeds, clients become increasingly active, completing various assignments and tasks. This approach contributes directly to reducing depression because it breaks the cycle of passivity and withdrawal. It may also foster skills to improve coping or self-efficacy, thereby reducing the probability of a recurrence of depression.

Contracting with Clients

Of course, encouraging depressed patients to be more active and having them do so are two different matters. A key part of the treatment is developing a contract with clients, through which they agree to perform certain tasks. Clients need to be engaged by the therapist through the use of basic therapeutic skills such as empathy that build trust. In the context of an empathic and accepting relationship, the therapist can then work with clients to develop specific plans for action and to gain their agreement to try out these steps. Although behavioral therapy can sometimes be presented in didactic ways, we have found it better to use a collaborative approach with clients. This type of approach is more likely to gain compliance and lead to clients taking more responsibility for their own behavior.

Developing Graded and Specific Tasks

A key feature contributing to the success of behavioral approaches is the use of graded and specific tasks. Initial tasks need to be planned very carefully, with the dual purposes of gaining compliance and having some initial, albeit small, success. Once clients successfully complete a task, it becomes easier to implement the next part of the treatment plan.

Tasks in a treatment plan should be graded; that is, they should proceed from simple steps that are likely to be successful to more complex and challenging behavior. Initial tasks should not be difficult or complex to perform and should have a high probability of success. For example, a depressed older person might be asked to exercise for 5 minutes a day. Although the client might have exercised previously for longer periods of time, the client and the therapist might decide that 5 minutes is an amount that the client can manage right now. In addition to keeping the task simple, it needs to be specific (e.g., what type of exercise) and scheduled for a definite time and place. Clients may say that they do not see how such simple tasks can help them with such a large problem as depression. They may also compare their performance to what they previously could do. When clients respond in those ways, the therapist can explain that these tasks are building blocks, the first steps that need to be taken in treatment, and that they will make it possible to address more serious problems.

Developing a thorough and detailed plan is very important. When first trying a behavioral approach, therapists sometimes do not spend enough time working out the details of assignments. A poorly specified task leaves an opening for the client to fail.

Monitoring Mood and Behavior

Clients learn to monitor their own mood and activities and to observe connections between what they do and how they are feeling. These steps are a central feature of treatment. They enable clients to take more control over their mood and to become active in the treatment of their depression.

Clients monitor their mood by providing a summary score each day for how they are feeling. Depression scales can be used during office visits to provide additional information on the course of symptoms. Clients also record specific behaviors, including pleasant and aversive events. Working with these records, the therapist can demonstrate how mood varies in relation to activities.

Increasing Pleasant Events

The central element of treatment is to increase the frequency with which clients engage in pleasant activities. There are two initial steps for planning this intervention. First, the clinician identifies what events or activities are potentially reinforcing, that is, events the client experiences as pleasant. This approach differs from simply telling someone to get more active or choosing a set of activities for them. Selection of activities comes from an individualized list, developed by clients, of activities that reflect their preferences.

Lewinsohn and his colleagues (Lewinsohn & Libet, 1972; Lewinsohn & MacPhillamy, 1974) developed the Pleasant Events Schedule, a list of over 300 activities that people experience as pleasant. Clients respond to each activity by indicating how frequently they have engaged in it recently and how enjoyable they find it. A shorter form has been developed specifically for use with older clients (Teri & Lewinsohn, 1982).

The second step is to obtain a baseline of the frequency with which clients engage in activities they find pleasurable. Usually the rate is quite low for depressed clients. Sometimes there are variations during the baseline period. The therapist may be able to use the records to point out that small increases in pleasant activities are associated with improved mood.

After establishing the baseline, therapist and client develop a plan to increase the number of pleasant activities. As noted, this plan must be specific and achievable by the client. Depressed clients avoid or postpone plans that are overly ambitious or vague. Written schedules and assignments are used as reminders for clients of any age and may be particularly helpful for older clients (Zeiss & Steffen, 1996b). Schedules serve as a concrete way for clients and therapists alike to monitor the progress of treatment.

As clients increase the frequency of pleasant activities, their mood generally begins to improve. This is often a critical point in therapy. Clients may come back after doing a behavioral assignment and say that they do not feel better, yet they look better and rate their mood as improved compared to prior ratings. What they are telling the therapist is that they do not yet feel as they used to. Client and therapist review together the records of mood and pleasant activities to confirm the association between what the client is doing and feeling. The therapist may reframe what clients are saying to reflect that they still in the early stages of treatment. By pointing out how mood has improved, the therapist can assure them that they are on the right track and that continuing in this direction will lead to further improvement. Once their mood begins improving, clients can go on to other tasks, which may be more difficult, including addressing aversive events in their lives, dealing with problems in social relationships, and treating cognitive features of depression.

Decreasing Aversive Events

Depressed people frequently have stressful or aversive events in their lives. In a comparable way to pleasant events, Lewinsohn and associates

(1986) assess which activities or events clients find unpleasant. Events are defined as aversive based on clients' perceptions, not on an arbitrary classification system. An activity such as housecleaning can be experienced differently by different clients. Some find it pleasant to clean the house, while others experience it as aversive. An instrument similar to the Pleasant Events Schedule has been developed for assessing aversive events (Lewinsohn et al., 1992).

The therapist focuses on reducing unpleasant or aversive events once a client's mood has begun to improve. Again, it is important to begin with problems that can be managed readily or problems over which clients have some control. For example, a client may want to have fewer arguments with her daughter. That is a goal that may require the client to change her behavior in complex ways, and it may be partly out of her control since her daughter must also respond differently to her. As a result, it might be better to start with a simpler task over which the client has more control (e.g., limiting the amount of time she cleans the house so that she has more time for other activities).

Cognitive and Social Skills

The behavioral model of treating depression also includes a focus on changing beliefs or cognitions that contribute to depression and improving social skills, such as becoming more assertive or learning how to communicate more effectively with other people. These features are dealt with extensively in the other two treatment approaches discussed.

Applications of Behavioral Treatment for Older People

Zeiss and Steffen (1996b) summarize the advantages of the behavioral approach for treatment of older people. The therapist is a collaborator with clients, developing a supportive relationship and encouraging them to be actively involved. The therapist brings one type of expertise into the relationship concerning treatment methods, but clients are the experts in their own experiences and skills. This approach is very useful with older people who are not psychologically minded. Behavioral treatment involves a very large element of common sense and an absence of psychological jargon, which appeals to many clients. For older clients, record keeping and scheduling can reduce concerns about failing memory. Finally, treatment is time-limited, which reduces the concern many older people have about the cost of treatment and counters the common stereotype of psychotherapy as open-ended and always long term.

Cognitive-Behavioral Therapy for Depression

Although sharing many elements with behavioral therapy, cognitive-behavioral therapy differs by giving primacy to the role of cognitions in the development of mood problems. According to Aaron Beck's classic formulation (1976; Beck et al., 1979), depressed people are likely to interpret the events in their lives in an excessively negative manner. They take pessimistic views of themselves, other people, and the future, interpret positive or neutral events as negative, and exaggerate the consequences of aversive events.

As in behavioral therapy, the cognitive therapist begins with an explanation of the rationale for treatment. Typically, the therapist explains that people's interpretation of events affects how they feel. Using an example from a client's own experiences can be useful, or the therapist can draw on general examples. In a pamphlet designed to orient clients to cognitive-behavioral therapy, Beck and Greenberg (1974) use the following example:

> Suppose you are walking down the street and you see a friend who appears to completely ignore you. Naturally you feel sad. You may wonder why your friend has turned against you. Later on you mention the incident to your friend, who tells you he was so preoccupied at the time that he didn't even see you. Normally, you will feel better and put the incident out of your mind. If you are depressed, however, you will probably believe your friend has really rejected you. You may not even ask him about it, allowing the mistake to go uncorrected. Depressed persons make such mistakes over and over. . . . They tend to see the negative rather than the positive side of things. And they do not check to determine whether they have made a mistake in interpreting events. (Beck & Greenberg, 1974, p. 2)

Also as in behavioral therapy, cognitive-behavioral therapy begins with a focus on daily behaviors and activities. Clients record activities and mood, and the therapist works with them to develop plans to increase activities or to solve immediate and pressing problems. The therapist starts with behavioral interventions for two reasons. First, increasing behavior is a good way to produce some immediate relief from depression. As a consequence, clients have more energy to work on cognitive dimensions of depression. Second, the focus on activities generates examples of the client's typical thought patterns or ways of interpreting events.

As in behavioral therapy, the cognitive therapist uses graded task assignments. After clients agree to a task, the therapist can have them cognitively rehearse the steps involved in carrying it out (Beck et al., 1979). The therapist asks, "What do you think would prevent you from being able to do this assignment?" As an example, a client who agrees to phone an old friend may realize she does not have her friend's phone number. Obstacles may also be cognitive. The same client may believe that it has been so long since she talked with her friend that her friend will reject her. Planning can be done to overcome these obstacles so that the assignment will eventually be carried out.

Characteristics of Cognitive-Behavioral Therapy

The main emphasis in treatment is on identifying characteristic thought patterns, that is, how clients typically appraise the events in their lives. In depressed people, thought patterns are marked by logical errors that lead to incorrect conclusions and consequently to feelings of depression. A depressed client may, for example, focus on the negative moments in a recent experience, ignoring the majority of the event that was positive. Other common patterns are to make incorrect inferences about the intention or meaning of an event and to exaggerate the negative consequences of an event.

As an example, an older woman had interviewed for a job and had not heard from the company. She concluded that she had not gotten the job, that companies preferred hiring only younger women, and that she would never get a job. The therapist encouraged her to test her inferences by calling the company. It turned out that they had been trying to call her back for another interview. This example illustrates how incorrect inferences (that she had not gotten the job) can lead to exaggerated or catastrophic interpretations and to intense feelings of depression. Without the therapist's intervention, the client would have acted on her incorrect beliefs (that she had not gotten the job and that her situation was hopeless) and would have remained mired in her depression. This example also illustrates the connection between clients' interpretations of events and effective behavior.

In cognitive-behavioral therapy, clients are taught to recognize and then record these "automatic" thoughts. These types of thoughts are "automatic" because they occur quickly and spontaneously as we evaluate a situation, and we are often not aware of them. The use of written thought records helps clients recognize how they are interpreting events. Focusing on situations in which they feel sad or depressed, clients write down what happened and what thoughts they were having at the time. By writing these thoughts down as close to the occurrence of an event as possible, clients learn to recognize thought processes that trigger depressed feelings.

Once dysfunctional thought patterns are identified, therapist and client work collaboratively to test the beliefs behind them. A lot of time is spent logically examining the assumptions made by clients and generating alternatives. Beliefs can be tested through experiments, such as in the example in which the client called her prospective employer. Other ways of examining thoughts include reframing, determining whether the evidence supports a particular conclusion, and generating alternative explanations. As clients generate more adaptive alternative thoughts, they begin substituting these new cognitions for dysfunctional ways of interpreting events.

The following dialogues illustrate the use of these techniques.

Reframing

CLIENT: I've been really depressed this week. I've barely exercised at all.

THERAPIST: How many times did you exercise?

CLIENT: Only twice, and I quit after half an hour each time.

THERAPIST: Well, you wanted to exercise a minimum of 20 minutes, three times a week, which would be 60 minutes. So you could look at what you have done as meeting your goal for how long you would exercise, even though you still want to work on how often you exercise.

CLIENT: That doesn't seem so bad.

In this example, the client has actually met part of his goals but has discounted his whole effort and gains no satisfaction from what he accomplished. The therapist examines what the client has actually done and suggests a way of reframing the situation. Part of this process involves examining the evidence, the second cognitive technique that we describe.

Examining the Evidence

CLIENT: I feel all alone in the world. My husband is gone, and since we never had children, I don't have anyone to look after me.

THERAPIST: Who do you see on a day-to-day basis?

CLIENT: Well, my neighbors in the apartment building, but they have enough problems of their own.

THERAPIST: Do you see any of your relatives?

CLIENT: I talk to my brothers every week and my niece comes by to take me out nearly every week. But they have their own families.

THERAPIST: Do you do anything in the community?

CLIENT: I want to go to Senior Citizens, but I haven't gotten there yet. When the weather is good, I go to church.

THERAPIST: So it sounds as if you really are lonely for your husband, but when you look at your day-to-day life, there are a number of people you are in contact with.

CLIENT: I guess I'm not completely alone, but I am lonely.

By examining the evidence, the therapist shows that the client's extreme statement that she is all alone in the world is not accurate. These types of extreme statements result in strong feelings of sadness. This example also illustrates that the therapist does not dispute with the client but instead uses questions to gather information and then summarizes the information in a way that gently reframes the conclusions the client has drawn about herself. Being lonely is still associated with negative feelings, but it is not as extreme a view of one self as being all alone, and it is a problem with many possible solutions.

Alternative Explanations

CLIENT: My son and his family don't care about me. That's why they didn't invite me along when they drove up to Massachusetts to pick up my grandson.

THERAPIST: I wonder if you can think of any other reason they might not have asked you?

CLIENT: No, I think they don't want to spend time with me.

THERAPIST: Could they have thought that such a long ride would be uncomfortable for you? Or might they have been looking forward to the drive to have some time alone to talk together?

CLIENT: I never thought about that. They *might* have some other reason.

As clients progress in treatment, they learn to generate alternatives by themselves and to recognize how jumping to conclusions without examining the alternatives often leads to feeling depressed. Once clients have considered the alternatives, they can test which explanation is correct, as in the earlier example of the woman who had interviewed for a job.

Therapists need to be able to differentiate exaggerated or negative thoughts from social stereotypes about aging (Blazer, 1993). A client may claim that she is too old to change or that her problems are due solely to other people or the situation she finds herself in. These types of beliefs may seem especially compelling if they are linked with physical disabilities. Therapists with limited experience with older clients may be willing to accept these conclusions uncritically, thereby maintaining negative beliefs that contribute to depression. Examination of these types of thoughts usually reveals that they represent overgeneralizations and that clients have alternatives they are overlooking. We return to this point later in the chapter.

The process of conducting cognitive-behavioral therapy is important. The early sessions are used to develop a therapeutic relationship with the client that is characterized by empathy and a nonjudgmental attitude (Beck et al., 1979; Gallagher-Thompson & Thompson, 1996). The relationship should be collaborative. As the focus of treatment turns to clients' beliefs, therapists should avoid turning these discussions into arguments. They should also avoid fostering excessive dependencies.

Closing sessions can be used to prepare clients for the possibility of relapses and how to deal with them. During the final session, cognitive therapists usually review the therapy, summarizing the problems presented, the techniques that were most effective, and predicting certain anticipated problem areas in the future. The therapist can promise a booster session, should something unexpected occur. Sometimes just knowing that this is possible eases the anxiety the client might have about termination. Because of the tendency for depressed people to exaggerate negative events, it is important to suggest that relapses are minor and expected events that they have the skills to manage, rather than evidence that the therapy has failed.

Modifications of Cognitive-Behavioral Therapy for Older Adults

The therapist may want to make some modifications in cognitive-behavioral therapy for older people, especially for clients who are frail or have disabilities (Gallagher-Thompson & Thompson, 1996; Grant & Casey, 1995; Zeiss & Steffen, 1996b). Among the modifications are (1) proceeding at a slower pace; (2) determining whether the client has an unrealistic or negative expectation about therapy (e.g., only crazy people go to a therapist); (3) taking a family systems perspective and involving families, when appropriate, in helping with compliance; allowing the focus to shift from the here and now to include life review; and (4) making referrals to appropriate professionals (e.g., physical therapist) to treat related problems.

Interpersonal Psychotherapy for Depression

Interpersonal psychotherapy focuses on interpersonal problems in the patient's life as the major source of depression. Developed by Klerman and associates (1984), interpersonal psychotherapy has been found to be an effective treatment with younger individuals (e.g., Elkin et al., 1989; Frank et al., 1990). Preliminary studies suggest that this approach can be adapted successfully with older clients (Miller & Silberman, 1996), including those who are also medically ill (Mossey, Knott, Higgins, & Talerico, 1996).

Characteristics of Interpersonal Psychotherapy

The central focus of interpersonal psychotherapy is relationship issues, which is a common problem for depressed older adults. They may have concerns about a husband or wife or more often about children or friends or difficulties meeting new people and forming friendships. Some older clients complain of loneliness yet act in social situations in ways that drive people away. Interpersonal psychotherapy explicitly examines these relationship issues and what older clients can do to improve them.

As with behavioral therapy and cognitive-behavioral therapy, interpersonal psychotherapy is structured and time-limited. The typical length of treatment is between 12 and 20 weekly sessions (Miller & Silberman, 1996).

Treatment begins with an assessment to identify depressive symptoms and their sources. The assessment includes a review of the client's past and current relationships. The therapist identifies who is or has been important in the person's life, which interactions are conflicted or problematic, and which relationships are associated with the current episode of depression or with prior episodes. As with behavioral therapy and cognitive-behavioral therapy, interpersonal psychotherapy emphasizes establishing rapport with clients and explaining how treatment works.

Four broad areas are considered critical in the development of depression (Klerman et al., 1984; Miller & Silberman, 1996): (1) grief, (2) interpersonal disputes, (3) role transitions, and (4) interpersonal deficits. Assessment determines which areas are involved. In each case, the therapist encourages clients to develop more adaptive behavior to overcome the problem. With grief, for example, the therapist encourages the mourning process and then works with clients to identify ways to replace or compensate for the loss. The therapist is active throughout treatment, offering reassurance and support.

A major focus of treatment is helping clients improve their communication with other people. The main emphasis is on current problems and relationships, not past issues or intrapsychic phenomena. Although past relationships are acknowledged for their influence on the present, clients are encouraged to work on their current situation.

Modifications of Interpersonal Psychotherapy for Older Clients

As with the other depression treatments, interpersonal psychotherapy is modified somewhat for use with older clients (Miller & Silberman, 1996). One such modification is the use of shorter sessions, if an older client cannot tolerate a full-length therapy session. Older clients may have more limited options for replacing problem relationships, so the therapist is more likely to encourage working out these problems rather than discarding relationships. The therapist may also need to role-play with the client to develop new interpersonal skills.

Similarities of the Three Psychotherapy Approaches for Treating Depression

These three treatments for depression share many points of similarity. All are structured and require active intervention by the therapist. The focus is generally on the here and now, that is, the immediate events and beliefs associated with feelings of depression. All have a strong psychoeducational component, teaching clients how their own actions affect their mood and how they can change their mood. Clients are helped to break out of the cycle of depression by changing behaviors in their daily life and thinking differently about themselves and other people. The emphasis is on changing habitual actions that have contributed to depression and replacing them with more adaptive behaviors. Clients are assigned tasks to perform between sessions as a way of either gathering data for treatment or implementing new actions. This convergence of techniques in the three approaches suggests that the method of treatment—direct, structured, focused on the here and now—may be as important to positive outcomes as the specific theoretical orientation.

Therapists using these approaches also concur on the types modifications that are helpful with older people: a somewhat slower pace of treatment, use of written assignments and other aids to offset memory problems, and the careful handling of the therapeutic relationship: the relationship is supportive without encouraging dependencies that might be difficult to reverse.

Given the similarities among the three approaches, therapists can probably draw techniques from each and develop a synthesis that uses interventions most suited to a particular client. They can focus on increasing or decreasing specific behaviors, on automatic thoughts, or on social relationships, depending on the client. As in any situation, therapists should monitor a client's progress closely and modify procedures that are not proving to be effective in altering mood.

Applications of Psychotherapy for Depression

The basic principles used in treatment of depression can be implemented in other formats besides traditional one-on-one psychotherapy. A group therapy protocol for cognitive-behavioral therapy has been found to be effective (Beutler et al., 1987) . Lewinsohn and his colleagues (1992) have developed a class called Control Your Depression, which has had promising results. Thompson, Gallagher, Nies, and Epstein (1983) have modified this approach specifically for older adults and report that participation in the classes resulted in reduced depressive symptoms, improvement in life satisfaction, and decreased negative thinking. Finally, bibliotherapy, which is often a component of behavioral therapy and cognitive-behavioral therapy, has been found to be effective with mildly and moderately depressed older adults (Scogin, Jamison & Gochneaur, 1989).

Little attention has been paid to the question of when group therapy might be more advantageous than individual treatment with older adults. Some older clients do not do well in groups or have strong negative feelings about being in group treatment. Indications that group treatment should not be undertaken include (1) hearing loss that is severe enough to interfere with understanding conversation in a group setting, (2) evidence of personality disorder, (3) severe depressive symptoms, and (4) a prior history of poor response to group treatment. Groups may be particularly helpful when people share a common problem or concern and can use the group to share information and build mutual support. An example is a group for people with a chronic illness or disability. Psychoeducational groups are particularly appropriate for primary prevention efforts and for reaching out to nontraditional clients who might not come for psychotherapy but are willing to attend classes about depression.

FIVE COMPONENTS OF TREATMENT WITH DEPRESSED OLDER PEOPLE

The three therapies for depression described here provide a basic framework for treatment of depression in later life. Treatment can sometimes be straightforward and uncomplicated, following the manuals that have been developed for each of these psychotherapies. More typically, the therapist is confronted by a complex picture that requires flexible responses drawing on other resources and approaches. Five issues that need to be considered when treating an older person for depression are (1) the use of medications, (2) electroconvulsive therapy (ECT), (3) the family's role in treatment, (4) comorbidities of health problems and depression, and (5) comorbidity of personality disorders.

Medications in Late-Life Depression

Medications have an important role in treatment of late-life depression. There is growing evidence of the efficacy of many of the antidepressant medications, especially the newer class of medications, the selective serotonin reuptake inhibitors. For some clients, antidepressant medications alone are sufficient to relieve acute feelings of depression. More typically, antidepressants form part of an overall treatment plan, relieving symptoms sufficiently so that clients can then work on the psychological and social dimensions of their depression.

In the following section, we review the use of antidepressants and antianxiety drugs, which are sometimes used in conjunction with antidepressants. When referring to drugs, the scientific literature uses generic names, while physicians and patients typically mention the brand name. We provide both the generic and brand name of a medication when it is first presented. After a medication is initially discussed, we refer to it subsequently by the brand name.

Antidepressant medications are effective by blocking the reuptake by brain neurons of neurotransmitters that are associated with depression, particularly, norepinephrine, serotonin, and dopamine. As a result of the medication's actions, the amount of one or more of these neurotransmitters that is available at neuronal synapses is increased. Some medications have a greater effect on norepinephrine, others act more on serotonin. Though used less frequently, antidepressants that act predominantly on dopamine levels also seem to be effective in some cases (Shuchter, Downs, & Zisook, 1996).

Antidepressants can be grouped into four broad classes (Table 8.1). The first generation of antidepressants were the tricyclic drugs (TCAs), such as amitryptyline (Elavil) and imipramine (Tofranil). Prior to the approval of fluoxetine (Prozac) by the FDA in 1989, the TCAs were the most widely used antidepressants. These drugs block the reuptake of norepinephrine and serotonin and have both antidepressant and sedative effects. There is considerable evidence that these medications reduce depression, but they also have high rates of adverse side effects, which makes it difficult for some people to tolerate them or to reach a therapeutic level with them. Many of the older TCAs have high anticholinergic effects (see Table 8.2), resulting in such symptoms as dry mouth, blurred vision, urinary retention, and constipation. Another anticholinergic effect is memory loss, which is particularly a problem in older patients because symptoms can resemble dementia. Severe reactions can include psychotic thinking, hyperthermia and worsening of glaucoma (Blazer, 1993). Another side effects of TCAs is orthostatic hypotension, which can lead to falls and serious injuries (De Leo & Diekstra, 1990). Other possible side effects include weight gain, motor tremor, liver toxicity, decreased sexual interest or impaired sexual functioning and a risk of seizures (Blazer, 1993). The sedating feature of the TCAs is an advantage when treating a depressed patient with anxiety and/or sleep problems, but it is sometimes difficult to achieve the proper balance of antidepressant and sedating effects. The amount of sedation is difficult for some clients to tolerate. Nortriptyline (Pamelor) and desipramine (Norpramin) are more frequently used with older adults because they have fewer anticholinergic and sedating side effects (Blazer, 1993).

The selective serotonin reuptake inhibitors (SSRIs) are largely displacing tricyclic medications in treatment of depression. These medications have three principal advantages. First, they mainly target one neurotransmitter, serotonin. As a result, it is possible to determine whether altering levels of serotonin alone is sufficient to alleviate depression. If that is not the case, medications that affect the other neurotransmitters associated with depression can be used. Second, the SSRIs have fewer side effects. They have minimal anticholinergic or sedating effects and can be tolerated more easily by most clients, including older people (Salzman, 1994). Third, patients feel symptom relief relatively quickly, typically from a few days to 2 weeks, compared to 6 weeks at maximum dosage for the tricyclics. Contrary to popular opinion, the SSRIs do not have a greater impact on depression than the tri-

TABLE 8.1. Antidepressant Medications and Their Side Effects

Medication generic (brand) names	Primary targets[a]	Anticholinergic effects	Sedative effects	Cardiac effects
Tricylcic tertiary amines	NE, SE			
Amitriptyline (Elavil, Endep)		High	High	High
Imipramine (Tofranil)		Moderate	Moderate	Moderate
Doxepin (Adapin, Sinequan)		High	Moderate–high	Moderate
Clomipramine (Anafranil)		High	Moderate	Moderate
Tricyclic secondary amines	NE, SE			
Desipramine (Norpramin)		Low	Low	Low
Nortriptyline (Aventyl, Pamelor)		Moderate	Low–moderate	Low
Other tricyclics	NE, SE			
Amoxapine (Asendin)		Moderate	Low–moderate	Moderate
Tetracyclics	NE, SE			
Maprotiline (Ludiomil)		Moderate	High	Low
Dopamine reuptake inhibitors	DA			
Bupropion (Welbutrin)		Very low	Very low	Very low
Selective serotonin reuptake inhibitors (SSRIs)	SE			
Fluoxetine (Prozac)		Very low	Very low	Very low
Sertraline (Zoloft)		Very low	Very low	None
Paroxetine (Paxil)		Very low	Very low	None
Monoamine oxidase inhibitors (MAOIs)	NE, SE, DA			
Phenelzine (Nardil)		Low	Low	Very low
Tranylcypromine (Parnate)		Low	Low	Very low
Serotonin–norepinephrine reuptake inhibitors	SE, NE			
Venlafaxine (Effexor)		Low	Moderate	Low–moderate
Trazodone (Desyrel)		Low	Moderate	Moderate
Mirtazapine (Remeron)		Moderate	High	Low
Nefazodone (Serzone)		Moderate	Moderate	High

Notes. Data from Alexopoulos (1994); De Leo and Diekstra (1990); Blazer (1993).

[a]NE, norepinephrine; SE, serotonin; DA, dopamine.

TABLE 8.2. Types of Side Effects with Antidepressant Medications

Anticholinergic	Antihistaminic
Blurred vision	Sedation
Dry mouth	Drowsiness
Memory disorders	Hypotension
Tachycardia	Weight gain
Urinary retention	Mental confusion
Constipation	Serotonergic
Glaucoma	
Speech blockage	Headaches
Decreased sweating	Nausea
	Gastrointestinal problems
Anti-alpha-adrenergic	Nervousness
Postural hypotension	Anxiety
Dizziness	Tremors
Reflex tachycardia	Insomnia
	Sexual dysfunction
	Weakness
	Dizziness
	Increased sweating

cyclics (Schneider & Olin, 1995). Their main advantage is fewer side effects, which allows more people to reach a therapeutic level of the medication.

Side effects, however, can still be a problem (Table 8.2). Among the serotonergic side effects, clients complain of difficulty falling asleep, poor appetite with weight loss (not always a problem!), a feeling of "jitteriness," and sometimes headache. While most of these problems disappear within a few weeks, people often need support to wait them out. Once the side effects disappear, they feel "better than good." Sertraline (Zoloft) and paroxetine (Paxil) produce fewer side effects and are generally better tolerated by older adults than Prozac.

As more people have taken SSRIs for longer periods of time, three other side effects have emerged. First, some people develop diarrhea to such an extent that the medication has to be discontinued. Second, some older patients become drowsy and hypersomnic, particularly those who are also taking antihypertensives. And third, patients complain of loss of libido. Despite these problems, the SSRIs are usually the first antidepressants that should be tried, unless there are specific medical contraindications or a prior history of a good response to another antidepressant.

A third group of antidepressant medications is the monoamine oxidase inhibitors (MAOIs), such as phenelzine (Nardil) and tranylcypromine (Parnate). These medications have a broad effect, increasing the availability of norepinephrine, serotonin, and dopamine (Shuchter et al., 1996). MAOIs have often been used for depressions that do not respond to other treatments. These medications are more difficult to administer because clients must avoid many common foods, such as cheeses and wines, that have a high amount of the amino acid tyramine. Interaction of an MAOI with tyramine can lead to a hypertensive crisis or a stroke. MAOIs also have adverse interactions with many common medications. MAOIs have been reported to worsen cognitive functioning and result in symptoms such as agitation and paranoid thinking, especially in people with some evidence of prior cognitive deficits (Blazer, 1993). They can cause orthostatic hypotension and, more rarely, hypertension (Salzman, 1993). These medications are generally not used with older people because of their higher risk of side effects and lack of therapeutic advantages over other available drugs (De Leo & Diekstra, 1990; Salzman, 1993).

Finally, a variety of other medications that do not fall into these broad categories are occasionally used for depression. One such medication is venlafaxine (Effexor), a serotonin–norepinephrine reuptake inhibitor that has fewer side effects than the tricyclics. It is generally tolerated better than the tricyclics but not as well as the SSRIs. Bupropion (Welbutrin) is another atypical antidepressant, and it has been found to be effective with older adults (e.g., Branconnier et al., 1983). This drug primarily blocks reuptake of dopamine. It has fewer sexual side effects than the SSRIs but can cause agitation, seizures, and Parkinsonian symptoms. Lithium carbonate (Lithane) and other mood stabilizers are used in bipolar disorders and can be tolerated by older patients (De Leo & Diekstra, 1990; Blazer, 1993). Salzman (1993), however, urges caution in their use with older patients, because their effectiveness and appropriate dosage have not been established. Patients also must be monitored carefully because of the risk of toxic side effects, cardiac problems, and a variety of other adverse symptoms. Finally, some stimulants (e.g., methylphenidate and D-amphetamine) have been used with older depressed and medically ill patients. The rationale for this use is that these medications have fewer cardiovascular side effects than tricyclic medications. Controlled studies, however, suggest that stimulants are not effective as antidepressants (Schneider & Olin, 1995).

Attention is being paid to the use of natural substances in treatment of depression. Recently, a substance called St. John's wort has been very popular among advocates of alternative medicine. Preliminary studies suggest that it has antidepressant properties (Linde et al., 1996). Unlike medications that are rigorously tested before being put into use, there is little information on side effects or possible harmful interactions with other medications or illnesses. Another cautionary note is that the purity of St. John's wort varies, so it can be difficult to regulate dosage.

The efficacy of psychotropic medications has usually been determined with samples of young and middle-aged adults. Most drug trials have not included older people, and only a few studies have focused specifically on older samples (see Salzman, 1994, for a review). As discussed in Chapter 7, older adults are more likely to experience adverse side effects with any medication, including the psychotropics. The interaction among the various drugs an older person may be taking or drug–alcohol interactions can minimize or exaggerate the effects of one or more of the medications involved or can lead to an adverse reaction.

Despite the potential complications, the antidepressant medications are reasonably effective with older people. In a review of the literature on the use of antidepressant medications with older people, Schneider and Olin (1995) found 30 randomized studies with placebo control groups. Summarizing the results across these studies, they report that 50% to 60% of patients improved with treatment, although many still had significant depressive symptoms at the end of the intervention period (see also Salzman, 1994). Approximately 30% of people in the placebo condition improved, as well. Additionally, many patients had significant side effects. Most of these studies involved tricyclic antidepressants. The few studies done with older patients using the SSRIs suggest that they are effective in lowering depression, with fewer side effects than the tricyclics (Schneider & Olin, 1995). Schneider and Olin (1995) also found that the best outcomes occur when medications and psychotherapy are used together.

Most drug studies focus on treatment of major depression. There is also evidence that antidepressant medications are helpful in treatment of dysthymia in older patients (Kocsis, 1997).

Some individuals do not respond initially to medications. It is estimated that between 18% and 40% of older depressed patients do not respond to standard medication protocols (Bonner & Howard, 1995). When the initial response to a medication is poor, the prescribing physician usually tries one of the alternatives. Differences among the SSRI medications result in somewhat different benefits. These differences are not always predictable, as there can be a great deal of individual variability in response.

In clinical practice, a certain amount of experimentation with medications goes on to identify which drugs are more likely to be effective for a patient and at what dosages. This approach can be successful. The main problem we have observed is prescribing physicians continuing treatments that are not effective or that are having significant side effects. On the other hand, switching rapidly from one medication to another without careful evaluation of the response can overwhelm the depressed individual and lead to resistance to the use of *any* treatment.

We find it very helpful to spend time with clients discussing the side effects of medications they are taking and also helping them recognize the positive benefits. When clients understand that side effects can be transitory and that it takes a while to experience the therapeutic benefits of medications, they are often more compliant and give the medication a chance.

Relapse of depressive symptoms is a common problem across the life span. In fact, as described in Chapter 4, many older people with depressive symptoms in later life have had prior episodes. Information about what treatments were effective for previous occurrences is useful in planning treatment for the current episode, because clinical experience suggests that treatment approaches (medication, ECT, psychotherapy) that were previously effective are helpful for the new episode.

One recent study explored ways of preventing recurrence of depression in older people with a history of prior episodes (Reynolds, Frank, Perel, Mazumdar, & Kupfer, 1995). This study was conducted in two stages. In the initial stage, people age 60 and older with a current episode of depression and a history of prior episodes were given treatment that included Pamelor and interpersonal psychotherapy, and 77% of the subjects responded. The responders were then assigned randomly into four maintenance groups: drug alone, drug and therapy, therapy alone, and placebo. Therapy maintenance consisted of one visit per month. Though this study is still in progress, preliminary findings indicate that 80% of people in the drug and drug with therapy groups had no recurrence of a major depression for a 1-year period, compared to 50% of people receiving therapy alone and 20% of placebos. These results suggest the value of longer-term treatment for people with recurrent depression.

Medications for Anxiety and Sleep Problems

The medications most likely to be used in conjunction with antidepressants are benzodiazepines, tranquilizers that treat anxiety and sleep problems (Table 8.3). It is not uncommon for depression and anxiety symptoms both to be present, and sleep disturbance is frequent in older depressed patients. Sometimes physicians prescribe a combination of antidepressant and tranquilizing medication to produce a specific therapeutic benefit that would not occur using either medication alone.

The benzodiazepines are widely used throughout the population, including with older patients (Salzman, 1992). Besides their effects on anxiety, these medications can reduce irritability and agitation. Side effects of the

TABLE 8.3. Short-Acting and Long-Acting Benzodiazepines

Short-acting medications	Long-acting medications
Oxazepam (Serax)	Clordiazepoxide (Librium)
Lorazepam (Ativan)	Diazepam (Valium)
Alprazolam (Xanax)	Prazepam (Centrax)
Triazolam (Halcion)	Clorazepate (Tranxene)
	Clonazepam (Klonopin)

Note. Data from Salzman (1992).

benzodiazepines can be serious. Salzman (1992) groups possible side effects into four categories:

1. *Sedation:* Patients can become overly sedated and, as a consequence, agitated or belligerent.
2. *Cerebellar symptoms:* These problems include ataxia, dysarthria, unsteadiness, and decreased motor coordination. Patients who are already unsteady or have other physical problems can become much worse on these medications.
3. *Slowing:* Patients have decreased reaction times and perform a variety of tasks more slowly. Slowing, along with poorer coordination, can lead to significant impairment in driving.
4. *Cognition:* Short-term memory can be significantly impaired. Some people appear demented, though full recovery occurs when the medication is withdrawn.

Benzodiazepines can be classified into short-acting and long-acting medications (see Table 8.3). Side effects are more likely in long-acting drugs. Short-acting medications build up to therapeutic dosages quicker and are eliminated from the body faster. Long-acting drugs stay in the body longer and can continue producing symptoms for several days or even weeks after they have been discontinued (Salzman, 1992).

Although short-acting benzodiazepines are generally recommended for older people, there are situations when long-acting drugs are preferable. They can be given less often and the effects last longer. A common problem with a short-acting drug that is given at bedtime is that it wears off before the patient would normally wake up, producing restlessness and anxiety. A long-acting medication could be effective in helping someone sleep through the night.

Another antianxiety drug, buspirone (BuSpar), is chemically different from the benzodiazepines. It is frequently used to treat anxiety symptoms in people with depressive disorders and may help potentiate the SSRIs. BuSpar is less sedating than the benzodiazepines and is less likely to cause cognitive symptoms, but it is also not as effective as an antianxiety drug.

When used as a sleeping medication, the benzodiazepines lose their effectiveness after 20 to 30 days (Regestein, 1992). With prolonged use, they can actually make sleep problems worse. As with other problems, insomnia should be carefully evaluated before medications are prescribed. Several factors can induce insomnia or make it worse, including use of caffeine, nicotine, or alcohol (Regestein, 1992). Many prescription and over-the-counter medications can also affect sleep. Daytime naps and lack of exercise frequently contribute to insomnia.

A variety of approaches can be used to treat insomnia, in addition to or as a complement to medications, including setting regular sleep and waking habits, avoiding daytime naps, increasing exercise, taking a hot bath before bedtime, and use of relaxation techniques (Engle-Friedman, Bootzin, Hazlewood, & Tsao, 1992; Regestein, 1992).

Collaborating with Physicians

Nonphysicians need to work collaboratively with physicians to coordinate use of antidepressant and other psychoactive medications. Therapists are in an ideal position to monitor effectiveness, compliance, and side effects of medications. They see patients weekly and listen in depth to their experiences. Thus, they can provide valuable feedback to physicians on the effectiveness of a medication. They can also discuss with physicians the experiences that other patients had with certain medications. In a successful collaboration, information flows freely between physician and therapist, so the patient perceives a united effort in treatment.

We strongly recommend that mental health professionals who work with older clients get training in psychopharmacology so that they gain a thorough understanding of the uses of medication. There are excellent programs sponsored by the American Psychological Association and the National Institute of Mental Health, among others, that provide the latest research on the uses of psychotropic medications.

Electroconvulsive Therapy with Older Depressed Patients

Electroconvulsive therapy (ECT) remains controversial, but it is widely used with depressed patients, including those who are older. In fact, older people are probably more likely to receive ECT than younger patients (e.g., Thompson & Blaine, 1987).

ECT may help patients who are deeply depressed when other treatments are not effective. It is generally used when a patient does not respond to a course of antidepressant medication. In medication-resistant cases, ECT has been reported to be effective about 80% of the time (Kramer, 1987). Patients who respond to ECT generally have more vegetative symptoms, such as sleep and appetite disturbance, and are also more likely to have delusional depressive symptoms.

The American Psychiatric Association (1990) has proposed guidelines for the appropriate use of ECT. ECT is recommended if (1) patients have had a poor response or cannot tolerate antidepressant medications; (2) they have a history of responding to ECT during previous depressive episodes; (3) the risks of antidepressants are greater than the risks of ECT; and (4) when a rapid response to treatment is needed, such as for a suicidal patient. Since some patients respond to psychotherapy but not medications, that should also be considered. Finally, the patient's preference should weigh heavily in the decision.

Studies of the effectiveness of ECT indicate that results are generally better than for the tricyclic antidepressants and MAOIs (Meyers & Mei-Tal, 1985–1986; Sackheim, 1994). It is not always clear, however, if drug dosage in these studies was optimal. There are no comparisons of ECT with the SSRIs. More patients can tolerate the SSRIs, so the difference with ECT may be smaller.

Relapses following ECT are high. About one-third of patients have significant recurrence of symptoms within 1 year and two-thirds relapse within 3 years (Blazer, 1993; Sackheim, 1994). That may be in part because patients receiving ECT are often unresponsive to other treatments and have a more intractable form of depression. It may also be that efforts have not been made to prevent relapses, for example, through the use of antidepressant medications and psychotherapy.

ECT is usually considered medically safe with older patients and, indeed, may have fewer side effects than some medications. The greatest medical risks involve cardiovascular problems and falls (Sackheim, 1994). Blazer (1993) estimates that one third of older patients are likely to experience some adverse effects (falls, cardiovascular symptoms, confusion) following ECT. Other side effects are headaches, nausea, and muscle pain. The oldest old (75 and over) are most likely to have medical complications and increased mortality (Cattan et al., 1990).

The possible effects of ECT on cognitive functioning are more controversial. It is clear that ECT results in some short-term memory loss immediately following treatment. Memory problems include both anterograde and retrograde amnesia. In fact, ECT may be effective to the extent that it induces a mild delirium. Patients have trouble remembering some events from prior to the ECT and have difficulty with new learning. These problems usually clear up within a month, but some patients have been found to have more persistent deficits (Sackheim, 1992). We have encountered people in our practice whose cognitive difficulties apparently originated with or were intensified by ECT.

There are competing explanations for these long-term effects. One possibility is that ECT may cause permanent brain damage, which results in deficits in cognition. This possibility is especially likely if the ECT is administered improperly. It is sometimes possible to establish through neuroimaging studies that ECT is the probable cause of the brain damage, usually in the form of a discrete infarct. An alternative explanation is that the patient's memory problems are associated with other pathologies or even normal aging, rather than ECT. Some depressed older people are at risk of developing dementia, especially if they have cognitive symptoms at the time of the depressive episodes (Alexopoulos, Meyers, Young, Mattis, & Kakuma, 1993). In these cases, the emergence of dementia symptoms is inevitable and unrelated to ECT or other depression treatment. ECT is generally regarded as safe even in patients with mild cognitive deficits, but the possibility that it may accentuate these problems should be considered (Gatz, 1994). While most of the available evidence suggests that ECT generally produces no permanent damage (Blazer, 1993), more careful investigation of long-term outcomes is needed.

The decision to use ECT is often related to social factors. Historically, people who were given ECT had less education and were believed to have little personal insight into their problems (e.g., Kahn & Fink, 1959). Families of older depressed patients play a major role in the decision to use ECT (Gatz & Warren, 1989). When family burden was higher, such as when the patient was no longer performing activities of daily living or was behaving in bizarre or deviant ways, ECT was a more likely choice. In many cases, families pressured the patient into giving consent for treatment. A review of case records indicates that little effort was made to prevent the buildup of stress on the families (Gatz & Warren, 1989).

ECT, then, should be regarded as a tool for use when other treatments are not effective and the situation is critical. Questions remain, however, about the long-term safety of ECT, as well as its acceptability to some older people. Consistent with the guidelines of the American Psychiatric Association, ECT should be considered only after other treatments have been used. The newer SSRIs mean that more treatment alternatives are available. We also want to emphasize the importance of evaluating both patient and family and considering when family interventions might play an important component of treatment. We expand on this theme in the next section.

Family Issues in the Treatment of Late-Life Depression

Family issues are frequently central in an older person's depression and successful treatment sometimes involves bringing in relevant family members. A study by Hinrichsen and his associates (Hinrichsen, 1992; Hinrichsen & Hernandez, 1993; Hinrichsen & Zweig, 1994; Zweig & Hinrichsen, 1993) demonstrates the effects that the family has on recovery and relapse rates in late-life depression. The sample consisted of people 60 years of age or older suffering from major depression, who had an involved spouse or child. Initial treatment was with medications or ECT and resulted in improvement in 72% of cases. A follow-up examination after 1 year indicated that 19% of the improved clients had relapsed. These figures on treatment response and relapse are fairly typical for both younger and older depressed patients.

Hinrichsen and Hernandez (1993) then examined predictors of recovery and relapse. Turning first to recovery rates, neither sociodemographic variables nor clinical characteristics of the depressed patient at the start of treatment were related to recovery. Instead, characteristics of the involved family member differentiated between people who improved and those who did not. Specifically, depressed older patients were less likely to have a successful response to treatment when their family member had higher psychiatric symptoms, reported more difficulty helping the depressed patient, and assessed their own health as poor. The type of psychiatric symptoms of family members that were associated with poorer outcomes were primarily depression and somatization.

Similar to recovery rates, relapse was not predicted by either sociodemographic characteristics or clinical features of the patient. Only one variable significantly distinguished relapsed cases from those with sustained improvement: the amount of difficulty the family member reported in caring for the patient. In this case, however, relapse was related to reporting *low* rates of difficulty at the outset of treatment.

This approach was extended to consider which patients attempted suicide during the 1-year study period (Zweig & Hinrichsen, 1993). Of the 126 people in the study, 11 (8.7%) made a suicide attempt. Factors associated with the suicide attempts included higher socioeconomic status, past history of suicide attempts, more suicidal behaviors at the time of initial assessment, and not having a remission in depression with treatment. Family variables also were associated with suicide attempts. Family members of people who later attempted suicide had more psychiatric symptoms themselves, reported more strain in their relationship with the patient, and had more difficulty caring for the patient than did family members in the non-suicide group.

These studies establish that the relationship between the depressed older patient and significant family member plays a major role in recovery from depression and perhaps also in risk for a suicide attempt. Given the prominence of families in the lives of older people and the role they play in depression, clinicians should consider when and how to bring families into treatment. The case examples later in the chapter give examples of involving families.

Comorbidity of Depression and Medical Illness

Depression is a frequent and important concomitant of medical illnesses throughout the life span. The relationship between medical problems and depression is complex. Depression, of course, can be a consequence of illness. Patients can become depressed for a variety of reasons: discomfort or physical distress, disabilities, or the life-threatening consequences of the illness. Illness and disability can cut people off from friends and family and reduce their ability to engage in usual activities. Complicating the socioemotional consequences of illness is the fact that many diseases and medications have physiological effects that can result in an increase of depressive symptoms. (See Chapter 4 for a list of illnesses that can lead to depression.)

As an example of the interaction of depression and illness, we recently consulted with a colleague on a case of an older woman she was treating for depression. We immediately noticed the woman's face, which had the masklike and expressionless quality typical of Parkinson's disease. On our recommendation, her physician began an investigation for possible Parkinson's and subsequently started her on an anti-Parkinson's medication. As a result, her overall functioning improved somewhat and she was able to make better progress in therapy.

It can be difficult to sort out whether depressive symptoms are a consequence of an illness or have been caused directly by the illness. There can also be synergistic effects. For example, some nutritional deficits can cause depressive symptoms. In turn, the depressed patient may eat less, thereby increasing nutritional problems (Blazer, 1993). Overeating can be a consequence of depression and can complicate other health problems, as well as contributing to a negative body image. Pain and depression are associated in a similar way. The experience of chronic pain can lead to depression, and depressive symptoms can worsen the experience of chronic pain (Blazer, 1993).

Whether the onset of symptoms is primarily medical or psychological, treatment of depression reduces the patient's distress and leads to a better medical as well as psychological prognosis. If a medication is suspected as a cause of the patient's depression, it should be eliminated when possible.

When someone with a chronic illness is depressed, the normal grieving over losses is intertwined with exaggerated negative beliefs about the consequences of one's illness or disability. Clinicians can acknowledge feelings of sadness over these losses, but they must avoid dwelling solely on loss or endorsing depressive thoughts that magnify the negative consequences of the illness. It is easy to feel overwhelmed by a patient's health problems. Identifying with the patient, the therapist may agree that life with a particular disability is not worth living, or that making an effort at rehabilitation is pointless because so much has been lost. These types of statements, however, represent typical depressive thought processes, which exaggerate the negative consequences of the patient's illness or disability. Therapists who agree with these statements do not know the alternatives or possibilities the patient might have.

Therapists need to learn about the illnesses their clients have and the possibilities for rehabilitation and retraining, including how other patients with similar illnesses to manage. With that information, it becomes possible to differentiate between the real and enduring losses clients suffer and their exaggerated reactions. Treatment involves helping clients identify realistic alternatives that allow them to compensate for their loss or make progress in the recovery of function.

Treatment of older people with significant visual problems provides an example of differentiating between real and exaggerated losses. Vision problems that cannot be corrected by ordinary eyeglasses are a frequent problem in later life. Among the vision disorders affecting older people are macular degeneration, which causes a loss of central vision, glaucoma, which is associated with a loss of peripheral vision, and diabetic retinopathy, which can have varying effects. Most of the time, older people with vision problems do not become totally blind; they have residual vision. Nonetheless, these disorders can be extremely upsetting. Visually impaired older adults may no longer be able to drive, read ordinary print with eyeglasses, or do a variety of other everyday activities. It is no wonder that depression is a common feature of eye disorders in late life (Horowitz et al., 1994).

While vision loss is extremely disturbing, rehabilitation efforts can help patients regain the ability to perform many different activities. People with vision losses are able to make successful adaptations by learning how to use their remaining vision and by making modifications in their environment that enhance their sight. A variety of visual aids can enable people to use their remaining eyesight for visual tasks. Examples range from simple and familiar devices such as magnifying glasses to technologically sophisticated equipment such as closed-circuit televisions that enlarge print and reverse the field (showing white on black, rather than the opposite), making it possible for some visually impaired people to read print (see Genensky, Zarit, & Amaral, 1992, for a discussion of vision rehabilitation in later life). Environmental modifications can also help people function more effectively. Using lamps that have high illumination and are focused directly on work or reading areas can help someone read print. Increasing the lighting in hallways and stairways can prevent falls. Another modification that prevents falls is placing contrasting color strips on steps. These interventions do not lead to recovery of certain abilities, such as being able to drive, but they enable vision-impaired people to perform a wide range of activities and to have a meaningful and fulfilling life.

Many patients with vision problems are understandably depressed. They may have been told that nothing can be done to help them, and they dwell on what they have lost rather than what may still be possible for them. They frequently complain that their life is not worth living without their vision and describe themselves in exaggerated terms, for example, calling themselves blind when they can, in fact, see. As in many situations in which depression is involved, clients' beliefs about the events in their life and their own abilities determine whether they will take the necessary steps to manage their problems more effectively. If they believe that their situation is hopeless, that nothing can be done to help them, or that the only change that would make their life satisfying again is to be able to see the way they used to, they do not take the steps necessary to learn how to use visual aids or environmental modifications that make it possible for them to carry out a variety of activities. Sometimes people with relatively good remaining vision make poor adaptations, while others with much poorer eyesight make good progress in regaining function. This discrepancy is frequently the result of differences in beliefs—one patient sees the situation as hopeless, another believes it is possible to improve. Treatment of depressive beliefs, then, is a necessary part in an overall rehabilitation program.

In addition to challenging and reframing beliefs that exaggerate the consequences of the loss, therapists use other strategies with visually impaired older adults, such as behavioral interventions that increase pleasant activities and treatment of family or other interpersonal problems that may interfere with rehabilitation efforts. Clients can benefit by talking with people who have similar disabilities, either in a group or in a one-to-one situation. A client may resist trying out a vision device when it is presented by an optometrist but ask to use the same device when another person uses it. In therapy groups we have run with visually impaired people, participants pass around and try out each other's visual aids, as well as talk about other techniques for improving functioning. This sharing of information speeds up the rehabilitation process.

Following is an example of treatment of depressive symptoms in a 69-year-old woman with a serious vision problem. The client, Phyllis, had glaucoma and cataracts. Surgery to correct these problems was only partly successful, leaving her extremely light sensitive. Under conditions of bright light, she was functionally blind. As a result, she could not see well enough outdoors during the daytime to cross busy streets safely. Phyllis had been virtually housebound for the past year, not leaving her apartment except for trips to the grocery store. Despite these problems, her vision was fairly good under conditions where glare and illumination were controlled.

Phyllis sought treatment in a comprehensive visual rehabilitation program. As a first step, an orientation and mobility specialist went to her house to teach her how to cross streets safely. She was also fitted with wraparound sunglasses that greatly reduced glare and made it possible for her to get around safely outdoors on sunny days. As a result of these interventions, she could take the bus to the vision center for her appointments, as well as resume other activities.

Despite these initial gains, Phyllis remained very depressed and was referred for psychological treatment. Her depression revolved around the belief that there was nothing she could do anymore that was satisfying or important to her. Treatment focused simultaneously on identifying pleasant activities and addressing the ways in which she exaggerated difficulties and minimized the value of things she was able to accomplish. After several sessions of exploring possible activities, Phyllis set a goal to learn how to paint. She had always been interested in painting but never had the opportunity to pursue it. She was able to locate a painting class for senior citizens and to figure out the bus routes for traveling there. She did quite well in the class, learning how to work around her vision difficulty. She discovered that the light in her kitchen was best for her in the morning, so she set up her easel then and painted. She got a great deal of satisfaction from painting and became quite good at it. She even gained recognition for her ability, winning a prize in a local art competition. Besides painting, Phyllis gradually became involved in other social activities, including serving as a volunteer at the vision rehabilitation center.

This example is both typical and exceptional. As in many cases, treatment involved challenging and reframing the client's dysfunctional beliefs that exaggerated the consequences of her loss and prevented her from getting the most out of rehabilitation efforts. Treatment also involved increasing pleasant activities and addressing family problems. What was unusual is that the main breakthrough involved a visual activity—painting. This example underscores how important it is not to identify with clients' statements that they cannot do anything anymore or do not see the sense of going on. Although vision loss is a major change, it is not an inevitable barrier for many activities.

This approach can be applied to many chronic disabilities. The opportunities and methods for rehabilitation and retraining vary considerably from one type of disorder to the next. When working with a client who has a particular illness or disability, the therapist needs to become familiar with the disorder and the possibilities for rehabilitation and recovery. An understanding of what is possible helps therapists identify and reframe depressive beliefs. Treatment may also involve increasing pleasant or meaningful activities and addressing family and other social concerns.

Comorbidity of Depression and Personality Disorders

By far, our most challenging clients are those who have depression and personality disorder (see Chapter 4). Although depression is the initial complaint, it quickly emerges that these clients have long-standing difficulties in many areas of their lives, such as anxiety, paranoid symptoms, and obsessive–compulsive symptoms. The particular pattern of problems depends on the type of personality disorder. Borderline or histrionic people, for example, have more dramatic symptoms, usually anxieties and fears, but on occasion paranoia. By contrast, people with a schizoid pattern may have an emptiness inside that makes it difficult for them to find pleasure in anything or to develop a relationship with the therapist. Of course, the distinctions among the different personality disorder diagnoses can become blurred and clients can have features of more than one.

These clients typically have good reasons to be depressed. Our experience has been that individuals with personality disorders are more likely to be alone in old age. Many are estranged from children or other relatives or have ongoing struggles with them. They want their children's attention but drive them away with their behavior. They characteristically place themselves in difficult situations, getting into conflicts and frustrating anyone who might help them. They have difficulty enjoying the positive events in their lives or experiencing positive feelings. Most important, their dysfunctional behaviors and cognitions are very difficult to change.

We often find ourselves doing long-term therapy with these clients. Treatment is a balancing act, trying to prevent crises while also building more adaptive behavior. We often work to prevent burnout of their children or other support sources. Suicide risk can be high in many of these patients. Initially, clients may be mistrustful and even critical of the therapy relationship. If good rapport is developed, they benefit from therapy.

Modifications of cognitive-behavioral therapy have recently been developed for long-term treatment of people with particularly rigid, underlying belief systems (Beck et al., 1990; Linehan, 1993; Gallagher-Thompson & Thompson, 1996). Cognitive-behavioral therapy for personality disorders emphasizes identifying the underlying themes or beliefs that give rise to automatic thoughts. Examples of these underlying themes are "I am no good" and "No one can ever love me."

These underlying themes emerge from the content of automatic thoughts. The therapist can also use an assessment instrument developed by Young (1994; see also Gallagher-Thompson & Thompson, 1996) called the Historical Test of Schemas to identifying underlying themes. Using this instrument, clients create a time line of significant events in their lives. Client and therapist then work together to identify how the client interpreted key events, as well as evidence that contradicts long-standing schemas. For example, someone who believes his life has been a failure often includes contradictory evidence in this kind of review. The therapist can use the information to identify the client's tendency to discount positive experiences or to believe that negative events outweigh them. New schemas are developed through a reformulation of the events in the person's life.

The relationship between therapist and client becomes a more important vehicle in conducting long-term cognitive-behavioral therapy. The relationship is used to test the validity of automatic thoughts and underlying themes, still with considerable emphasis on how clients respond to current events in their lives and on monitoring thoughts and feelings.

Just as therapy is more difficult with these clients, so is the use of medications. Compared to other depressed clients, these clients get only limited relief from medications. In our experience, they make up most of the cases that do not respond well to medications. Often psychiatrists use combinations of medications with them, but the side effects can outweigh any therapeutic benefits. The right combination of medications can greatly facilitate therapy. But unlike the unequivocally positive response we see in many depressed patients, those with personality disorders never feel that good in treatment with SSRIs.

Another problem these clients have is dealing with their physicians. We often have to interpret their behavior to the physician and the physician's findings to the client. When they have a serious medical problem, these clients may not get the treatment they need because they alienate physicians and other medical personnel.

Termination of a client with personality disorder can be problematic because it may represent the severing of the only truly positive relationship in the person's life. When we are able to develop a good relationship and address the more immediate and pressing problems, we decrease the frequency of visits gradually to once or twice a month. By maintaining regular but infrequent contact, the therapist can ensure that the gains made in treatment can be maintained. It is also possible to detect signs of deterioration before the problem is too far advanced.

We believe it is possible to make slow progress, but these patients will continue having difficulty and crises. For the therapist, treating this patient is emotionally draining. Therapists need to be realistic about the prospects for improvement and to make sure they keep proper boundaries.

LONG-TERM OUTCOMES OF LATE-LIFE DEPRESSION

Studies of late-life depression suggest that outcomes are generally positive. Over the long term, between 60% and 80% of patients do fairly well (Baldwin & Jolley; 1986; Frank, 1994; Murphy, 1994). Some people may have repeated episodes between interludes of good functioning. As discussed earlier, maintenance treatment involving medications, psychotherapy, or a combination of both improves the rate of long-term recovery (Frank, 1994). Factors associated with a poorer prognosis include evidence of cognitive impairment or a chronic physical illness (Murphy, 1994). Because depression often accompanies the onset of Alzheimer's disease and other dementing illnesses, the poor outcome in these cases is the result of the underlying degenerative illness, not depression per se. Age, however, has not been found to be related to a poorer long-term prognosis.

CLINICAL EXAMPLES OF LATE-LIFE DEPRESSION

The controlled studies that have established the effectiveness of various treatments for depression in late life follow logical and strict protocols. In clinical practice, the therapist is often confronted with complex cases that would not necessarily have been included in clinical research trials because of medical or psychiatric comorbidities. Rather than a straightforward depression, the client may have mixed symptoms (e.g., anxiety or paranoid symptoms), features of a personality disorder, and/or be suffering from a chronic health problem. These are situations where it is best to employ all the treatment tools available (for example, using both medications and psychotherapy), rather than to test one approach at a time. The practicing therapist should draw on clinical research in selecting approaches with known effectiveness. But it is also important to respond flexibly, providing an optimal mix of treatment approaches suited to a particular situation.

The cases described here illustrate situations likely to be encountered in an outpatient or private practice setting. They illustrate many of the issues discussed in this chapter: how therapists must consider and coordinate therapy with medications and/or ECT, how to involve family members to facilitate treatment and the role of chronic illness.

Case 1. Recurrent Major Depression

Jean was 78 years old and had nine adult children. She had seen several other psychologists, usually for a single visit. She was soft-spoken and reluctant to reveal too much about herself initially. She reported that she had her first major depression at the age of 64, several years after an uneventful menopause, for which she did not take hormone replacement. She was prescribed Trazodone (Desyrel; see Table 8.1) at that time, which she said helped her with her mood but slowed her down. She had recently seen a psychiatrist, who had started her on venlafaxine (Effexor) and a sleeping medication. The current depression was triggered by two strep throat infections, for which she took antibiotics, and a fall that resulted in a fractured leg and arm. Depression is not an uncommon aftereffect of an infection, and antibiotics can trigger a depressive reaction in some individuals.

Jean described herself as an excellent homemaker, very perfectionistic and extremely hard working. She had cared for eight of her nine children at home by herself much of the time, as her husband had a job that required a lot of traveling. The other child was severely retarded and resided in an institution. She had not seen him in many years. Jean had grown up on a farm and had a high school education. She married young and helped her husband through college. Most of their children had finished college, and several had professional degrees. Jean had always felt ashamed of her meager education. When all the children were grown, she took a housecleaning job, since cleaning was something she felt competent to do. Her husband was embarrassed by her work, but she persisted because she received a lot of praise from her clients. When she fractured her arm and leg, she was unable to work and had to quit her job. Her mood plummeted, leading her into a major depressive episode.

The night before her second session, Jean took an overdose of Effexor and aspirin—only a few pills—with the hope that she would not wake up in the morning. When she did wake up, she was worried that she had damaged her brain with the medication. She came to the session worried and fearful. She felt more worthless because she couldn't even commit suicide right. We increased her visits to twice a week, and her husband accompanied her about half the time. She was unhappy with the psychiatrist she was seeing for medication; she felt that he was not interested in her. When she told him about the overdose, he did not seem concerned. We arranged for her to see a different psychiatrist. Since she had responded to Desyrel before, the new psychiatrist started her on that.

Over the next two weeks, Jean's depression remained severe. She continued to be very negative in her thinking, very ruminative, and lethargic, and the suicide risk remained high. As it did not seem possible to stabilize her on an outpatient basis, we discussed hospitalization. Her husband had just signed their Medicare benefits over to a managed care plan, which complicated the decision making. Jean would have preferred to return to the hospital she had been to 12 years earlier, which she had found to be much better than the local psychiatric hospital. She now revealed that she had received ECT 12 years ago and that it was helpful. However, by joining an HMO, she had given up Medicare as her primary insurance, and the hospital she preferred was not covered. Instead, eventually she was admitted as an inpatient at the HMO hospital. Treatment there consisted of bilateral ECT (which is no longer standard practice because of the high incidence of memory impairment) and medication. There was no individual therapy, no group therapy, and minimal therapeutic milieu. She was happy to leave the hospital at the end of the maximum stay of 10 days, as she did not feel that she was getting much treatment there, and she could as easily have had ECT as an outpatient.

She was again seen twice a week for structured cognitive-behavioral therapy for depression. She had been started on an SSRI, Paxil, in the hospital, and it helped considerably with her ruminative thinking. She responded well in therapy to written thought records, particularly because she could take a copy home with her and reread it between sessions. We would often include clarifying or affirming statements on the thought record, like "My full-time job right now is fighting my depression."

Several important historical antecedents to her depression were revealed as we worked on the thought records and she came to trust me more. Her mother had died when Jean was 16 years old, and she became the only woman on the farm. One of the farm hands took advantage of the situation and raped her. She did not tell anyone but always felt damaged and inadequate because of it. Her third son became brain damaged when he was born precipitously and with such force that he slipped out of the midwife's hands and landed on his head. He was so severely retarded that Jean was unable to care for him, so they institutionalized him. She felt guilty and responsible for this decision. We reframed this choice as one that allowed her son to have all of his needs well met, which might not have been the case in their home. She described the hospital where he lives as a good place for him and said that the staff are quite consistent and caring with him. Subsequently, she and one of her daughters went to visit him and found him clean and well cared for, although he did not recognize them or have any idea who they might be.

In her marriage, she had often felt overwhelmed with the care of all of the children when her husband was gone for extended periods of time, and she compensated for this by being overly close to her oldest daughter. This closeness led to significant sibling rivalry among the children that continues to affect family relationships. Her husband was now semiretired, but he was continuing to travel and would be absent for weeks at a time.

During the joint sessions, Jean's husband was able to see that she was lonely with the children gone and that his absences were a problem for her. He began including her in his trips, and since they often would go to places near one or another of the children, Jean enjoyed the trips. She did not drive, so she had not been able to visit the children before. Her husband also started working on being more supportive of the things Jean did well, and when she was occasionally asked to clean for a client, he no longer was critical of her. Ironically, on the Paxil Jean became much less obsessive about cleaning their own home and started to postpone unpleasant cleaning tasks, allowing some clutter to accumulate. This is not an unusual reaction to an SSRI. People describe a feeling of "just not caring as much" if something gets done.

Treatment continued for 8 months, twice a week for 2 months during the acute phase of her depression, then once a week for about 3 months, then every other week. Jean now no longer felt depressed. Then we received a telephone call canceling an appointment because her husband had been in a terrible automobile accident. A young woman had been driving too fast for the road conditions and crossed over the center line, hitting Jean's husband's car head on. He had multiple fractures of every extremity and spent 3 months in the hospital. When he returned home, he was wheelchair bound, though determined to walk again, and within 4 months he was walking with a cane. Jean now had to deal with the fact that he was at home all the time and with the anger and irritability that accompany chronic pain and disability. She managed it quite well, and as of the present time, she has not had a recurrence of her depression. She continues to take Paxil and to have maintenance therapy sessions once or twice a month.

This case illustrates many of the elements involved in late-life depression, such as coordination of therapy with medications and, in this case, ECT, the prominence of family issues, and the occasional involvement of a spouse in therapy sessions. Therapy addressed long-standing issues, such as the rape when she was 16 and the institutionalization of her son, as well as current concerns. The common thread in treatment was the negative beliefs Jean had about herself. Once the initial crisis was handled, she made excellent progress. Long-term outcome was good, due to the combination of medications and therapy. One other point in this case, which we encounter more and more frequently, is the limited choice available to Jean for psychiatric inpatient treatment as a result of joining an HMO. That plan, however, was generous in its outpatient therapy coverage.

Case 2. First Major Depression at Age 67

Emily's daughter called initially and told me she had been given my name by a former client and family friend. She told me that her mother, who had always been a dynamo, getting up at 5:30 A.M. and cleaning the house and starting the laundry before anyone else was up for breakfast, was now not getting out of bed. Emily had seen a number of psychiatrists and a psychologist and had not felt that any of them understood her or were at all helpful. Her family physician had hospitalized her on a medical ward of the local hospital because she refused to go to the psychiatric unit, but the 3-day hospitalization had done very little for her. Since Emily was not getting dressed or going outdoors, I decided to do a home visit to assess the situation. This would also give me an idea of the home environment and allow Emily to feel somewhat "special." Luckily, she lived between my office and home, so I could arrange to see her at the end of the work day with little inconvenience.

Emily's home was not only immaculate, it was tastefully and expensively decorated. Her husband, Harry, was very attentive and often finished her sentences for her. Both of them were very worried about the changes in Emily, and both were fairly sophisticated psychologically. They were college educated and very well read. They had both been widowed at early ages and had found one another at about the time their children were grown. Emily's husband had been killed during a robbery, and Harry's wife had died of cancer. Between them they had seven children, ranging in age from 30 to 45. Their children would have problems from time to time, and Emily and Harry would handle the situations as they arose.

Emily's symptoms included poor sleep, with early, middle, and late insomnia, poor appetite, loss of libido, loss of interest in activities, anhedonia, lethargy, and an anxious and depressed mood. She described a rapid heartbeat, episodes of sweating, tightness in her chest, and a feeling of impending doom. It seemed to her that these feelings came out of nowhere. She was constantly afraid that the feelings would return, adding to her overall sense of dread and hopelessness. When her husband was murdered, Emily had been given diazepam (Valium) to take as needed. For the next 20 years, she took it once or twice a week. When she became more depressed in the past few months, she began taking the medication more often, eventually taking it daily. Then she became worried that she had become addicted to it, so she sought medical advice on how to stop. She was switched to lorazepam (Ativan), which is a simple substitute for Valium. She took it twice a day until she ran out. At that time, the doctor who had prescribed it was on vacation, so the back-up physician told her to just stop. When her regular doctor returned she was agitated and upset, and so he restarted her on Valium. She did not improve, so she was referred to a psychiatrist. The psychiatrist started her on risperidone (Risperdal), a major tranquilizer, and lithium carbonate (Nardil), which is used for bipolar disorders. The psychiatrist perhaps interpreted her lack of sleep and agitation as mania. She had severe side effects from the Nardil, but when that doctor was called, he had gone on vacation. His back-up psychiatrist discontinued those two medications and put her on alprazolam (Xanax), which seemed to help. However, he then switched her to clonazepam (Klonopin), supposedly to wean her from benzodiazepines, but she still had significant side effects, especially gastrointestinal distress. She saw a psychologist at this time who said she needed long-term counseling and started some behavioral stress management exercises. Her depression was steadily worsening through all of this, and she felt more and more hopeless about ever feeling better.

The early sessions were spent with both Emily and Harry, allowing them to describe in detail exactly what was happening and what benefits and side effects the medication she was taking was having. It was clear from the history that what was important initially was spending enough time with them both so that they felt heard and understood. Initially, I saw them twice a week for about a 3-month period. A considerable amount of time was spent explaining exactly what each medication was, when it would normally be indicated, and what the side effects were. As more and more of their experience was explained to them, both Emily and Harry became involved in problem solving to find the best medication, and Emily was referred to a different psychiatrist, one who was willing to work closely with a psychologist.

The new psychiatrist started Emily on an SSRI antidepressant, Paxil, with Klonopin in the morning and at bedtime to address her anxiety. Gradually she was weaned from Klonopin (which is a benzodiazepine) to BuSpar. She started to experience tremors as the Klonopin was withdrawn, and the psychiatrist prescribed propranolol hydrochloride (Inderal) to take as needed for the tremors. Inderal is an antihypertensive medication also used in the treatment of tremors. Emily used the Inderal sparingly, but one day she felt shaky and took the prescribed dose. I saw her shortly afterward, and she seemed fine. By this time, she was no longer severely depressed, and she was busy making plans for the holidays. Two hours after my visit, Harry called me, very upset, because Emily had what he called "amnesia." He put her on the speaker phone, and I asked her if she remembered seeing me earlier. She not only did not remember seeing me, she had no idea who I was. She was not distressed, just completely disoriented. I told them to call the psychiatrist immediately and follow his instructions. He told them she was "overstimulated" from the weekend and that she would be fine in the morning.

I was unsatisfied with this answer, so I consulted with a geriatrician, who said that this is a known response to Inderal in the elderly and that it should not have been given on an as-needed basis. Rather, if the intention was to wean her from the Klonopin and treat the tremors, the medications should have been given together and decreased together. Luckily, the delirium cleared by the next day, and Emily had no memory of the episode. Harry decided to throw away the Inderal, and Emily decided she could tolerate the tremors without medication.

At the present time, Emily is doing well, continuing to take Paxil daily, with minimal use of BuSpar as needed. In this case, onset of depression did not involve any clear precipitants except possibly her dependency on tranquilizers. However, the old, unfinished business from Emily's past that had to be dealt with might have been influential. Emily continues to have psychotherapy sessions twice a month to deal with these issues and as insurance against a recurrence of depression when it comes time to discontinue the Paxil.

Although the outcome of this case was ultimately successful, it was complicated by a litany of prescriptions for various psychotropic medications, some involving questionable judgment and having adverse consequences. We should like to say that this type of problem occurs rarely, but that is not the case with older clients. That is why the geriatric mental health specialist needs to be familiar with medications and their effects and, when possible, to work collaboratively with prescribing physicians.

We prefer to see patients at least once a month as long as they are taking antidepressants, particularly if they are being prescribed by an internist or by a psychiatrist who only spends a brief time with them discussing side effects. On a number of occasions, we have been able to head off a recurrence of depression when we have "caught" patients discontinuing medication on their own, usually because they had so few side effects with SSRIs that they underestimated what the medication was doing for them. In these instances, it was a relatively simple matter to get the clients back on course; if they had not been followed, they might have ended up back in a major depressive episode.

Case 3. Dysthymia

Betty is an 81-year-old divorced mother of four, who suffers from chronic symptoms of depression. She recently moved to a new city to live near her only daughter. She was referred to us by her geriatrician after several trials of antidepressant medications were unsuccessful due to her complaints about side effects. Her symptoms of depression were not severe enough to warrant a diagnosis of major depressive disorder, but they were distressing and disruptive in her life. This pattern of chronic depression meets DSM-IV criteria for dysthymia.

Betty is the oldest of five children who grew up in poverty. She was the babysitter, assistant mother, and housekeeper for the family. She married young to escape the home and had her own children right away. Her husband was a civilian employee of the military, and when he left her after 30 years of marriage, she was not even eligible to collect Social Security benefits. She lives on the small amount of support her ex-husband sends her, around $400 per month. Her children try to help her financially, but she is very proud and refuses most of their offers.

Betty has a negative cognitive style, anticipating the worst in every situation, and using her life experiences to justify her thinking. She has lived with financial insecurity her entire life, although she actually has more security now than she has ever had: she has Medicare for her medical expenses and a subsidized apartment. Still, she turns every situation into a negative scenario. Her children surprised her on her birthday by paying her cable television bill for her for a year. Rather than being pleased or accepting their intention, she complained that it wasn't what she wanted, that the cable company would not know what to do with it, and that she would much rather have had something else. That something else is their time. She has never asked directly for them to spend more time with her; this longing came out after considerable probing in therapy. What she would really like is for each child to call her weekly and have a leisurely conversation with her, letting her be a part of their lives. She has a hard time realizing that her negative style causes them to limit their exposure to her.

Apart from her depression, Betty is healthy and lives independently. Her biggest problem is that she is a chronic complainer, which drives her children away, rather than getting them to give her the attention she wants. She travels across the country to visit some of her children, and although she enjoys traveling, she does not allow herself to enjoy the visits. Her children's affluence makes her uncomfortable, and she criticizes their life styles. In therapy sessions, Betty has recognized that she turns her children off with her complaining, but that was as far as she could get. Her insight does not translate into more positive behaviors.

A main focus of treatment was dealing with the side effects of the medications she was taking for her depression. When Betty took Prozac she got diarrhea, a common side effect (see Table 8.2), so it was discontinued. Then she tried Paxil, and for about a week she felt as if she had been reborn. She was no longer depressed, ruminative, or negative in her outlook on life. The benefit did not last, however. Ultimately, she tried all the SSRIs and Effexor, but with little relief. Finally, I referred her to a new psychiatrist, who spent time listening to her history and all the past medications that she had tried. He started her on Pamelor, and when she complained of lethargy, he gave her Ritalin to take in the morning. This combination proved to be effective, helping her feel somewhat better and facilitating some progress in therapy.

Betty has continued in therapy for over 2 years, though like other older clients, she limits the number of sessions to one a month. The work in therapy, combined with a better drug regimen, has led to a small amount of progress. She now recognizes that her negative beliefs contribute to her dissatisfaction with her children and with life in general. She will say during a session, "I know I have to be more positive in my outlook. Help me do it." This awareness is a major step forward for her, as she had shown very little insight into her problems at any point previously in her life. It has not, as yet, led to a change in her behavior, in part due to the low frequency of her visits.

This case is fairly typical of older people with dysthymia. Though not meeting criteria for a major depressive disorder, symptoms are fairly constant and related to the person's cognitive style. Progress in treatment is slow and often involves preventing decline rather than achieving a major breakthrough.

Case 4. Coming to Terms with the Past

John is a retired economist. The youngest of four children, he was born just before the Depression. His father worked episodically during the Depression, and his oldest sister, who never married, also helped support the family. One brother, who was very much a loner and may have been paranoid, died of a heart attack. John was estranged from his remaining brother because of what he perceived as poor treatment of his wife by this brother. John thinks his father may have suffered from episodic depression and that his mother was depressed for the last 15 years of her life.

John's wife, Mary, is an artist, who helped found a nonprofit art school. John and Mary have been married for 40 years, and they have three children, a son and two daughters. The children are scattered around the country, none closer than a 4-hour drive. John feels some difficulty in these relationships, some of which he attributes to himself and some to Mary. He describes both himself and Mary as people who don't like to be told how to do anything, people who think they know the right way to do things. This has led to some tension in the marriage, and at times Mary has threatened to leave. They are very active in the community, although not without some pain because of perceived slights and grievances during their working years. About 2 years ago, they returned to John's family's hometown in southern Indiana and purchased a historic home, which they have been gradually restoring. They both feel much more relaxed in this community and enjoy the work they are doing on the house.

John retired in 1985 and had an episode of depression at that time. In

1986 he saw a psychotherapist for a year, but he felt he did not make progress with him. He had just finished a 4-year project, a book that he had not only written but typeset and published himself. He had also gotten involved in the stock market, developing theories that he had worked on during his career. John had irritable bowel syndrome, which had historically worsened in the fall. He also had high blood pressure, for which he took medication.

Just before the initial interview, John's internist had started him on Prozac. He reported a long history of morning anxiety, which he felt was a little better with the medication. He had tried Desyrel with his previous physician, but it had given him a dry mouth and constipation, so he had discontinued it.

John entered therapy with a determination to get to the root of his problems. He recognized that he was depressed and that he had been uncomfortable with people all his life. With some help, he was able to identify several areas that he worked on gradually over the next 2 years. First, he reviewed his career, in which he felt both an imposter and a failure. Using cognitive therapy techniques, he was able to examine and reframe many of his experiences and reach a measure of peace with what had been an active and primarily successful working life. Having been born during the Depression may have led to a pervasive sense of insecurity about the stability of work, and it certainly caused him to be very conservative financially (a common trait in this cohort). Further, there was a fair amount of psychopathology in his family, which may have colored his interpretation of people and events around him.

The second main focus in therapy was John's relationships with his children. John acknowledged difficulty getting close to his children, particularly his son. As he examined the relationships, he realized that both he and Mary were very critical of their children and that many of their visits ended in unpleasantness. Some of it was his fault, but much of it was Mary's. They had unvoiced expectations of how the children should treat them, then became angry and unpleasant when their expectations were disappointed. Over the course of treatment, and in collaboration with Mary's therapist, these expectations were identified, and John and Mary were able to be much more direct with their children. By the second year of therapy, John was reporting much less tension during visits and that the children were all talking directly to him, rather than avoiding him as they had in the past.

The third problem area was the marital relationship itself. John felt that he had been very self-absorbed during the course of his working career and not as supportive of Mary as he could have been. Both of them had experienced frustration and burnout in their careers simultaneously, and they had not been able to support one another. During the time this issue was discussed in therapy, John and Mary began to talk about it at home, and they gradually were able to resolve their past disappointments.

While John initially had a positive response to Prozac, after a few weeks he was having a hard time falling asleep. His physician prescribed

BuSpar at bedtime, but it did not help very much. After about 3 months on Prozac, John was switched to Zoloft. He was quite willing to stay on medication because he was experiencing not only a lift in mood but a marked reduction in ruminative thinking. He found himself waking without anxiety, wanting to begin the day, and with a much more optimistic outlook on life. He reported intense dreams that seemed very real, and he used them to help him think about the issues he was working to resolve in therapy. All the SSRIs can cause intense dream experiences and the likelihood that people remember their dreams. John has been on Zoloft for almost 2 years now with no adverse reactions. In his words, he had always been overly sensitive to rejection. On Zoloft he has been able to tolerate looking at his own role in creating situations where he feels rejection and to change his responses. By the end of therapy he had developed a sense of satisfaction with what he had been able to accomplish in his career, and he was optimistic about continuing to improve his family relationships. He had also begun to explore an artistic side of his nature through photography, which in the past he had been too self-conscious to try.

This case underscores the potential for growth in older clients. As in the other cases, treatment involved addressing current problems, as well as coming to terms with critical events in the client's past. Medication was again important, making possible the progress that took place in therapy. Over the course of treatment, John improved his relationships with his wife and children and developed a sense of satisfaction with himself and his life that he probably never had had before. He was also able to develop new interests and abilities.

CONCLUSIONS

In this chapter, we have examined treatment of depression, looking at psychotherapy approaches, medications, and ECT. We also consider the role of family in treatment of older depressed people and how illness and depression interact. Depression has been the most studied of any mental health problem of later life. With classic, uncomplicated cases, a variety of treatments have been found to be effective, including behavioral, cognitive-behavioral, and interpersonal psychotherapies, as well as medications and ECT. With clients who have a more complex clinical picture, for example, a mixture of depression and anxiety, a chronic illness, or a difficult family situation, therapists must find the combination of approaches that best addresses affective symptoms and their correlated cognitive, behavioral, and interpersonal dimensions. Medications are a valuable asset when used judiciously with older adults and a liability when not. Although there is little improvement in some cases, many older people can make significant gains and remain symptom free for long periods of time.

9

Coordination of Mental Health and Aging Services

An overriding goal of treatment of older adults is to support their continued independence and autonomy. Timely use of community services can make it possible for older people with mental and physical problems to remain in their own home. For older people who have chronic mental health problems, such as schizophrenia or personality disorders, or who are suffering from dementia, use of community resources is often the best strategy for providing help and preventing burnout of family or other providers. When home care is not feasible, clinicians can help in selecting the most appropriate and least restrictive alternative.

Knowledge of aging services is an indispensable part of geriatric practice. Clinicians are frequently called on to make complex judgments about an older person's ability to remain at home. To do so, they must be familiar with the types of services that are available and how to access them. In this chapter, we begin by examining why staying in the least restrictive setting should be a goal for interventions. Next, we look at the range of social and health services that can support older people living in their home. We then explore the types of specialized housing available to the elderly. The chapter concludes with a review of model mental health programs for older people.

MAINTAINING INDEPENDENCE: USING THE PRINCIPLE OF MINIMUM INTERVENTION

When older people's independence is threatened, minimum intervention means supporting them in their own home or in the least restrictive setting possible There are many threats to the independence of older people. The frequent comorbidity of physical and mental health problems in later life combined with negative expectations about old age lead to widespread acceptance of custodial care as an appropriate solution. When confronted with patients who have prominent physical and mental disabilities, many physicians and other health professionals encourage placement in nursing homes without considering other alternatives. Nursing homes are what people are familiar with. It also requires less effort to place someone in a nursing home than to arrange for care in the home. There are, however, reasons to maintain someone at home for as long as possible, as well as hidden costs associated with placement.

As an example, an older woman living alone might be prone to dizziness and falls. Since she lives alone, she could potentially injure herself and not be able to get help. One solution would be to place her in special housing, such as an assisted living facility, a board and care home, or even a nursing home, where there would be someone to check on her. That would be a reasonable solution, if it were preferred by the client and there were no other alternatives. But while addressing the main problem, this solution would place restrictions on this woman that have nothing to do with her problem. Depending on the facility, she might have to give up her furnishings and share a room with a roommate not of her choosing. She might not be familiar enough with the neighborhood to go out for walks or shopping. Or the facility might be reluctant to let their clients go out, for instance, if the neighborhood is unsafe or if they are concerned that clients might wander off, fall, or get into other difficulties. In addressing one problem, the risk of falling, the move to a protected setting can set off a chain of other changes in her life that restrict the client, compromise her independence, and possibly set a downward course in physical and/or emotional functioning.

Alternatives to moving this woman would be to provide her with an emergency call system, which she could use to get help, or to find a neighbor or volunteer who could check on her at regular intervals. These approaches are consistent with minimum intervention; they address the main problem or concern, the risk of falling, but do not compromise the woman's independence in other ways.

Kahn (1975) contrasts minimum intervention with the usual approach to treatment of older people, which he characterizes as "custodialism." Custodial approaches emphasize an older person's dependency while failing to identify or support remaining areas of competence. Much of our long-term care system is custodial in nature, stressing security over independence, maintenance over rehabilitation. By contrast, treatment guided by the principle of minimum intervention identifies strengths of the client or situation, as well as resources that can be drawn on to reduce the risks or problems.

The decision to place someone in an institution is usually based on the judgment that the person is not safe to remain at home or will not receive adequate care at home. Focused on the risks associated with remaining at home, the decision fails to take into account risks associated with placement. The move itself is stressful and can lead to some loss in functional ability for a frail older person. The stresses of nursing home placement have been well-documented and include, under some circumstances, increased rates of mortality (see Schulz & Brenner, 1977; Aneshensel, Pearlin, Mullan, Zarit, & Whitlatch, 1995). A move to a new home or apartment, to a child's home, or into a retirement complex are typically less disruptive but still can be stressful. The degree to which a move is stressful depends on the amount of change between the old and new environment. Healthy older people who move into planned retirement or life care communities usually experience few problems or difficulties (Préville et al., 1996). A move from the community to a nursing home, however, is much more stressful than moving from one community setting to another. The degree of control the older person has over the decision to move also is related to postrelocation adjustment (Schulz & Brenner, 1977).

The other main risk associated with institutional care is that it will induce unnecessary dependencies, or what Kahn (1975) termed "excess disabilities." Excess disabilities is a term that has come into wide use in geriatrics. It often is applied to the results of not treating potentially treatable conditions, for example, failing to identify and treat depression in a person with a chronic health problem. As a result of not providing appropriate treatment, the patient remains depressed and does not maximize remaining abilities or take full advantage of rehabilitation efforts. Failure to provide adequate treatment is a very important source of excess disabilities. Kahn (1975) was also concerned about the opposite situation, that providing too much treatment or care would induce unnecessary or excess disabilities. He believed that excess disabilities develop from interactions in which helpers support dependence and discourage independence. As an example, if an older person needs a lot of time to get dressed in the morning, and a helper, whether family or staff of an institution, gets frustrated with how long it is taking and instead dresses the person, that can lead both to psychological dependence on the helper and a loss in the range of motion needed to dress oneself. In this example, the helper does too much for the older person, thereby encouraging dependence. In other situations, a helper might restrict independent behavior to reduce any risks associated with it, for instance, discouraging an older person who might fall from walking. Without regular exercise, however, muscles weaken and the person becomes even more frail or may stop walking altogether.

These kinds of interactions can occur at home as well as in an institutional setting. An overprotective or controlling spouse or child can unwittingly undermine independent functioning or recovery from disability. A patient who is depressed or dependent to begin with may elicit responses that encourage further dependency and disability. But while there is potential for excess disabilities in any setting, they are more likely to occur in an institution than at home.

Several features of an institutional setting lead to excess disabilities. First and foremost, institutions inadvertently reinforce dependent behavior. In a series of elegant studies, Margaret Baltes and her colleagues (e.g., M. Baltes & Wahl, 1992; M. Baltes, Neumann, & Zank, 1994) have studied the interactions of nursing home staff with patients. Staff consistently reinforce dependent behaviors while ignoring or discouraging residents' independence. They do so out of a mistaken view that residents are helpless and incompetent, so they provide too much assistance with dressing, bathing, and the like. It is also easier and quicker to take over tasks, for example, dressing or feeding. To cite another example, staff find it more convenient and quicker to put patients into adult diapers than to take them to the toilet on a regular basis. Despite continued warnings about the risks of overprotection, excess helping is found in most institutional settings.

A second factor in the development of excess disabilities is that nursing homes restrict independence out of a concern that they would be liable for falls or other accidents. If someone walks unsteadily and might fall, the institution discourages walking, even though that leads to a decrease in the ability to walk. An older person living at home may be willing to accept the risk of a fall, but in an institutional setting, the responsibility for the decision is taken away.

Third, institutional settings take control away from residents in a wide range of domains, not just in areas where they need assistance. Such choices as when people get up and go to bed, what they eat, when they bathe and go to the toilet, what activities they engage in, and who rooms with whom may be made by the institution. Think for a minute about your own food preferences, and then imagine a situation in which all your meals are planned according to the lowest common denominator, sufficiently bland to be served to everyone in a facility. It is easy to see why people feel a loss of control over their lives in institutional settings.

Personal control is an important psychological component of well-being and has been found to have sweeping consequences for functioning and health. Loss of personal control is related to poorer health and psychological distress and even to higher mortality among older people (Rodin, 1986). Restoring even small amounts of control to nursing home residents, such as letting them care for plants in their rooms, leads to better functioning and, remarkably, reduced mortality.

Control is an issue for community programs as well. Even when keeping people out of nursing homes is their stated goal, service programs can have the opposite effect, because they do not give elders or their families any control over treatment decisions (MaloneBeach, Zarit, & Spore, 1992).

The principle of minimum intervention does not imply that institutions are always inappropriate or should be avoided at any cost. Specialized housing has a place in a continuum of services for disabled elders. Institutionalization is frequently necessary and the results can be positive. Some older people do better after moving to a protected setting, because they receive adequate assistance and social support. The nursing home environment can be preferable to the home that a patient came from, such as in cases of abuse or neglect. Given their limited resources, most nursing homes do a creditable job. New approaches to nursing home design and programming are also reducing some of the inadvertent dependency. Mental health consultants can intervene with staff and patients to minimize the adverse consequences of institutional life (see Chapter 13).

Rather than asserting that one type of intervention is always better than another, we stress that all treatments have potential risks associated with them. Instead of thinking only about the problems that an intervention might solve, clinicians need also to consider the problems it can create and to weigh the gains against the possible losses. From this perspective, minimum intervention guides us to select an approach that effectively addresses the client's major problem in the least disruptive or destabilizing manner possible.

The Decision to Move an Aging Parent

The decision to move an older adult is usually complex, and a clear best choice is not immediately obvious. A particularly complicated situation is when children and their parents live in different communities, and the children grow increasingly concerned that their parents can no longer care for themselves. The parent or parents may live alone with a shrinking nearby support network, and with diminishing ability to manage by themselves. Sometimes their house and/or neighborhood have deteriorated. Children may be frustrated trying to coordinate medical care or social services at a distance. They may have tried to arrange for home help only to have their parent fire the helpers after a short trial. As a result of these concerns, children may consider moving their parents close by or even into their home. This decision assumes urgency if the parent has frequent health crises or other emergencies.

In some circumstances, the decision to relocate is straightforward. Some older people may choose to move to be closer to their children. When an older person actively participates in the decision, there are likely to be fewer post-relocation problems. In situations where there is clear risk if the parent continues living alone, for example, the parent suffers from dementia and does not eat regularly or wanders away from the house and gets lost, then relocation is necessary. The decision becomes complicated when the risks associated with remaining in place are not clear-cut or immediate and the older person is reluctant to move. In those situations, the decision process should take into account not just the perceived benefits of the move but also the possible risks associated with relocation—and the older person's competence to make the decision.

One cost of moving is that the older person loses contact with neighbors and friends. Families may underestimate the extent to which their parent depends on these interactions. After moving, their parent may become totally dependent on them for social interactions. The assumption that a frail older person can replace friends of a lifetime in a short time is unrealistic. Children may encourage their parent to meet new people at a senior center or similar program, but a newcomer may not be accepted quickly in these programs. An older person who is demoralized or depressed over the move or who has limited mobility is likely to have a very difficult time making social contacts outside the family.

Another drawback to relocation is that the familiarity of one's home and neighborhood may enhance some competencies. An older person may be able to drive safely on familiar streets but may not be able to learn his or her way around a new locale. Other daily routines, such as cooking and shopping, can become disrupted by a move, especially if the elder is now sharing a house with children. A move is especially disruptive to someone with cognitive impairment, who has difficulty learning new routines. On the other hand, an argument can be made for moving dementia patients earlier in their disease, rather than later, because they may still have adequate cognitive resources to make an adjustment.

There is no perfect solution to this dilemma. Arguments can be made on boh the sides of moving and not moving someone. The clinician's role is to help older people and their families explore their alternatives, not to make the decision for them. Any decision ultimately needs to reflect the older person's values and preferences, not what we as mental health professionals might want to see. Over the years, we have worked with families who keep a relative at home despite a burden on them that we would be unwilling to accept for ourselves. We have also encountered the opposite situation, where the family relocates a frail older person despite adequate resources to continue at home. Our role is not to tell families what we think they should do. It is to present them with information and to help them weigh the pros and cons of their alternatives.

AGING SERVICE NETWORK

The key to supporting frail older people in the community is access to services that can assist them and provide relief for family caregivers. Most communities in the United States have a network of aging services designed to provide assistance to older people. Many services are authorized under provisions of the Older Americans Act, which was passed by Congress in

1965 and renewed several times since (see McConnell & Beitler, 1991, for an overview). Services are funded from a variety of other sources as well, including federal, state, and local funds and private donations. The result is a patchwork system of services that can vary from one locale to another and that is not always coordinated within itself or with mental health services. The method of paying for services can also vary considerably. Some programs require partial or full payment by clients, others are free or involve minimal costs. We describe a typical array of services and also strategies for identifying how clients can obtain the services.

A starting point for identifying services for older people is the local Area Agency on Aging (AAA). AAAs were authorized by the Older Americans Act and are found in every part of the United States. In some places, the AAAs run services for well elderly, such as senior citizens centers and nutrition programs, and in a few states, they also provide case management, that is, helping match client needs to the available services. In most states, however, the AAAs do not provide services directly but serve as a clearinghouse, providing information about what type of help is available.

Another valuable source of information about local services is voluntary organizations, such as the Alzheimer's Association, or similar groups that focus on a specific problem or illness. Local chapters of these voluntary organizations maintain lists of agencies that provide assistance and may even be helpful in identifying physicians or other professionals who work well with people suffering from a particular disorder. In some parts of the country, there are unique arrangements for providing information and assistance. In California, for example, a statewide network of Caregiver Resource Centers provides information and services to families of adults suffering from brain injuries and illnesses, including dementia and stroke (Feinberg & Kelly, 1995).

Some community programs support the well elderly, older people who are living independently and who do not have significant mental health or physical problems. Other services target people with disabilities or who are at risk in other ways. Among programs for the well elderly, the most visible and best known are senior citizens centers. Senior centers typically provide social and recreational activities for healthy older people. In most instances, senior centers do not have sufficient staff to assist people with significant disabilities, nor is their programming geared for that population. A long-time senior center participant who becomes disabled may be able to continue attending, often with the help of other participants, but it is usually very difficult for someone new who has significant disabilities to get involved in a center. Some senior centers provide information about support services for the disabled elderly and may even help arrange for services.

Nutrition programs are also widely available, usually through senior centers, but sometimes at other community locations as well. Older people can get a hot lunch at these programs at a low cost. Like senior centers, nu-

trition programs are designed for people who are at least partly independent and do not require supervision or assistance during the meal. Home-
bound older people can take advantage of meals-on-wheels programs,
which deliver a hot middle-of-the-day meal and a cold evening meal. Cost
varies but is usually subsidized so that lower-income people can afford the
service. Meals on wheels are provided through many different agencies. Local AAAs have information on how to obtain meals on wheels in a particular community.

A service that is usually available for both well elderly and those with
special needs is transportation. Rides are typically provided to medical and
mental health appointments and to other services and programs. In some
locales, elderly can arrange for rides to the grocery store. Transportation services are organized at the local level and vary considerably from one part of
the country to another. Rural areas may have very limited coverage.

For people who need assistance with everyday tasks, an extensive array of services is available in most communities. Home health programs
provide nurses to assist with health care in the home or nursing aides to
help with activities of daily living, such as dressing or bathing. Home health
care is reimbursable under Medicare if it follows hospitalization for an
acute health problem and is ordered by a physician. Medicaid or special
state programs sometimes pay for this kind of assistance when Medicare
runs out or in chronic care situations that Medicare does not cover. Most
home health costs, however, are paid privately.

One of the major needs for families taking care of an older person is
respite services, that is, programs that provide supervision for a disabled elder to relieve the family caregivers. Respite can be provided by home health
aides, through adult day services, or in overnight programs.

The number of adult day service programs has increased greatly during the past 10 years. These programs are designed to provide structured
activities and supervision for older people who have physical and/or mental disabilities and to give relief to family caregivers. Programs can vary
widely in how they are organized and what populations they serve. Some
are organized on a medical model, are staffed by nurses, and have allied
health services such as physical therapy available as part of the program.
These programs are eligible for Medicare and Medicaid reimbursement.
While often geared to people making the transition from hospital to community, they also serve elderly with chronic disabilities, though Medicare
does not usually apply in those situations. In contrast to medical day care
programs, social models emphasize the benefits of social and recreational
activities for their clients.

Some day service programs are designed only for people who are cognitively intact. Others specialize in care of dementia patients. Most day programs serve both cognitively intact and impaired older people and have
varying amounts of special programming and activities for people with de-

mentia. Some centers conduct almost all activities separately, and in other programs, cognitively intact and impaired patients will spend most of the day together doing the same activities (Steiner & Zarit, 1995). These different ways of organizing services for people with dementia cut across the medical–social model distinction.

Adult day service programs vary in their hours of operation. Some programs are designed to assist a working family caregiver by offering services Monday through Friday, with extended hours to accommodate work schedules. A few centers even offer Saturday hours as well. Other programs are open for a shorter period of time during the day (e.g., 10:00 to 3:00) or only 3 or 4 days a week.

There is no consensus on which models of adult day services—medical or social, dementia-specific or integrated—work best. Families' reports of satisfaction with adult day service programs are generally high and show no difference between the various models (Steiner & Zarit, 1995; Greene & Ferraro, 1996). A more important consideration is that prospective clients and their families often misunderstand the purpose of the programs. Equating these programs with child day care, they believe that elders receive nothing more than baby sitting. Good day service programs offer highly varied, structured activities that can maximize functioning in people with a variety of disabilities.

Another way families can obtain respite is by hiring a home health aide or similar worker to come into the older person's home. Sometimes that person will also do some chores, such as prepare a meal. The in-home aide can supervise the elder but usually does not have training to structure activities appropriate to the person's level of functioning. The level of experience and competence of home health aides is quite variable, especially when it comes to care of dementia patients (MaloneBeach, Zarit, & Spore, 1992). In some places, Alzheimer's Association chapters or other advocacy groups have organized respite care services to meet this need.

Many families prefer in-home help to adult day services. They are sometimes able privately to hire someone, who can provide good-quality care. The cost of this service can become prohibitive, especially when solicitated through an agency. Another limitation of in-home help compared to day care is that it is more unreliable. A worker can be sick or quit or decide not to show up for some reason on a particular day. Aides have sometimes taken advantage of older people living alone, stealing money or other items from them, or physically abusing them. In contrast, day services are consistently available. The program operates even if a staff member is ill. The presence of several staff members and the comings and goings of families protect against abuse.

One other type of respite service is overnight care. The least developed of these alternatives, overnight respite can be provided by hospitals, nursing homes, and, on occasion, adult day service programs. Families can place their relative in these programs for short stays that range from 1 day to a few weeks.

There is a great deal of variability from one community to another in what services are available and how they are organized. It should be no surprise, then, that services have been developed to help families through the maze of programs and agencies. These services go under the names of case management, care management, and similar terms. Case managers identify available services and assess an older client's eligibility for particular services. Some AAAs provide case management, but this service is usually available in other community agencies. Increasingly, independent, fee-for-service providers offer care management. These providers usually offer more extensive care management than agency or public programs. We routinely work with a private care manager who helps older people and their families identify appropriate services to bring into the home.

The other main entry point for community long-term care services is the hospital, which is mandated to conduct discharge planning. In theory, there should be a lot of coordination between hospital social workers and community programs, but they often operate independently (Wiener, 1996). Since the early 1980s, hospitals have been under pressure to discharge older patients as quickly as possible as a way of controlling costs. One consequence of shorter hospital stays is that hospital social service personnel may not have the time to work with the family or to develop adequate discharge plans.

Paying for Community-Based Long-Term Care Services

Although community services can be instrumental in keeping an older person in his or her own home and out of an institution, these services are not routinely covered by Medicare or by any other third-party payer. Medicare will pay for home health services following hospitalization for an acute medical problem if the services are deemed medically necessary and are ordered by the physician. Care for chronic problems such as dementia is not covered, though patients with dementia who were hospitalized for other medical diagnoses can sometimes receive Medicare for home health services on discharge. Home health care has been growing faster than any other part of Medicare in recent years, mainly because people stay in the hospital for shorter periods of time. Services provided under the auspices of the AAAs, such as nutrition programs and senior centers, do not charge fees but ask for donations.

Many people carry private Medigap policies, which are designed to provide insurance for the portion of costs for medical services not covered by Medicare, such as copayments. Medigap policies pay for home health services when Medicare does, not in situations when a charge is not eligible for Medicare reimbursement. Coverage of these services by most Medicare HMOs is limited.

Some individuals may have coverage for home health care through long-term care insurance. This type of insurance is designed to provide coverage for nursing homes but usually includes benefits for services designed to keep someone at home. Private long-term care insurance is expensive and is not widely used.

People with low income who qualify for Medicaid may be able to receive some community-based services at minimal cost to them. What services are covered varies from state to state. States may also have special programs for lower-income people who fall above the minimum income levels for Medicaid eligibility. New Jersey, for example, provides assistance to families using adult day care for a relative suffering from dementia, while California helps families pay for respite care in cases of dementia, stroke, or other causes of brain damage. Finally, many nonprofit or charitable agencies provide scholarships or other financial assistance to people who cannot pay the full fee.

The system of reimbursement for community services, then, is piecemeal. Coverage of the costs for services is not universal and can vary considerably from one state to another or even within different regions of a state. The absence of a comprehensive system of insurance for community-based long-term care is a major barrier to service use for many older people. It also has probably slowed the development of a more effective network of services.

SPECIALIZED HOUSING FOR OLDER PEOPLE

The programs we have reviewed so far are designed to assist people living in ordinary community housing. Many different kinds of specialized housing are available for older people. Some housing is designed specifically for well elderly, some is for people with varying degrees and types of disabilities, and some facilities include both.

The well elderly have many different options for specialized housing. Retirement communities are planned developments that provide housing for independent older people. These communities usually provide a great deal of autonomy. People have their own apartment or house, but there are also shared facilities and social activities. Retirement communities do not routinely provide help to a disabled older person. That must be arranged by the individual and his or her family. People who require assistance to continue living in their home or apartment can remain in these communities as long as they are able to arrange for the help they need.

The term "retirement home" covers a wide range of facilities, but most also target the well elderly, or those people who can largely care for themselves. Social and recreational activities are usually available, as are meals and housekeeping. Some facilities bring in services as their residents age in place and need help to remain in their apartments. In some parts of the country, retirement homes are evolving into assisted living or board and care facilities. As residents decline, the facility arranges for help with activities of daily living. That approach is widely used in the Scandinavian countries, where residents can have their own apartments in a senior citizens building but can get assistance as needed (Malmberg, Sundström, & Zarit, 1995).

Many retirement homes are private, and those catering to the wealthy older population are quite luxurious. Housing for low-income seniors is also available, with eligibility and rent tied to the person's income. As with other retirement housing, residents must largely be independent, and little or no assistance is routinely available on the premises.

For people with significant disabilities, nursing homes are the best known alternative, but there is an increasing number of other facilities that provide care, particularly, assisted living or board and care facilities (the title varies depending on state regulations and traditions). They differ from nursing homes in emphasizing the social environment rather than medical care. Some programs offer innovative services that support the autonomy of disabled elderly, while other facilities are little more than warehouses. These programs are described in more detail in Chapter 13.

Finally, continuing care retirement communities (CCRCs) represent a unique part of the spectrum of senior housing. These communities provide a full range of housing, from independent living to nursing home care. Residents pay a substantial entrance fee when they move into the community and then pay a set monthly fee. If they subsequently need nursing home care, it is provided in the community for little or no extra charge. CCRCs admit only people who are still independent. Because of the high entrance fee, these programs are limited to the more affluent elderly, although some CCRCs are sponsored by religious organizations, unions, or other nonprofit groups and have reduced fees for some residents.

Paying for Housing

As with community-based long-term care services, the various housing alternatives are not routinely paid by Medicare. Medicare will cover nursing home stays for short periods of time (up to 120 days) if the older person has come from the hospital and has medical problems that can respond to continued treatment. With the trend toward shorter hospital stays, it is increasingly common for older people to be discharged to subacute care units in nursing homes, which provide follow-up medical care and rehabilitation services. But long-term residence in nursing homes is not covered by

Medicare. Long-term care insurance is specifically designed for nursing home costs, but, as noted, it is still quite rare and expensive. Some Medigap policies cover the copayment for nursing home care when Medicare is the primary payer. Other types of specialized housing for people with disabilities, such as assisted living, may be covered by long-term care insurance but not by Medicare.

Who, then, pays for nursing homes? The biggest payers are the residents themselves or their families, who pay 57% of the costs, while Medicaid payments account for 40% of the costs. The remaining amount comes from Medicare or other sources (Wiener, 1990). People become eligible for Medicaid coverage when they spend down their assets paying for care. They can retain a minimal amount of assets (about $2,400, a small amount of insurance, and personal possessions), but all other resources need to be used up before they can qualify for Medicaid. In the past, some people avoided the spenddown requirement by transferring assets to children, but current laws require a 3-year look-back period. If assets were divested by the person during that period, they are counted toward the amount that must be paid privately for nursing home care before the person becomes eligible for Medicaid.

When a nursing home patient is married, his or her spouse has protection against impoverishment. Under rules established by the 1987 Omnibus Budget Reconciliation Act, a spouse can retain one half of an estate up to approximately $67,000, as well as a home. The remaining assets are used to pay for nursing home care, with the patient becoming eligible for Medicaid when those assets run out. It is estimated that 43% of elderly in nursing homes are either initially on Medicaid or spend down their assets and require Medicaid (Spillman & Kemper, 1995).

Another consideration is that not all nursing homes accept Medicaid. A patient who uses up his or her assets paying for a private nursing home may then have to move to another facility that accepts Medicaid. This possibility needs to be considered in the choice of a facility.

Clearly, the absence of universal long-term care insurance has serious consequences. Families face a severe financial burden when they place a relative in a nursing home. This burden is particularly hard on spouses, even with the protection they now have. This is one more reason why it is important not to recommend placement to families in a casual way or without considering all the alternatives.

COORDINATION OF COMMUNITY AND MENTAL HEALTH SERVICES

An important step in providing support to frail elderly in the community is coordinating mental health services with the help available from the aging network. Someone suffering from chronic physical or mental health problems typically has multiple needs, and so several agencies may need to be involved. Coordinating this effort is critical to its success. Failure to provide adequate coordination can result in a breakdown of community care and subsequent institutionalization.

While there is widespread recognition of the need for coordination of services, the service system remains disorganized and confusing (McConnell & Beitler, 1991). There is no central entry point for services and little coordination among programs. Often, the task of getting two programs to cooperate with one another is monumental. They may have different eligibilities, assessments, and reimbursement procedures. Clients find themselves dealing with multiple bureaucracies, each with rigid rules about service delivery.

The ideal would be a user-friendly system that brings services to the older person and makes access easy and understandable. One promising strategy is development of links between community mental health programs, AAAs, and key providers of support services. These links lead to increased referrals of older adults to community mental health centers as well as access for mental health clients to appropriate community services (e.g., Knight, 1989; Lebowitz, Light, & Bailey, 1987; Raschko, 1985).

Advocates for the mentally ill elderly have long argued the need for a coordinated system of services to identify cases and support independence. A pioneering program was developed by British psychiatrist Duncan Macmillan (1967). Taking over a traditional geropsychiatric inpatient unit, he devised a program of short-term inpatient care followed by ongoing community treatment. A particular innovation he used was that inpatient staff followed up patients after discharge. The result was adequate coordination between inpatient and outpatient care. Coordinated outpatient care made it possible to keep most people in the community and out of nursing homes.

Several innovative programs of community mental health care for the elderly have been reported over the years (e.g., Glasscote, Gudeman, & Miles, 1977; Knight, 1989; Perlin & Kahn, 1968; Raschko, 1985, 1992; Whitehead, 1970). A number of common features can be identified. First is an outreach program to find cases before the problem is so severe that little can be done. Second, home assessment is critical. Many clients are reluctant to go to an office. Home assessments, as we stressed earlier, also provide valuable information about clients' ability to care for themselves. A third factor is building effective bridges between aging services and mental health care. Regular meetings or sharing staff between agencies can go a long way to reducing the problems of coordinating services.

One of the most successful programs serving older clients has been developed by the Spokane Community Mental Health Center (Raschko, 1992). This model program serves both traditional and hard-to-reach clients, such as those suffering from chronic mental health problems. Several unique features of this program contribute to its success. First is the method of case identification, called the gatekeepers program. The gatekeepers program is designed to identify high-risk older people. The program provides training to personnel in a variety of service roles who might have contact with older people in need, such as meter readers from the electric, gas, and water companies, property appraisers from the county assessor's office, bank personnel, apartment and mobile home managers, postal carriers, pharmacists, police and fire department personnel. The "gatekeepers" are taught how to identify older people who may be having difficulties.

Once a client is identified through a gatekeeper or traditional referral, a multidisciplinary team conducts an assessment. In-home assessments are routinely made. An emphasis is placed on developing rapport and building trust, which is critical in order to gain access to the home of a suspicious or frightened older person. The assessment leads to development of a detailed treatment plan. Implementation of this service plan is overseen by a clinical coordinator on the service team.

Agreements with the AAA and other organizations facilitate coordination of mental health and aging services. Regular meetings are held with other agencies to enhance coordination of services and deal with problems as they arise. The program is successful in overcoming the resistance of typically hostile or suspicious clients and in developing a coordinated effort to maintain people in their own homes when doing so is safe and appropriate.

A similar program that provides comprehensive community mental health services is described by Knight (1989). Through a model of community outreach and coordinated mental health and aging services, Knight found it possible to reduce in-patient admissions and to support people in community settings.

The need for multimodal interventions underscores the importance of multidisciplinary approaches for working with older people. Building treatment teams in hospitals and community mental health centers or between mental health programs and aging service programs is very important. Many disciplines have valuable roles to play in treatment of older people. While it is not necessary for all disciplines to be involved in treatment of each case, the potential for consultation and collaboration is critical.

Zeiss and Steffen (1996a) describe the theory of team building and its implementation in a health care setting. They emphasize the need for interdisciplinary teams because the problems older people have are complex and require attention from people from several disciplines. A team approach assures that care is not fragmented and does address consistent and appropriate treatment goals.

A particularly significant feature of interdisciplinary collaboration is mutual respect among disciplines. The perspective of one discipline should not be seen as primary over another. In our current system, too much emphasis is usually placed on medical solutions, with the consequence that appropriate psychological and social interventions are overlooked.

Wattis and Church (1986) described a geriatric mental health treatment team that had a unique arrangement designed to provide better integration of multidisciplinary perspectives. In this approach, the multidisciplinary team conducts and then reviews the assessment. Following their review, one member of the team is placed in charge of the case to carry out the treatment plan. This person can be from any discipline and is not necessarily the psychiatrist or geriatrician on the team. This procedure acknowledges that the main focus of treatment will sometimes appropriately be nonmedical. It also assures fuller representation of each disciplinary perspective.

CONCLUSIONS

In this chapter, we have presented a framework for treatment of the elderly that emphasizes coordination of mental health and aging services in order to support continued independence. Treatment that allows clients to make choices consistent with their values and that maximizes opportunities for appropriate levels of independence should be emphasized. Supporting the independence of older people depends on coordinating efforts among professionals and agencies. Effective coordination can often be difficult but is typically the key to maintaining someone in an optimal community setting. Placement in a protected setting such as a nursing home or boarding home is sometimes necessary, despite the best efforts to arrange community resources, and may represent the optimal intervention when compared to the available alternatives. Before taking that step, however, we encourage considering the alternatives and the client's own values and preferences. A frail older person encounters risks while struggling to remain in a community setting but faces other risks in a protected setting. The decision should never be made quickly or mechanically, such as matching the client to a setting based solely on level of functional impairment. These situations require clinicians to draw on a full range of assessment, treatment, and consultation skills for working with the client, the client's family, and other professionals and service providers, as well as the ability to examine values and choices in complex situations.

10

Paranoid Disorders

An older man complains that he is awakened during the night by a light shining on him through his bedroom window, but his wife maintains that the room is dark all night. A woman claims that she hears music playing wherever she goes. She moves from one apartment to another to get away from the music, but it has started to bother her in her new home, making her nervous and upset. Another woman believes that an intruder has been coming into her home, messing it up and stealing things, but there is no evidence that anyone has broken in.

Paranoid symptoms such as these are very disruptive, both to older patients and to the people around them. People with paranoid symptoms are often upset and frightened but usually have little insight about how they are distorting reality. This combination of delusional beliefs and lack of insight is very disturbing to other people. It can weaken family supports and make professionals angry with patients or refuse to help them. A person who has paranoid symptoms is more likely to be stigmatized as crazy than someone who is depressed. Much can be done to help older people with paranoid symptoms. Interventions can often reduce or eliminate symptoms and make the problem more manageable for both patients and the people around them.

We have devoted considerable attention to paranoid disorders for a couple of reasons. First, many of the patterns of paranoid symptoms encountered in older people are not found in younger adults. Second, paranoid disorders call forth all the special skills clinicians need to work effectively with older adults: conducting a differential diagnosis, forming a therapeutic relationship with a person who may be frail or difficult, coordinating psychological and medical treatment, working with families, and working with community resources to help patients stay in their own homes.

Paranoid symptoms in late life can have several distinct patterns and etiologies (see Chapter 4). Clients with long-standing symptoms may be suffering from paranoid schizophrenia or paranoid personality disorder. Treatment would be similar to that for other people with these disorders, with attention to appropriate age-related issues (e.g., comorbidity with physical illness, death of key support person). When the onset of symptoms has occurred in late life (after age 45), the etiology may be due to sensory losses or stresses that increase social isolation and bring out or exacerbate long-standing personality problems.

The current consensus is that late-onset paranoid disorders are a form of schizophrenia, and they are classified that way in DSM-IV. We prefer the older term "late-life paraphrenia," because there are substantial differences in symptoms and treatment from more typical cases of paranoid schizophrenia. There is usually little evidence of loose, tangential, or circumstantial thought patterns or other characteristic schizophrenic symptoms. From a treatment standpoint, viewing these late-life disorders as schizophrenia can lead to an overreliance on antipsychotic medications, which sometimes is not the best approach. We believe reserving the term "schizophrenia" for more classic cases encourages careful evaluation of older clients with paranoid symptoms and formulation of a multifaceted treatment plan that includes more than just medication. Symptoms can also be due to dementia or delirium. Even in people with a prior history of paranoia, organic causes should be ruled out carefully.

Treatment depends in part on the etiology of the paranoid symptoms, but there are elements that are common to every type of paranoid disorder. Psychological treatment takes place on several levels: building a relationship with the client and, when appropriate, working with family, community, and/or institution staff so that they can respond in ways that help contain the symptoms. A basic step is for the clinician to establish a trusting and accepting relationship which is a challenge because clients are suspicious and their symptoms are often blatant and disturbing distortions of reality. It is possible, however, to enter into the paranoid person's world, to identify the pain that lies behind their distortions, and thereby to establish the trust needed to make treatment successful. Another important feature of treatment is coordination of medical and psychological approaches, especially when medications and health problems are involved in onset of symptoms or when medications are part of the treatment plan.

Treatment of paranoid symptoms should follow the principle of minimum intervention. The goal of treatment is to identify and treat any reversible components, and if that is not possible, to reduce the negative ramifications of paranoid beliefs, allowing a person to function as well as possible despite some paranoid thinking. When possible, paranoid clients should be helped to stay in their homes, because an unwanted move usually only heightens their symptoms. This type of approach can prevent the breakdown of a fragile system.

The number of clients with paranoid symptoms a clinician sees varies by the treatment setting. In university-affiliated clinics, few clients with paranoid symptoms are willing to fill out all the forms and go through the thorough evaluations that are often required by a teaching facility. Clients with paranoid symptoms are more likely to be encountered in community mental health programs and occasionally in private practice. Paranoid symptoms can also be a problem in institutional settings.

We illustrate the different patterns of paranoid symptoms and their treatment with case examples.

LONG-TERM PARANOID SCHIZOPHRENIA

People with paranoid schizophrenia earlier in life grow old, and their problems sometimes continue or are exacerbated by losses and other stresses in later life. With long-standing paranoid schizophrenia, the main issues for clinicians are to continue treatments that were effective in the past, to help the person's support network cope with symptoms, and to identify and address any new problems or stressors that may be upsetting the client and exacerbating symptoms. Treatment that focuses on these new problems and stressors can lead to an overall improvement in functioning.

The following example illustrates treatment of a woman suffering from paranoid schizophrenia. She had a long history of delusions and hallucinations, which she reported as being continuous but which also worsened periodically. She first sought help because she believed she was being harassed by people who lived in the apartment next to her. She said her neighbors had computers that were constantly making noise and were reading her thoughts. She asked for help in finding another apartment so that she could escape the computer people. Although we did not think a move would necessarily reduce her symptoms, we provided information about available housing, and she arranged a move for herself and a daughter who lived with her. The therapist who had initially seen her was accepting and empathic, so when the computer people "tracked down" the client at her new residence, she went back for treatment. Treatment focused on giving her support and empathy and helping her build adaptive skills to resist the intrusions by the computers. Her symptoms were never contradicted. Reality testing dealt with alternatives on how she could cope better, never on whether the computer people were really tormenting her. The goal of treatment was to minimize the disruption the symptoms caused in her life and to prevent decompensation that might lead to hospitalization or even nursing home placement.

This client was seen at a teaching clinic, so her therapists changed about once a year. Despite her suspiciousness, she was able to tolerate new therapists because of the supportive relationship that was established and continued with each new person.

During the course of treatment, the woman frequently talked about her daughter, a woman who was in her late 30s, whom the client described as mildly retarded and needing her care and supervision. At one point, the client became ill and needed hospitalization. Although the hospitalization went smoothly, the client was increasingly symptomatic following discharge. Her therapist identified that she was worried about what might happen to her daughter if she should die, and that the woman expressed this concern in part by worrying more about the computer people. We have observed in other clients with paranoid symptoms this pattern of an exacerbation of delusional ideation masking a real concern.

The therapist suggested working with the woman and her daughter to identify programs that might take care of her daughter, including special housing and employment. Both mother and daughter welcomed this intervention. We met with the daughter and conducted a psychological assessment to determine her level of functioning. Based on the test results, it was concluded that the daughter was not retarded but had low normal functioning (full scale WAIS-R in the mid-90s). She had never worked and had always been dependent on her mother, but that appeared more due to their enmeshed relationship than to limited cognitive abilities. With that in mind, the therapist identified appropriate job and skills training for the daughter and helped her make contacts with the programs. Both mother and daughter were pleased with this outcome, and the mother's paranoid symptoms decreased to a lower level. Resolution of a reality-based and age-related concern—what would happen to her daughter when she died—led to a stabilization of the situation. Although never symptom free, the client was able to continue functioning at home at probably the best level possible for her.

Antipsychotic medications have typically been part of the treatment of people with long-standing paranoid problems. Long-term use of these medications becomes increasingly problematic in later life, because the possibility of tardive dyskinesia increases with age. Haloperidol (Haldol) is frequently used with older patients as it has low anticholinergic effects, but it is hard to dose it low enough and still get a therapeutic effect. Often the result is oversedation. Risperidone (Risperdal) is now being used more frequently than Haldol, but it does not control the symptoms as well and there is still a tendency toward oversedation. Thioridazine (Mellaril) in low doses, despite its anticholinergic effects, is sometimes helpful. The potential gains in symptom relief from use of these medications must always be weighed against side effects (see Lohr, Jeste, Harris, & Salzman, 1992, for a thorough discussion).

PARANOID SYMPTOMS AND PERSONALITY DISORDERS

More common than people with paranoid schizophrenia are people with paranoid symptoms who have a long-standing personality disorder. There is often a history of paranoid beliefs. Based on their history, some of these cases meet the criteria for paranoid personality disorder. In other cases, however, paranoid symptoms were intermittent in the past or occurred only during stressful situations. For these people, the onset of symptoms in late life marks a change rather than continuation of old patterns.

The most common feature in these cases is a history of poor social adjustment. Patients are usually estranged from their family and do not have close friends. As they grew older, their social isolation increased. Employment often provided structure and social contact in their lives, lost with retirement. Most of these patients are women. When they were younger, they had been able to get attention from men because of their physical attractiveness. Now, however, like other older women, they are largely invisible and feel ignored. Clients have even described being bumped into by someone as if they were not there and not being waited on in restaurants. Depression is often mixed with their suspiciousness and delusions. Treatment involves developing a supportive relationship, addressing age-related issues and concerns, and appropriate use of medications.

The following example describes a client who had a long-standing history of paranoid symptoms and met the diagnostic criteria for a paranoid personality disorder. The client, Marie, was in her late 60s when we saw her. When she was younger she was very attractive and as a result got a lot of attention from men. The physical changes with aging meant that men no longer noticed her and she became increasingly isolated. She had married a man who was probably a paranoid schizophrenic. The marriage was short-lived and explosive, but they had a daughter whom Marie raised. Once the daughter reached adulthood, she tried to have as little to do with her mother as possible. Now, however, Marie's health was failing, and she moved to the small town where her daughter lived to be closer to her and to get help from her. Her daughter was upset with having her mother so close to her, and Marie, in turn, was upset by her daughter's ambivalence toward her.

Treatment had three goals. The first was to provide Marie with support and acceptance to lessen her isolation and fears. A second goal was to help set boundaries with her daughter. Her compliance with these efforts was gained by reframing the situation. We discussed the importance of not burning her daughter out so that she could provide Marie with assistance when she really needed it. As is the case with people suffering from other personality disorders, Marie required many repetitions of this reframing before she was able to use it to control her behavior. A third goal was to prevent Marie from becoming overly upset or suspicious about everyday occurrences in her life. When she became too upset, her functioning deteriorated and she needed hospitalization, which she did not tolerate well. Marie frequently struck up conversations with strangers and easily made a lot of new acquaintances. But then she would dwell on something that had been said during a conversation, taking an innocuous statement and reframing it as threatening or hostile. A lot of time in treatment was spent helping her reinterpret these interactions.

As with many paranoid clients, the therapist sometimes became the target of Marie's suspicions. It was important to check with her periodically how she was reacting to what the therapist said. She would frequently dwell on an innocuous statement made during the therapy session and give it a hostile interpretation. The therapist had to spend considerable time and effort helping Marie reinterpret these statements. Complicating the situation was the fact that Marie's attacks on the therapist sometimes did produce hostile or angry feelings, which Marie readily detected because of her hypervigilence.

Overall, treatment was used to sustain Marie at her current level of functioning. There was little progress in reducing her paranoid symptoms, and antipsychotic medications that had been frequently used in the past had little effect, either. Though Marie did not improve with treatment, exacerbations of symptoms were short-lived, and it was possible to prevent psychiatric hospitalization on several occasions. There was also some improvement in her relationship with her daughter.

We have generally found that the best approach with older paranoid clients is to be very accepting of how they view the world, not challenge it. To help us develop empathy for them, we conceptualize their complaints as a problem in living rather than paranoid thinking. It is not possible to convince them that their beliefs are distorted, for example, that people are not out to harm them. Instead, we can help them feel a bit more secure and reduce the worries associated with their paranoid beliefs. We join them and try to see the world through their eyes. In doing so, we find a lot of depression and pain associated with their fears and preoccupations. When there is a depressive component, antidepressant medications can sometimes be useful as part of the overall treatment.

ENCAPSULATED PARANOID DELUSION

Encapsulated delusion is a very interesting pattern of late-life paranoid symptoms. This pattern can be seen in someone who has functioned well in life, with steady employment and possibly a long-term marriage, and then experiences an event that triggers the encapsulated delusion. Some people with borderline personality disorders also have encapsulated delusions.

In this example, Lilly was an older woman veteran who was having chronic migraine headaches. She was referred for treatment of these headaches. The treatment involved relaxation training, and Lilly had been doing very well with this approach. At that point, we asked her about doing a training videotape to demonstrate the use of this treatment. She got very frightened and mistrustful and explained, "I can't do that, because the CIA is after me. You know they send messages at the bottom of the TV screen. And you can always tell which cars they have because there is a little mark on the bottom of the license plate." This was astonishing to us, because we had seen no indication of paranoid tendencies until that point. This was, in fact, the first time she had mentioned her belief to anyone. It only came out because of the request to videotape a session. We discussed her belief in a few subsequent therapy sessions, and then she did not want to talk about it anymore.

Lilly had had a successful career as a teacher. She had been married briefly, had a son, and raised him. Her son had been involved in drugs as a teenager and died of a drug overdose in his early 20s. He had been the focus of her life and his drug-related death was unacceptable to her. Much of her delusion had to do with her son's death. She maintained that the CIA had murdered him because he knew something he should not know.

The therapy relationship continued for some time around the original problems, with Lilly experiencing continued improvement for her headaches and related health problems. The therapy relationship was supportive and she had a great deal of trust in the therapist. She stopped treatment when she moved out of the area to be closer to relatives. We continued to receive Christmas cards from her every year until her death, with no indication that the delusion had ever come out again or that her functioning had become impaired because of it.

Lilly's delusion was very important because it helped her accept her son's death. Most of the time, the clinician does not encounter this type of delusion. Clients complain about problems such as depression or, in this case, migraine headaches. When a delusion is brought up, the therapist needs to be accepting, not challenging. As in this example, an encapsulated delusion does not necessarily interfere with functioning, as long as the client does not dwell on it or talk openly about it to family and friends. If the delusion becomes public and upsets the client's family, the therapist can encourage them to accept rather than challenge the disputed belief. There usually is little harm in these beliefs, and they can recede into the background.

PARANOID BELIEFS AND OBSESSIVE–COMPULSIVE DISORDERS

One issue in differential diagnosis is to identify people whose preoccupations might be part of an obsessive–compulsive disorder. People with obsessive–compulsive disorder can be so hypervigilant that their obsessions take on a paranoid quality. The following example illustrates this pattern. Sarah, a client in her 50s, had long-term psychological problems and at least one psychotic episode during which she was hospitalized. She had been treated for many years with a major tranquilizer, thiothixene (Navane), and had developed mild symptoms of tardive dyskinesia, mainly excessive mouth movements. As a result, her psychiatrist was trying to lower the dosage. When he did, she became extremely sensitive to the things people around her were saying. These symptoms initially seemed paranoid, but on closer examination revealed an obsessive–compulsive component. She was worrying excessively about whether her boss thought she was doing a good enough job, if he would give her a good evaluation, and if she would be fired. There was no apparent factual basis to these worries, as she had been receiving very positive work evaluations. Her worrying was more like obsessive–compulsive disorder than a paranoid disorder, though her worries included suspiciousness and hypervigilence. The hypothesis that her problems might involve obsessive–compulsive disorder led to a change in medication: the amount of the tranquilizer she was taking was reduced, which helped control her tardive dyskinesia, and an SSRI was introduced to help with obsessive–compulsive disorder. She responded positively to the new medication with a reduction in worrying about her work performance.

A similar pattern in which obsessive and paranoid thinking are intertwined is found among hoarders. Hoarders are people who fill their homes with possessions or objects, never throwing anything away. They usually do not seek help for this problem, so clinicians encounter them in the process of community outreach or home visits or when neighbors or health authorities complain about the condition of their home. The most extreme instance of hoarding we have seen involved a couple who had collected newspapers and magazines for many years and had so filled their house that there were only small passageways left between one room to the next. Everywhere else were piles of newspapers stacked high. The clutter had piled up to such an extent that the house had become unlivable, and the couple lived in a trailer parked in the driveway.

There is an obsessive component to this kind of collecting, but it often also indicates a suspiciousness toward other people. In one case, a man saved virtually every piece of paper that came into the house, including junk mail. He was convinced that he could not throw anything away because he might need it in the future. His house had not been cleaned for many years. He did not want anyone to come in because he was ashamed about what they would find and because he was mistrustful of having someone in the house. At one point, a neighbor came in to clean. Afterward, whenever the man could not find something, he accused the neighbor of having stolen it. The suspiciousness is obvious, but the main problem was obsessive–compulsive disorder. He was also depressed, and when treated with an SSRI, both his depression and hoarding improved somewhat, although he still accumulated excessive amounts of paper in his small and dirty home.

SENSORY LOSS AS A CONTRIBUTING FACTOR

A common trigger of paranoid thinking in later life is sensory loss. Hearing loss is more typically involved, though vision loss can also play a role (Rabins, 1992). The mechanism by which sensory loss leads to paranoid thinking is that the person misinterprets and distorts input. A person with hearing loss who is having trouble understanding conversations may come to believe that other people are talking about him. A person with vision loss may believe that she cannot find things around the house, because someone has come in and moved them.

We take a similar approach to treatment of paranoid thinking associated with vision and hearing loss, that is, emphasizing the development of a trusting relationship and the judicious use of medication. An additional component is to identify ways of correcting or compensating for the sensory loss. With hearing loss, for example, it may be possible to fit the person with a hearing aid. More commonly, environmental modifications can help improve hearing. Background noise is particularly problematic for people with typical late-life hearing loss. Cutting down on background noise in the home (e.g., turning off televisions or radios when no one is listening to them) can help. Perception can also be improved by speaking slowly and distinctly and using complete sentences. Talking in a low range is more important than talking loudly. Encouraging family and friends to talk one at a time and to talk individually with the person with hearing loss can also help. For vision loss, a variety of aids are available that can improve functioning (Genensky, Zarit, & Amaral, 1992). Improving lighting and contrast can also be helpful.

The following example illustrates paranoid beliefs in a man with severe hearing loss. John was brought to a clinic by his family because of their concern over his increasingly bizarre and troubling behavior. He was 80 years old and had a significant hearing loss, and he believed that he heard on television that the bank was going to repossess his house. He became increasingly preoccupied and disturbed by this thought. He insisted that his wife turn out all the lights during the evening, and he prowled the house with a knife to prevent the bank officials from breaking in and seizing his house. He had also become suspicious of two of his sons, whom he thought were plotting against him. John's family was concerned that he would mistake his wife for a bank official in the dark and injure her. They were also concerned about the poor quality of her life as a consequence of his eccentric behavior. As in many of these cases, John had no prior history of paranoid thinking.

When the family brought John to the clinic, the family physician had already prescribed Haldol, but they were reluctant to try it. We conducted an interview with the man, letting him tell his story and empathizing with the distress that he was feeling over the perceived threats. We then introduced the medication. Following the suggestion of British psychiatrist Felix Post (1973), we told John that it was important to take the medication because it would make him stronger.

We also encouraged the family to make some environmental modifications. This was a big family, and family gatherings tended to be large and noisy. Some of John's paranoid beliefs toward his sons developed during these gatherings, when the amount of background noise caused him to misinterpret what his sons were telling him. His sons had also tried to argue with him over his fears about the bank repossessing his house. We recommended that everyone be reassuring about the house, but in a general way, without disputing John's belief that the bank was a threat. We also recommended that everyone talk to John one-on-one and in situations in which there was a minimum of background noise.

John was willing to take the medication and experienced an immediate decrease in symptoms. His family also made the recommended changes. Follow-up a few months later indicated that the situation was stable, and John had no recurrence of paranoid thinking.

MULTIPLE ETIOLOGIES FOR PARANOID SYMPTOMS

Multiple problems are often involved in the onset of paranoid symptoms. The experience of losses, such as death of a spouse or retirement, can be a trigger. We have often observed that when one partner in an enmeshed couple dies, the other is vulnerable to developing paranoid thinking. The surviving partner may not be skilled at interpreting what other people do in relationships. Add to that a little vision or hearing loss and there is considerable potential to misinterpret social communications. For example, a widow goes to a senior center. If no one makes a place for her to sit, she might interpret that as hostile. She might also misperceive gestures and expressions. She might say, "I saw the look on that woman's face. She doesn't really want me here. I'm not wanted."

We once were involved in supervising a case where we observed the onset of paranoid symptoms following the death of a spouse in an enmeshed relationship. The client in this case, Donna, was a woman in her 50s. She had married young and had been very dependent on her husband. She had never been employed and did not have many friends or interests outside the home. When her husband became severely ill with cancer, she traveled 3 hours each day by public transportation (she did not know how to drive) to see him at the Veterans Administration Hospital where he was receiving care. After a long illness, he died, leaving no insurance and few assets. Donna was referred for therapy by the chaplain at the hospital because of his concern over her depression and grief.

Treatment initially focused on depression and on identifying and building skills that would help Donna become more independent. After a few months, she felt ready to get involved in social activities and identified dancing as something she enjoyed. She started going to a social club that held weekly dances and obviously enjoyed the activity and the attention she received from the men there. One of the men she danced with developed an interest in her, and at one point she rebuffed him after he made a sexual advance. In her recounting of the event, it appeared that he had made a comment that had a sexual innuendo, which upset her and caused her to rebuff him. The prospect of getting involved sexually was very frightening to her. She then became preoccupied with the belief that he and the other men were all talking about her and saying bad things about her because she would not sleep with him. She became increasingly distressed and reluctant to go back to the group.

Were the men actually talking about her? It is likely that Donna was the subject of conversation among them as a single, attractive woman who enjoyed dancing. But they probably were not conspiring against her, as she believed. Moreover, in reaction to her fears, it appeared that she was going to isolate herself and dwell on the thought that all the men in the group were talking about her. Using the supportive relationship they had developed, her therapist encouraged her to look at the situation in other ways. Though Donna's beliefs did not change, she was able to identify another dance group and began going there with no recurrence of the problem. Her therapist worked with her on developing better social skills and reality testing so that she was less likely to overreact to advances from men at the dances. Gradually, she became more skilled at taking care of other issues in her life (e.g., managing her finances, getting part-time work). She continued to attend dances and to enjoy them as a social outlet. She liked the attention from the men she danced with but continued to maintain a distance from them.

In this example, the key factors were the client's long dependence on her husband and her lack of social sophistication. When dancing led to sexual interest by her partner, she overreacted and then felt that all the men had turned against her. The therapy relationship was used to help lower her fears and to build more adaptive social skills.

PARANOID SYMPTOMS IN DEMENTIA AND DELIRIUM

Paranoid symptoms are often observed in dementia and delirium. A delirium should be suspected when delusions or other paranoid symptoms develop suddenly. The clinician must first ask what has changed recently—medications, the client's health, or anything else. Although delirium can have many different causes (see Chapter 3), the most common triggers are medications and illnesses. We have observed that heart and antihypertensive medications, antibiotics, and steroids frequently are involved in development of paranoid delusions and other delirium symptoms, though many other medications can be involved as well.

This example illustrates a delirium that was precipitated by a change in heart medications. The client had been prescribed propranolol (Inderal), (a medication used in heart disease and for hypertension) after a heart attack 20 years earlier. She became psychotic and had to be hospitalized in a psychiatric facility. With discontinuation of the medication, the psychotic symptoms disappeared and she was discharged, with no further problems over the next 20 years. Her current physician did not have this history, and although the woman remembered the episode clearly, she did not recall the name of the medication. When he made a change in her medications, prescribing Inderal, she developed homicidal thoughts. She believed she was going to kill her daughter who was living with her. Because of these beliefs, the physician referred her to us. Taking her through her history revealed the psychotic episode 20 years earlier and the fact that the current onset of symptoms coincided with starting the heart medication three months earlier. Stopping the medication made the symptoms go away.

There are a couple of points that should be emphasized about this example. First is the importance of history. In this case, the events of 20 years ago provided a clue to the present episode, as did the sequence of events (i.e., change in medication) leading up to the onset of symptoms. We are continually surprised at how often history is overlooked. Careful reconstruction of the sequence of events leading up to the sudden onset of paranoid delusions or other delirium symptoms typically provides valuable information about the cause. Second, this case clearly illustrates the role of medications. Unless trained in geriatrics, physicians are not familiar with the mental changes associated with medication reactions and can easily ascribe these symptoms to other causes. Over the years, we have encountered older patients with medication-induced deliriums who have been labeled as schizophrenic or demented. By developing good working relationships with physicians, we have found we can encourage them to review the medications as possible contributing factors to a sudden onset of paranoid symptoms.

The following case illustrates onset of a delirium with paranoid symptoms following treatment with steroids. This older woman had been a smoker and developed bronchial problems. She was hospitalized for these problems and placed on prednisone, and she became increasingly suspicious and fearful while on the medication. She was discharged on a decreasing dosage of the medication. Once she was discharged from the hospital, we dealt with her fears by talking with her daily on the telephone. We gave her reassurance that the bad things that she feared would not happen. We explained that her fears were the result of the medication, not how people felt about her. By hearing this frequent reassurance, she was able to tolerate the suspiciousness until the medication was reduced and the symptoms diminished.

In this case, the patient had some degree of insight and could use verbal reassurances that her fears were due to the side effects of the medication. Her insight contrasts with cases of paranoid beliefs due to other causes. In both lifelong and late-onset paranoia, there is little or only fleeting awareness of the distortions that are involved in the beliefs. Even with a reversible delirium, insight may be limited.

As an example of the lack of insight, we once supervised the treatment of a woman who was accusing her husband of having an affair with a young girl. According to the patient, her husband would sneak out at night after she was asleep to see this girl. The girl would also keep her awake at night by whistling outside the bedroom window and sometimes would come into the apartment. She did not see the girl, who ran away when she heard the woman coming. Her husband, who was a very religious man, was mortified by the accusation. He denied ever having an affair in the past or in the present. His daughter confirmed that he was not going out at night and that no strangers were coming into the apartment. When the daughter tried to reassure her mother that there was no affair or intruder, her mother dismissed her as always having been a "daddy's girl."

The woman was in good health except for severe arthritis and macular degeneration; she had poor vision, especially when there was poor illumination. The accusations began soon after she began taking a new medication for arthritis, salsalate (Disalcid), a nonsteroidal anti-inflammatory agent. We reviewed the case with her physician, and he switched her to another arthritis medication. With the change in medication, her accusations gradually stopped. She continued to insist, however, that her husband had had the affair and that he had broken it off. She was much calmer now that she believed the affair was over. No amount of explaining by the family or therapist changed her belief. Her husband remained upset by the false accusation, and so the therapist worked with him to understand why she could not let go of this belief.

In this case, the combination of a new medication and the woman's visual impairment probably led to the delirium. What is interesting is how the client insisted that what she imagined happening during the delirium actually took place. We have encountered other people who maintained that the delusions and hallucinations they had during a delirium actually happened. Little can be done to change these beliefs. Fortunately, that is not the typical outcome.

As these examples illustrate, sudden onset of paranoid delusions can be due to treatable causes. Identification of a delirium and its probable etiology is very important, since treatment should begin as soon as possible. Removal of the offending medication or treatment of other causes usually results in full recovery.

Paranoid symptoms are very common in dementia, especially in the earlier stages of an illness. In some cases, the patient's dementia first comes to the family's attention because of the paranoid complaints. The psychological process leading to paranoid symptoms in dementia is similar to that of people with vision or hearing loss. With sensory problems, patients fill in stimuli they do not perceive adequately. With dementia, patients fill in the things they cannot remember by blaming other people. When they cannot find a wallet or purse, they say it must have been stolen. Thus, there is an adaptive component to these beliefs, helping patients explain to themselves why they are having increasing problems finding and remembering things and why events seems to be swirling around them in a bewildering pattern.

Another common symptom that dementia patients report is imaginary visitors who come into the house. Occasionally, these visitors are benevolent, for example, a child who comes to visit. More often, the visitors are threatening and frightening, and they steal things from the patient. These types of problems should be differentiated from the illusions that are experienced later in the dementia process. A later-stage patient may report seeing small animals running across a dimly lighted room. These illusions are not experienced as frightening and do not have a malevolent or threatening component. They are primarily upsetting to the family.

The main diagnostic issue is to rule out a comorbid delirium. Dementia patients have an increased susceptibility to delirium, and so this possibility should always be considered when there is a sudden change in functioning or when symptoms suggest a delirium. Once a delirium is ruled out, treatment takes place at several levels: patient, family or other involved people, and environment. When the patient's dementia is not too severe, the clinician can develop a supportive relationship and, as in other cases of paranoid symptoms, use the relationship to provide reassurance and reduce fears. As with patients with other forms of late-life paranoia, we do not confront dementia patients or try to get them to change their beliefs. Rather, we respond to the affective components of their delusions—the fear, anxiety, or depression that accompanies the belief that someone is stealing from or threatening them. Medications can be considered, but the problems associated with them are even more pronounced when there is dementia. Antipsychotic medications such as Haldol are typically used for these symptoms in dementia, but we have found that determining therapeutic dosage is very difficult. Haldol can be effective, but reduction in the paranoid symptoms often comes about only by producing pronounced sedation, thereby restricting verbal output. Though not widely advocated in dementia, the minor tranquilizers sometimes have benefits in treatment of paranoid and other symptoms (see Chapter 11).

Intervention is often necessary with the family or other caregivers. In many instances, the problem is not the paranoid belief but the family's reactions to it. It is especially problematic when the patient makes accusations against someone in the family. Family typically respond to paranoid symptoms by trying to change the patient's beliefs. Arguments over the facts, however, are not successful, because the patient's beliefs are embedded in the diminished ability to process information. These beliefs help patients understand their increasingly confusing world, and they hold onto them in the face of obvious and repeated contradictions. We work with the family or other caregivers to avoid confrontations and arguments over the facts. Instead, we encourage them to respond to the emotions the patient conveys in these communications (see Chapter 12 for a more detailed discussion).

Finally, changes in the environment or in daily routines can be helpful. A structured routine can keep patients occupied while minimizing opportunities to misplace or lose valued objects. Keeping patients busy also tires them out, reducing their anxiety and agitation. Simplifying the environment can also be beneficial. Caregivers, for example, might be encouraged to straighten up a messy home. In a neater setting, patients may still lose objects, but families have an easier time finding them. Good illumination in the home is also helpful, especially in late afternoon or early evening when these problems can be greatest.

PARANOID OR REAL?

In many of the cases we have encountered, the patient's paranoid beliefs are plausible, and it is important to consider whether some of what has been described might actually be occurring. In the case described earlier, we considered whether the woman's husband might actually be having an affair. When clients complain that someone is stealing from them, we assess whether that has happened. We have worked with clients who have been taken advantage of by strangers or even family members. The situation can be very complicated, as when a client's complaint has a basis in reality *and* an exaggerated, paranoid component.

We once saw a client who complained about intruders who had vandalized her house and property. We had recently seen two other clients who reported intruders who turned out to be imaginary. One of those clients suffered from long-term paranoid schizophrenia and the other had dementia. The details of the story the new client told were quite similar to the other cases. She was very upset when talking about the intruders and so her story was disjointed and many of the details were not clear. Rather than assume that she was delusional, however, we conducted a home visit, which revealed that there were gang activities in the lot next to her house and that gang members had, indeed, vandalized her property just as she described. Needless to say, treatment was quite different than intervention for a paranoid disorder.

CO-OCCURRENCE OF LIFELONG AND
LATE-ONSET PARANOID SYMPTOMS

We conclude this chapter with one of the most complicated cases we have ever followed. This case illustrates the importance of assessment in cases of paranoid beliefs and the potential for multiple etiologies. It also illustrates how a multifaceted treatment approach can enhance a client's strengths and support independent functioning.

Eleanor, a single woman in her early 70s, was seen at a clinic specializing in problems of older people. She initially said that she needed help in finding a job. When the interviewer questioned her about it, she told a fragmented story about a recent hospitalization. According to Eleanor, she had gone to the county hospital for treatment of a medical problem and had been held against her will on the psychiatric ward. She described a nightmarish sequence of being wheeled into the deep recesses of the hospital and put through an apparatus that examined her brain (probably a CT scan). She was afraid the doctors had put something into her brain during that procedure. Despite this odd story, Eleanor had no current overt psychotic symptoms and no gross cognitive impairment, as determined by brief mental status testing. She lived alone and claimed to have no living family.

A treatment plan was developed to explore her concern about working and her financial worries (she was afraid she would be evicted from her apartment for failing to pay the rent). The sessions would also be used to assess her further to understand better what had happened during the hospitalization and to respond to her fears that it might happen to her again. While medical records might have clarified what happened during the hospitalization, Eleanor did not want us to contact the hospital and would not sign a release so that medical records could be obtained.

A few treatment sessions were held, during which some progress was made toward developing a therapeutic relationship and exploring her concerns about money. From these sessions, her counselor learned that Eleanor received a small Social Security check as her only income and that her landlord wanted to evict her because she was sometimes late with the rent. The counselor inferred that her behavior made the threat of eviction more likely, but her stories were disjointed and difficult to follow.

Eleanor then failed to keep an appointment and did not answer telephone calls. After failing to contact her, her counselor visited her apartment building. When there was no answer at her apartment, the counselor talked to a neighbor, who described how Eleanor had been taken away in an apparently psychotic state by ambulance. For a few nights before this incident, she had been coming out of her apartment and waking neighbors by yelling loudly and in an incoherent way. The neighbor did not know where she had been taken.

After about a month, Eleanor phoned the clinic to speak to her counselor. She was now residing in a nursing home, where she had been brought by the ambulance. She wanted the counselor to help her get back to her apartment. After talking with the nursing home staff, the counselor agreed to make visits there.

From discussions with Eleanor, the sequence of events leading to this episode—and possibly to the previous one—became apparent. Her financial concerns had been quite serious; she ran out of money toward the end of each month. As a consequence, she had no money for food and stopped eating, which preceded her bizarre behavior. Our provisional diagnosis was that the episode was a delirium, given her psychotic and disorganized symptoms, their episodic pattern, the association with poor nutrition, and her apparent full recovery. She did, however, remain somewhat suspicious of other people, including the nursing home staff, whom she felt were trying to keep her against her will.

The staff at the nursing home felt that Eleanor could not live independently and were annoyed when they found out about her efforts to move. The physician at this facility had diagnosed her as having Alzheimer's disease, though once again our cognitive testing revealed no obvious deficits.

She had by now lost her apartment but had persuaded her brother (she had previously denied having any relatives) to move her possessions into storage. We talked with her brother, who indicated that he was involved reluctantly and that he preferred to leave her in the nursing home where she would not be a bother to him. He described his sister as having led a marginal life, able to support herself in the past by working at low-paying jobs but otherwise isolating herself and being suspicious of others.

When the social service staff of the nursing home resisted her requests to move, we provided Eleanor with names and phone numbers of low-cost retirement homes. She preferred that type of housing, because meals would be provided. We made weekly visits to be supportive in the face of her growing suspicions about the nursing home. In a few weeks, she was able to locate a retirement home she liked, and she arranged a move.

After the move, she functioned well for awhile. The retirement home provided meals and a small amount of supervision, allaying our concerns about a possible recurrence of a delirium. Nonetheless, Eleanor soon became suspicious of the management at the home. She was also having difficulty tolerating the close contact with other residents in the home. We were worried about the risks involved if she went out on her own, but she was insistent. Again taking the initiative, she found an apartment and arranged the move. To address our concerns about her nutrition, her counselor looked into the possibility of having meals delivered to her and, with Eleanor's consent, arranged for home-delivered meals. The counselor also visited Eleanor in her new apartment every other week, focusing the sessions on adaptive skills.

After a couple of months a new crisis developed, this time over the home-delivered meals. The agency that delivered the meals asked for donations to offset their cost. When Eleanor determined that donations were voluntary, she refused to give any money. The agency told us that the donation was indeed voluntary but that they expected everyone to contribute something. They were about to stop the meals because of her refusal. At that point, the counselor called the program's supervisor and reported that the meals were keeping Eleanor out of a nursing home and how important it was to continue deliveries. With that information, the supervisor agreed to continue, despite Eleanor's refusal to make a contribution.

We followed Eleanor for several more months, including through a medical crisis involving severe back pain. Although remaining suspicious of many people, Eleanor had a good relationship with her counselor and would call when she needed help. Retesting indicated that cognitive functioning was stable.

This case illustrates many important features of late-life paranoid disorders. The history provided by Eleanor and her brother suggested that she had a long history of poor social adjustment and suspiciousness toward other people. This suspiciousness became obvious in her relationships with the staff in the nursing home and with staff and residents in the retirement home. Complicating the situation, however, were the two episodes of apparent delirium. In retrospect, these episodes were triggered when Eleanor ran out of food and stopped eating. The bizarre behavior was never observed in any other situation. Thus, this case involved both lifelong paranoid beliefs *and* recent episodes that were part of a delirium.

The contribution of several different factors to paranoid symptoms underscores the importance of a careful assessment. Knowing only Eleanor's history, we might conclude that her problems were long-standing, possibly due to paranoid schizophrenia, and thus ignore the immediate antecedents of each recent episode. In turn, the physician at the nursing home responded to her disorganized behavior at admission by labeling it Alzheimer's disease and ignoring its sudden onset. The implications of diagnosis should be evident. If Eleanor had Alzheimer's disease and declining cognitive functioning, then keeping her in a protected setting might be justified. But our testing showed no evidence of dementia. Furthermore, she demonstrated the competence to make decisions and to live independently by locating places to live and carrying out two moves (one from a nursing home).

Given Eleanor's suspiciousness and history of fragile interpersonal relationships, our first emphasis in treatment was development of a supportive, trusting relationship. A counselor could not become too close or intrusive yet had to be perceived by Eleanor as a strong enough ally to be her advocate. As it became apparent that poor nutrition had triggered the delirium episodes, we emphasized helping Eleanor find a stable living situation in which she had adequate food. We had strong misgivings when she decided to move from the retirement home but recognized that she was competent to make that decision. Besides, she could not tolerate the close proximity of other people in the retirement home.

This case also illustrates how clinicians can identify strengths and build on them to focus on treatable problems. Some problems in functioning change slowly or not at all. Eleanor's general mistrust of people would, in all likelihood, be extremely difficult to treat, especially because this tendency was long-standing, and because of the absence of any stable personal relationships in her life. It was also not a problem for which she sought help. Her main concern throughout was maintaining independence, and we responded by reinforcing her adaptive abilities. She had, in fact, initially sought help in finding a job. In the end, we responded to this initial request in an indirect way, helping her find a stable living situation where she could afford food and rent. We supported the practical skills that she used in locating housing and that came into play in carrying out many daily tasks.

Helping Eleanor remain independent depended on coordinating with community agencies. Our role was to help her find resources and, on occasions, to run interference for her. Eleanor often alienated potential helpers. Home-delivered meals played a valuable role in helping her remain in an apartment, but we had to intervene with the program's director in order to keep this service. The aging service system is not used to dealing with people with serious psychopathology. Irritating people such as Eleanor easily fall through the cracks. This situation is the type where cooperation between mental health and aging services is especially valuable.

Eleanor's case illustrates the often delicate balance between independence and dependence in older clients. A clinician's primary goal should be to design interventions that are consistent with clients' values. There are many circumstances when taking protective actions are necessary, of course. But when the older person is competent to make a decision, the clinician should value and support independence to the extent possible.

The decision to place someone in a protected setting is frequently couched as a medical decision, much like a prescription for medication. Often, however, this decision concerns values about life style and quality of life, including the risks that someone is willing to take by continuing to live in a less protected setting. Clients may prefer to live in ways that clinicians or family disapprove of, accepting the accompanying risks as the best way to live out their lives. The pressure on the client and clinician in these situations can be tremendous. But it is important to keep in mind that there are risks associated with protected settings as well, and the best decision involves balancing risks in the broader context of the client's values.

In Eleanor's situation, the argument could be made that she would be better off and safer in the nursing home. Her brother and the attending physician both held that view. It was not medically necessary, however, as long as she was able to get regular meals. She valued her independence, and living in an apartment posed no immediate threat to her or anyone else. Remaining in a nursing home would also have been risky for her. Her suspiciousness and eccentricities, which did not bother anyone when she lived alone, might have provoked negative reactions in the nursing home staff. Eleanor's life style had not been, nor would it be in the future, one that her brother or anyone involved in her case would value for themselves. But the proper course was to support her right to continue making decisions for herself as long as possible.

CONCLUSIONS

Paranoid symptoms in later life are a complex and challenging problem for the geriatric psychologist. Cases require careful assessment, drawing on specialized knowledge of differential diagnosis with older people. There are several possible etiologies for paranoid symptoms in later life. Symptoms can be a manifestation of a lifelong disorder (paranoid schizophrenia, paranoid personality disorder) or a worsening of a long-standing personality disorder with little or no prior history of paranoid symptoms. Symptoms can also be a response to sensory loss, dementia, and delirium. Identification of the probable etiology is always the first step in treatment; interventions depend in part on the etiology. Successful treatment requires a full range of treatment skills, including developing a supportive therapeutic relationship with the client, the client's family, and other professionals, bringing in aging services when needed, and examining values and choices in complex situations.

11

Treatment of Dementia

Dementia is a devastating disorder, affecting not just patients but also their families and other caregivers. Trapped by their memory loss in an increasingly bewildering present, patients become unable to recognize their surroundings and the people around them. Though needing help, they sometimes lash out at people trying to assist.

Families, in turn, are faced with around-the-clock care demands from an increasingly unreasonable person. Not surprisingly, dementia is the major reason families place an older person in a nursing home or similar institutional setting. Just as care of these patients can be overwhelming for families, it also places considerable burden on institution staff, who all too often have insufficient resources and training.

Despite these catastrophic consequences, the geriatric mental health specialist can have considerable impact. Although treatment of the underlying disease is still limited, timely and well-planned interventions can help patients, their families, or institution staff function as well as possible. Interventions can reduce excessive strain on caregivers and lead to development of optimal care arrangements that maximize patients' remaining abilities while maintaining their dignity and autonomy.

This chapter provides an introduction to treatment of dementia. We present a framework for treatment of dementia, and then focus on four approaches: (1) medications, (2) cognitive stimulation, (3) behavioral interventions, and (4) counseling. We continue the discussion of treatment of dementia in subsequent chapters. Chapter 12 addresses family caregiving and how families can learn to manage the stresses associated with caring for people with dementia and other disabilities. Chapter 13 explores consultations in nursing homes and other institutional settings, many of which involve clients with dementia. We also consider issues pertaining to the design of special environments to enhance functioning in dementia.

FRAMEWORK FOR TREATMENT OF DEMENTIA

How a problem is conceptualized determines expectations for treatment. If we view dementia as a medical illness for which no treatments are available to stop or reverse the course of the disease, then it follows that mental health professionals can do very little. Dementia, however, can best be understood as an interaction of biomedical, psychological, social, and environmental processes (Figure 11.1). While the underlying disease causes massive changes, specific behaviors result in part from how people respond to patients and how the environment is structured. Even though the biomedical components of dementia cannot currently be altered to any significant degree, we can make changes in how we interact with patients and in other aspects of the situation that can lead to improvement. These changes do not, of course, restore a person to health, but they can make a substantial difference in a patient's functioning and in how well caregivers are able to manage.

Dementia can be viewed as increasing the probability that problematic behaviors will occur. The illness reduces thresholds for disturbed or agitated behavior in several ways. Neurons are lost in key regions of the brain, leading to corresponding deficits of neurotransmitters involved in regulation of mood and behavior (Kirby & Lawlor, 1995). Cognitive deficits associated with dementia also make problem behavior more likely. Patients may misunderstand or miscommunicate with other people or become frightened by their inability to recognize people, places, or things. They also have more difficulty initiating activities and keeping themselves occupied. Nonetheless, behavior problems do not originate in a vacuum. Patients remain responsive to the surrounding environment and their behavior makes sense

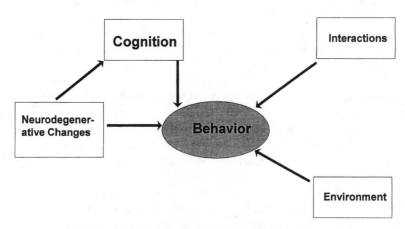

FIGURE 11.1. Model of behavior problems in dementia

when viewed in context. Even in advanced dementia, events trigger problem behaviors, and how people respond can reinforce them. The dementing illness, then, increases the likelihood of a variety of problems, but when and how often they occur are related to patterns of interaction within a particular setting.

We illustrate this process with an example that is familiar to people experienced in dementia care. If someone walks up behind a dementia patient (suffering from moderate or moderately severe impairment) and begins talking without making eye contact first, a frequent response is that the patient startles and swings out to hit. Some people would take that behavior as evidence that dementia patients are violent, in other words, that the disease causes the behavior. Yet if the person had walked around and made eye contact before speaking, the patient would not have struck out. The role of the disease in this example is not to cause violent behavior but to lower inhibitions against striking out when startled. This behavior might further be altered by characteristics of the setting, such as the noise level or number of other activities.

Sleep problems provide another example of the complex relation of disease and environment. Sleep disturbances are very common in dementing illnesses. Changes in sleep are in part due to damage in regions of the brain that regulate sleep and waking (Bliwise, 1994). Sleep problems, however, are more common among patients who nap during the daytime. Interventions that increase activity during the daytime can be an efficient and effective way of improving sleep at night. As an example, dementia patients who go to adult day care programs sleep better at night after they have attended the program (S. Zarit, Stephens, Townsend, & Greene, in press). A combination of structured activities and decreased opportunities for unscheduled naps may improve sleep during the night for dementia patients (as they do for the rest of us). Removal from settings conducive to napping to settings that encourage activity can contribute to establishing of appropriate sleep patterns.

Viewing the behavior of dementia patients as the outcome of an interaction creates the possibility for many types of intervention. Sometimes it is possible to intervene directly with patients, for example, by using medications or even psychological interventions. More often, we can change how other people respond to the patient or make alterations in the environment that lead to better functioning. The main goal is to identify treatable or modifiable aspects of the situation.

MEDICATIONS FOR DEMENTIA

Medications for dementia can be divided into two broad categories: those that treat the primary, underlying disease and those that treat associated symptoms, such as behavior problems and depression. Several different medications are currently being tested for their possible benefits in Alzheimer's disease (see Chapter 3). The first drug approved for use in the United States is tacrine (Cognex). This medication acts on the cholinergic system, making the neurotransmitter acetylcholine more available. In extensive trials conducted under the auspices of the National Institute of Aging, Cognex has been found to have limited benefits for between 20% and 30% of mildly to moderately impaired Alzheimer's patients (Committee on Aging, 1994). These benefits involve improvement of a few points on a composite measure of functioning. Families report a variety of improvements anecdotally, but these findings have not been substantiated. Benefits may last 6 months to a year, with progression of symptoms resuming at that point. Among substantial drawbacks, many patients cannot tolerate the medication and some develop distinct adverse effects, especially liver damage. To guard against possible liver damage, patients are required to have a weekly blood test to monitor liver function, which is costly, painful, and time-consuming and is not practical for some patients and their caregivers. Another disadvantage of Cognex is that it must be administered four times a day to sustain therapeutic levels, a regimen that is difficult for non-cognitively impaired people to maintain, let alone by someone with dementia.

A newly approved medication, donepezil (Aricept), has a similar profile of modest benefits without the extensive problems associated with Cognex. Aricept is taken once a day and does not result in liver toxicity or require regular blood tests. Patients taking Aricept show improved performance in activities of daily living such as dressing and feeding themselves. Some areas of cognition may also improve. Some families have reported to us that patients who previously did not recognize them were able to do so after starting on Aricept. Increasing patients' cognitive abilities, however, has a downside. Some patients become more aware of their own deficits and, as a consequence, get more depressed and angry. Another side effect is that some patients become excessively somnolent after using Aricept for a few months. The improvements associated with Aricept last from a few months to a year.

Aricept was put on the FDA's fast-track program for approval, so long-term controlled studies are not yet available. The drug was originally developed for patients with early Alzheimer's, yet clinically it is often used with people in middle and later stages. Its effects at different stages in the disease are not well known, nor is there a consensus on the optimal time for using it.

Reports of small benefits in cognition and behavior have been reported for several other medications, including estrogen and vitamin E supplements (see Chapter 3). Systematic trials, however, have not been conducted, and the benefits are modest.

The other main use of medications with dementia patients is for treatment of behavior problems, such as agitation or aggression. The judicious use of medications for managing behavior can be very helpful. A comprehensive treatment plan that combines medication with behavioral and environmental modifications is a powerful tool. The use of psychoactive medications with dementia patients, however, can be very tricky. Because of their increasing brain dysfunction, patients have a narrow therapeutic window; that is, it is difficult to determine dosages that will be effective. As a result, treatment often vacillates between dosages that are too low and do not have any benefit and those that are too high and result in significant side effects, such as excessive sedation or, paradoxically, excessive agitation. Medication-induced deliriums are also a problem.

The most widely used medications are the neuroleptics or major tranquilizers. These medications can be used in the treatment of behavior problems such as agitation, aggressive behavior, restlessness, hallucinations, and delusions. They also can reduce sleep problems.

The neuroleptics also have significant side effects and should be given not routinely but only when indicated by the presence of behavior problems. The main side effects are (1) excessive sedation; (2) hypotension; (3) anticholinergic effects (dry mouth, constipation, urine retention, increased memory impairment); (4) extrapyramidal symptoms, such as akathisia (motor restlessness and muscular tension), and Parkinsonian symptoms (bradykinesia, rigidity, tremor, and loss of postural reflexes); (5) acute dystonic reactions (spasms of the face, neck, back, or extraocular muscles); and (6) tardive dyskinesia (random jerking of facial muscles, which impairs talking and eating) (Lohr, Jeste, Harris, & Salzman, 1992).

Haloperidol (Haldol) is widely regarded as the treatment of choice because it has fewer anticholinergic side effects and does not reduce levels of cholinergic neurotransmitters, which are already deficient in Alzheimer's disease. We have found, however, that it is difficult for physicians to find the therapeutic window for Haldol. As a consequence, it is often not effective in reducing behavior problems, such as agitation. A new antipsychotic medication, risperidone (Risperdal), is now being used widely because it also has few anticholinergic side effects. Like Haldol, however, it is difficult to find the therapeutic window with dementia patients. Thioridazine (Mellaril) is an older medication that has greater anticholinergic effects, so some geriatric psychiatrists do not recommend it in dementia cases. We have found, however, that low dosages, especially before bedtime, can be sedating and can reduce agitation and induce sleep.

Overall, the major tranquilizers do not have consistently positive effects on behavioral disturbances in dementia (see Lohr et al., 1992; Schneider, 1996; and Schneider, Pollock, & Lyness, 1990, for reviews). These medications should be used cautiously because of their inconsistent benefits and potential side effects. They can provide considerable help when behavior problems are lessened but can increase a patient's difficulties when side effects or paradoxical reactions are ignored.

The benzodiazepines (see Chapter 8) often can have positive benefits. These medications should be used with caution in dementia, because they can produce excessive sedation and make cognitive functioning worse (Salzman, 1992). Lorazepam (Ativan), however, can lower anxiety and agitation in some dementia patients. Another antianxiety drug, buspirone (BuSpar), can also have positive benefits (Sakauye, Camp, & Ford, 1993. BuSpar is less sedating than the benzodiazepines and is less likely to cause cognitive symptoms (Salzman, 1992). Alprazolam (Xanax) is widely preferred for use with older people because it has a short half-life (i.e., it is eliminated by the body quickly). The downside of its short half-life is that Xanax wears off quickly, causing a rapid rebound of anxiety.

Finally, there has been increasing exploration of the use of antidepressant medications with dementia patients who are depressed. Early studies using tricyclic antidepressants found improvements with treatment (Reifler et al., 1989). The newer antidepressants (e.g., the SSRIs, trazodone [Desyrel], BuSpar; see Chapter 8) have fewer side effects and can be tolerated more easily by dementia patients. These medications represent a promising avenue for treatment. We have observed patients who do well on an SSRI during the daytime and a low dose of a tranquilizer at night to help with sleep. These patients are less depressed and less agitated. Some, patients who are not depressed have had improved behavior on these medications. Like any other medication, however, these antidepressants can have adverse effects.

Medications, then, are an important part of treatment, but their inconsistent benefits and the sensitivity of dementia patients to the effects of any medication mean that they should be used cautiously. It is helpful to maintain a trail-and-error attitude toward any psychotropic medication, with the idea that medications need to be changed as the disease progresses. Periodic reviews should be done to be sure that the medications being used are still effective. Another problem is adding one drug on top of another, until patients are taking several psychoactive medications. It is then not possible to tell which medication is helpful or harmful, or if each is needed. Of course, multiple medications also increases the likelihood of adverse reactions.

COGNITIVE STIMULATION

Cognitive symptoms are such a prominent part of dementia that it is logical to try to train patients to compensate for these deficits. Cognitive training strategies have had some success with head trauma patients. Several types of cognitive stimulation and training have been used with dementia.

In the 1960s, one variant of cognitive stimulation, reality orientation (RO), gained wide acceptance, and some aspects of this approach are still found in most nursing homes. RO involves providing dementia patients with information on the questions they typically get wrong on mental status examinations, such as today's date or the name of the president. Classes are held, which go over this information; orienting information, such as the date and season, are located in visible places in the nursing facility. RO has been found to have little or no effect on cognitive symptoms. Even modest cognitive improvements do not translate into improvements in activities of daily living or interpersonal functioning (Zepelin, Wolfe, & Kleinplatz, 1981).

The absence of positive findings from RO classes is understandable, because RO confuses a symptom of the disorder (e.g., not knowing what day it is) with the disease process. On the other hand, providing orienting information on a bulletin board is probably helpful, because the design of many homes makes it difficult for patients to see outside and tell the time of day or even what season it is. Orienting information may be particularly useful for patients without cognitive deficits or with mild difficulties. (We could also question why facilities designed for long-term care have to look like hospital wards and do not provide places for residents to look outside and get firsthand information about time of day and season.)

Other approaches have emphasized training people in cognitive skills that can enhance memory. Controlled studies of cognitive training have found that mild and moderately impaired dementia patients can make significant improvements, often to the same or greater extent than with drug use (e.g., Quayhagen & Quayhagen, 1989). Camp and his colleagues (Camp & Schaller, 1989; Camp & Stevens, 1990; Camp et al., 1993; Camp, Foss, O'Hanlon, & Stevens, 1996; Hayden & Camp, 1995) developed one of the most successful programs of cognitive intervention, using spaced retrieval to improve memory in dementia. This method involves training patients in a behavior (e.g., checking the calendar) and then gradually increasing the interval between trials until patients can perform the action independently. Studies have also investigated the use of external memory aids, such as reminders that patients carry with them (e.g., Bourgeois, 1990).

Although these approaches have resulted in statistically significant improvements, patients' cognitive gains may not generalize to everyday situations and may not make things easier for their caregivers. In a memory training study that involved both dementia patients and their caregivers, we found that patients improved significantly in memory performance, but caregivers were more depressed at the end of the intervention (S. Zarit, Zarit, & Reever, 1982). The reason for this paradoxical finding is that the training program brought out for caregivers how much patients could not do. Rather than giving caregivers hope or helping them manage everyday situations better, the training program confirmed the seriousness of their relative's illness. Although memory training had little practical value to them, caregivers said that the opportunity to get together with other people in their situation was helpful, a point we will come back to when we discuss support groups in Chapter 12.

Cognitive training, then, is not a panacea for the problems of dementia. In individual cases some cognitive training may be useful. External aids such as calendars and reminders are the easiest to use, but it is important to understand that dementia affects patients' ability to remember to use aids or reminders. They cannot be expected to check the calendar automatically but must be trained to use these types of aids. Spaced retrieval training such as developed by Camp and colleagues (1993) is useful for training patients to use reminders. Patients who have always used various reminders or memory aids can be encouraged to continue, to the extent possible. But it is important to monitor cognitive training carefully, since the limited gains can easily be offset by increasing frustration of both patient and caregiver.

BEHAVIORAL INTERVENTIONS

Behavioral strategies are a promising and powerful approach for managing problem behaviors in dementia. They have been used over the years in management of a variety of problems, including agitation, verbal disruptions, and urinary incontinence (Burgio, 1996; Hinchliffe, Hyman, Blizard, & Livingston, 1995; Stokes, 1996; Teri & Logsdon, 1991; S. Zarit, Orr, & Zarit, 1985). Although the number of controlled trials of behavioral approaches has been limited, results have been very positive.

Over the years we have used a basic framework for developing behavioral interventions in dementia. We describe the basic elements of this approach here, then expand on its use with caregivers in Chapter 12 and in institutional settings in Chapter 13. We begin with assessment. Assessment is the foundation on which subsequent interventions are based. From the assessment, we want to pinpoint the targeted behavior carefully. Staff or family may not describe a problem in a clear or precise way. By asking questions or instructing caregivers to observe the behavior over the course of a couple of days, we can get a more specific description of what actually happens. We also want to learn at what time of day a problem takes place and what events might be taking place at the time. Finally, the assessment tells us how often the problem occurs, which provides a baseline for evaluating the effects of the intervention.

Using the information we obtain, we next identify possible antecedents or consequences of the problem behavior. Antecedents are events that trigger the behavior, and consequences are actions that reinforce the behavior. Problem behaviors may be triggered by many different events. We have found, for example, that agitation and restlessness frequently follow periods of inactivity or daytime naps. Another common antecedent of behavior problems is an episode of discomfort. Behavior problems are often an indication of some kind of distress or pain. The consequences of problems are how caregivers respond. Caregivers may inadvertently reinforce problem behaviors. They may ignore patients when they are not causing any problems but give them attention when they act out. Some of the common antecedents and consequences of problem behavior in dementia are shown in Table 11.1.

Based on these analyses, we develop a behavioral intervention. The intervention is usually designed to disrupt the pattern of antecedents and consequences. Often, we try to prevent the antecedent event from occurring. If patients become agitated following a period of inactivity, a solution is to increase the amount of activity prior to the time when they usually become agitated. If the behavior is triggered by a particular person (e.g., a staff member at a nursing home), we would try to restructure the patient's schedule to minimize contact. Similarly, we work with caregivers to reinforce positive behaviors when they occur, not just respond to problems. Some general strategies for behavioral interventions are shown in Table 11.1.

Interventions are usually carried out by a caregiver, that is, a family member or staff person at an institution. A basic premise of behavioral approaches is that patients have limited ability to make changes in their behaviors. They cannot exercise willpower or in some other way gain a better control over their behavior. Caregivers, however, can change how they respond to patients or how the patients' environment is structured. It is critical, then, to gain the active support of family or staff in making interventions.

Interventions need to be practical and doable. As an example, we may

TABLE 11.1. Common Antecedents, Consequences, and Solutions for Behavior Problems

Common antecedents	Common consequences	Frequent solutions
Interactions with caregiver or other people	Attention	Activity
Boredom	Stimulation	Prevent naps
Napping	Contact	Reduce noise
Frustration	Food	Reassurance
Stress	Comfort	Comfort
Anxiety		Attention to positive behaviors
Noise		Food
Hunger		Treat pain or illness
Thirst		Change medications
Pain		Distraction
Illness		
Medications		

decide that increasing the patient's activities is likely to reduce agitation, but the family caregiver is too exhausted or angry to go along. In that case, we need to identify other resources that can be used, for example, enrolling the patient in a structured adult day care program or finding someone who can take the patient out for walks. Interventions should also be specific and detailed, that is, caregivers should know exactly what do and when they should do it. They should of course, actively participate in development of the plan, understand it, and be willing to carry it out.

Finally, the intervention is implemented and evaluated. Since the intervention is often made by a family caregiver or by staff in an institution, the clinician should check that it is implemented in the planned way. If the caregiver implements the plan adequately, does it then reduce the problem? The targeted problem should decrease as a result of the intervention. If not, we return to the starting point, gather more information, and develop a new plan. Usually, however, a carefully planned behavioral intervention does reduce targeted behaviors.

One of the most promising applications of behavioral methods has been for treatment of depression among dementia patients (Teri, 1994; Teri, Logsdon, Uomoto, & McCurry, 1997). As in behavior therapy for depression (see Chapter 8), this approach emphasizes increasing pleasant activities. Working with family caregivers, therapists teach them to identify and increase the number of pleasant events that dementia patients participate in. Caregivers also learn to modify other antecedents and consequences of the patient's depressed behavior. Caregivers play an active role in arranging for and structuring these activities. This intervention, then, addresses the patient's difficulties in initiating and sustaining satisfying activities.

This approach has been found to reduce depression in both patients and their caregivers, compared to control groups receiving usual care or on a wait list. The amount of improvement among patients is similar to that found with antidepressant medication (Teri et al., 1997). The benefits for caregivers are particularly surprising. By learning how to interact more effectively with patients, caregivers themselves may experience pleasant interactions and perhaps a greater sense of competency as caregivers. (A treatment manual and caregiver reader are available by writing to Linda Teri, PhD, Deptartment of Psychiatry and Behavioral Sciences, Box 356560, University of Washington, Seattle, WA 98195-6560.)

COUNSELING DEMENTIA PATIENTS

In the interventions discussed so far, dementia patients have been relatively passive recipients. Patients with early and mild impairments and even some with more extensive deficits can take an active role in their own care. One of the most promising ways of involving patients is through counseling. Programs of individual, couple, and group counseling for mildly impaired patients have been described (e.g., Yale, 1989, 1991). The goal is not to reverse the dementia symptoms but to give patients the opportunity to come to terms with their disabilities. Some may be able to make decisions about their subsequent care when they still have the ability to do so.

Individual treatment of the dementia patient can provide support, build coping skills, and address feelings of depression or anger over the illness and its symptoms. An empathic relationship can help patients address their fears and concerns. The implications of a diagnosis of Alzheimer's disease are catastrophic, so a frank discussion with patients about their illness can have adverse consequences. Some families, in fact, do not want to tell patients about the diagnosis and even some physicians advise families not to tell patients what is wrong. We find it better to answer patients' questions about what is wrong with them truthfully. It is their right to know, and they are either able to handle the information or conveniently forget it.

That is not to say that patients cannot react badly to the information. Suicidal thoughts may arise, and clinicians should respond as they would in any other situation, providing a non-judgmental framework for discussing suicide but seeking alternatives to it. If the clinician's assessment indicates a serious risk of a suicide attempt, it would be necessary to take steps to hospitalize the patient, but this is rare, perhaps because dementia patients no longer have the ability to plan and carry out the complex sequence of events that would be involved in a suicide attempt (see Chapter 4).

We have found that couple therapy can be helpful when one member of a couple is suffering from dementia. We have often alternated between conjoint and individual sessions with each person. This pattern allows us to hold shorter sessions with the dementia patient when his or her attention span would preclude an hour-long session anyway. It also allows us to build a strong relationship with the caregiver, which is important for the long haul. The sessions away from the patient allow the caregiver to express the full weight of his or her frustration with the patient and despair over the diagnosis.

The conjoint sessions are useful in other ways. They provide the clinician with direct evidence of how the couple is interacting. The patient's memory deficits can be exacerbating existing communication problems. There is also a shift in power in the relationship toward the caregiver. Clinicians need to be aware of this change and avoid allying solely with the caregiver, which will only increase the growing imbalance in the relationship. Instead, interventions should bolster and validate the patient's position in the relationship while allowing his or her spouse to take over responsibilities as needed.

One frequent source of tension is the caregiver taking over activities the dementia patient used to do. Patients are often threatened or upset when this happens, or they resist and argue with their spouse over whether they can continue performing a task. Conjoint sessions can help clarify which activities the spouse really needs to take over. Patients can sometimes identify what they would like their spouse to say or do when they need help. If the well spouse approaches the patient differently, problems can be avoided. In time, the patient's ability to participate in conjoint or individual sessions decreases, and the focus shifts to the primary caregiver and other family members.

Group treatment has been reported to be very helpful for patients with mild impairments (Yale, 1991). As in other group treatments, a major benefit is the opportunity to interact with other people going through the same process. Patients overcome the sense of being alone and isolated and gain support from one another. They may also learn better ways of coping with their problems, for example, discussing what to tell other people about their illness. Other topics covered in these groups include discussions about possible treatments, looking at how the disease has affected their lives and family relationships, concerns about the future, attitudes toward death, and how to maximize one's remaining abilities to engage in satisfying activities (Yale, 1991). A major focus can be reminiscing, which draws on memories not yet affected by the disease. Reviewing prior accomplishments and activities can build esteem in the face of this catastrophic process.

Yale (1991) recommends using here-and-now experiences in the group to build coping strategies. For example, if one member loses track of the topic being discussed, she asks other participants if that happens to them. Group leaders also need to be prepared to address communication and behavior problems. Denial is a common response in dementia patients. Group leaders should view denial as an adaptive response, not as an objective to be assaulted through a frontal attack. Patients should be helped to deal with information they cannot handle in a gentle and sometimes indirect way. The group can be used to explore these difficult areas, taking the focus off the individual. The clinician should consider carefully if anything valuable will be gained by overcoming a patient's denial. Often the answer is no. Finally, summaries by the leader at the start and end of the session can help participants orient themselves to the group and help them recall previous discussions. Although careful evaluations remain to be done, groups are becoming increasingly popular and have been promoted widely by community organizations such as local chapters of the Alzheimer's Association.

CONCLUSIONS

This chapter has introduced a framework for treatment of dementia patients. Behavior of patients should be viewed as an interaction. While the underlying disease alters the likelihood of disturbed behavior, the occurrence of problems depends in part on how people respond to patients and on the environmental setting. Using this framework, we have explored the role of four specific treatments; medications, cognitive stimulation, behavioral interventions, and counseling. Although there is as yet not much that can be done to alter the degenerative course of dementia, interventions can minimize behavioral disturbances and maximize patients' remaining abilities.

12

Family Caregiving

When people develop disabilities in later life, families are the first line of defense. Family caregivers provide extensive care, often at considerable sacrifice of their own health and well-being. To understand the stresses of caregiving, it is necessary to take a broad perspective that encompasses the care recipient's current problems and disabilities, how the disabilities have affected relationships in the family, how providing care places strain on caregivers and interferes with other activities or responsibilities they have, and what tangible and emotional resources the family can draw on to help meet the demands they face.

Families have always provided care for their disabled elders, but caregiving has received much more attention in recent years. The growing importance of family caregiving is due to the convergence of several social trends. First and foremost is the aging of the population. In the past, most people did not survive to old age, so family care of elders was relatively rare. Now more people live into their 70s and 80s, ages when rates of disability and the need for assistance steadily rise. Second, while the amount of active and independent life has increased, so has the period of morbidity. The same factors that have improved the health and functioning of the healthy elderly population are also extending life expectancy after disabilities develop. This notion is called the "expansion of morbidity hypothesis" (Cassel, Rudberg, & Olshansky, 1992). While unequivocal data to support this hypothesis are not available, a lot of evidence suggests that people with chronic illnesses survive for longer periods of time than was the case 20 years ago or even 10 years ago. Dementia patients, for example, once had a relatively short period of morbidity. Old textbooks describe life expectancy of Alzheimer's disease as 2 to 4 years following diagnosis. Now it is not uncommon for people to live 10 to 15 years or even longer after the onset of this illness (Aneshensel et al., 1995). Even allowing for the fact that diagnosis was more imprecise in the past and probably occurred later in the course of the illness, it appears that patients are living longer after the onset of symptoms, and they therefore require care for longer periods of time.

While demands placed on families have been increasing, their resources for providing care have shrunk. The most frequent person who provides care is the spouse of the older person (e.g., Stone, Cafferata, & Sangl, 1987). Spouses are older themselves and may be coping with their own limitations. Daughters are the next most frequent group of caregivers, providing assistance to their parents. With women's increasing participation in the workplace, however, care of an older parent often represents one more demand on top of an already overfull schedule of work and family responsibilities. Other trends, such as smaller family size and reduced economic opportunities for younger generations, also limit the family's ability to provide help.

As a result, the situation for families is unprecedented: more people require more extensive assistance for longer periods of time than ever before, while the family's resources for providing this help are often limited. It is no wonder that family caregiving has captured the interest of the general public and the media and has been the focus of intensive research over the last two decades.

This chapter is divided into two main sections. The first part is a review of research on family caregiving. As a first step in planning interventions, it is useful to understand the stresses of caregiving, particularly factors that seem to increase or decrease the problems caregivers experience. If we understand better how some families can manage caregiving responsibilities without extensive stress, we can draw on that knowledge in planning interventions. The second part of the chapter describes a comprehensive treatment program for family caregivers. Much of the emphasis is on families of dementia patients, which is the most challenging and stressful of care situations. Many of the approaches, however, can be applied to other caregiving situations.

FAMILY STRESS AND ADAPTATION

Over the past two decades, extensive research has been conducted on family caregivers. At the risk of oversimplifying the complex research findings on family caregiving, we have identified six points that capture the major themes and results of this work.

Caregiving Is Stressful

First, an obvious point: care of a disabled older person is very stressful, especially when the person suffers from Alzheimer's disease or another dementing disorder. Caregiving involves chronic stress, which exacts a considerable toll on families. Study after study has documented the negative effects that caregiving has on the health and well-being of family caregivers (e.g., Anthony-Bergstone, Zarit, & Gatz, 1988; Friss & Whitlatch, 1991; Wright, Clipp, & George, 1993; Kiecolt-Glaser, Dura, Speicher, Trask, & Glaser, 1991; Schulz, O'Brien, Bookwala, & Fleissner, 1995). Caregivers are more likely to be depressed and angry and possibly also to have poorer health than age-matched controls not involved in caregiving (Anthony-Bergstone et al., 1988; Gallagher, Rose, Rivera, Lovett, & Thompson, 1989; Wright et al. 1993; Kiecolt-Glaser et al., 1991).

Stressors and Outcomes Are Multidimensional

The second main finding from caregiving research is that the stresses and outcomes of caregiving are multidimensional. No single or key stressor or burden defines caregiving. Rather, multiple processes are involved, on which families can differ considerably from one another and from themselves over time.

One useful framework for viewing the stressors of caregiving differentiates between primary and secondary stressors (Aneshensel et al., 1995). Primary stressors are the problems embedded in the patient's disease and disability. They include the amount of care needed for daily activities and any behavioral, cognitive, and emotional disturbances that caregivers must cope with. A particularly poignant stressor in dementia is the growing sense of loss of the afflicted person among caregivers (Aneshensel et al., 1995).

Secondary stressors, in turn, represent the impact that the primary stressors have in other areas of the caregiver's life. Examples include the extent to which primary stressors interfere with the caregiver's employment and with other family relationships and the financial pressure care places on the family.

The number of primary and secondary stressors can vary considerably in caregiving situations. The particular constellation of stressors in any situation depends on the care recipient's disabilities and the caregiver's other involvements and responsibilities. The combination of primary and secondary stressors can lead to depression, poor health, or other outcomes for caregivers.

Adaptation to Stressors Varies with the Situation

That brings us to the third point, variability in adaptation. This is the most interesting and important finding to emerge from caregiving research. Caregivers respond differently to similar events or stressors, and they follow different patterns of change over time (Aneshensel et al., 1995; S. Zarit, Todd, & Zarit, 1986; Schulz, Williamson, Morycz, & Biegel, 1993). Some people manage reasonably well over time. Others are overwhelmed from the outset and do not adapt or recover. Still others fluctuate in their functioning over time.

We often assume that certain problems or behaviors of the care recipient are always experienced as stressful by caregivers. Incontinence, for example, is often viewed as a problem too difficult for family caregivers to manage that leads to placement into a nursing home. Although incontinence can be burdensome for family caregivers, both physically and emotionally, some caregivers respond to this problem with little or no stress. We followed one caregiver through the long course of his wife's dementia. Early in her illness, he struggled with having to take over managing the family finances. He tried everything he could to get her to continue paying the bills, even though she was now forgetting to pay some bills and was paying others twice. Finally, after much emotional distress and with considerable trepidation, he took over paying the bills. Much later in his wife's illness, she became incontinent. In contrast to his struggles with finances, he managed her incontinence with little difficulty.

Caregivers respond to other stressors in varying ways. Behavior problems such as agitation or not sleeping at night are often very difficult to manage, yet some caregivers manage even these problems well. Their calm response, in turn, may lead to a lessening of the behaviors.

Research confirms this varying impact of behavior problems on caregivers (e.g., S. Zarit et al., 1986). Measures of primary stressors, such as the extent of disability or number of behavior problems, account for a surprisingly small portion of variance of subjective strain and well-being. Even when the constellations of stressors are similar, for example, similar patterns of disability and behavioral problems in dementia patients, the outcomes can be quite different. Perhaps the best test to date of the impact of disabilities and behavior problems is a study that followed caregivers longitudinally over a 4-year period (Aneshensel et al., 1995). Using a longitudinal perspective, it was possible to evaluate how increases or decreases in stressors affected caregivers' emotional well-being. Stressors such as behavior problems accounted for a significant but surprisingly small proportion of changes in well-being over time.

We see a similar pattern with secondary stressors. Some employed caregivers find the added demands and pressures of caring for a spouse or parent overwhelming. Other caregivers, however, report that their employment gives them a break from caregiving. Research generally indicates that working caregivers are not worse off than comparable people who are not employed (e.g., Scharlach, 1994; Brody, Kleban, Johnsen, Hoffman, & Schoonover, 1987), though the amount of strain may depend in part on the ability of working caregivers to find paid help to supplement their efforts.

In a sense, disability creates the context in which severe distress may develop, but whether or not a family experiences distress depends on other factors. Caregiving events become stressful through their interface with other factors in the caregiver's life. That is important for intervention: while we may not be able to do much about a disability or underlying disease, some of the personal and social determinants of caregiving stress are potentially modifiable.

Some Factors Associated with Caregiving Stress Are Modifiable

What are some modifiable dimensions of caregiving? Identifying factors associated with reduced stress has been a major theme in stress research. Caregiving research has focused on two domains that have been found to buffer the effects of stressful events in other situations: social support and coping.

In contrast to other stress situation, social support has not consistently been associated with positive outcomes for family caregivers. There are some important reasons for this finding. First, caregivers often get very low levels of help, either from their families or from paid services (Aneshensel et al., 1995). A related issue is that formal services sometimes do not provide the help that families need and may even make care more difficult. Caregivers are often grateful for any help they get, but they often find the help provided by community agencies unpredictable and unresponsive to their needs (MaloneBeach, Zarit, & Spore, 1992). They do not understand how agencies decide what type or how much help is appropriate, and they do not understand the complex reimbursement system. They are also upset that they have no say over when help is provided or who provides it. In other words, formal agencies provide help to people who are faced with uncontrollable stress in a manner that makes them feel an even greater lack of control over their situation. When service personnel complain that caregivers do not use available services, it is important to understand that more is involved than just a reluctance to get help. Sometimes reluctance is a realistic appraisal of the help that is available.

The caregiver's family is a very important source of support and assistance, but along with the help family members provide can be disagreements or conflicts over how care should be provided (MaloneBeach & Zarit, 1995; Semple, 1992). Caregiving can also intensify conflicts between a parent and children or reawaken sibling rivalries. Findings suggest that the area of social support is complex, and that the attractively simple notion that more help is always better is not correct.

The other main focus of research on modifiable aspects of stress has been coping. Again, the picture is complex. Some measures of coping, such as having a sense of mastery, have been found to predict positive outcomes for caregivers (e.g., Aneshensel et al., 1995). Studies of other dimensions of coping have found contradictory results (e.g., Pruchno & Kleban, 1993; Williamson & Schulz, 1993).

Clinical observations have identified some promising coping strategies. Treating patients in a calm way and knowing how to distract them can lower rates of behavior problems while lessening strain on caregivers. By contrast, caregivers who respond to behavior problems in confrontational or controlling ways may actually increase the patient's agitation or disruptiveness.

As an example, one caregiver was awakened at 2:00 in the morning by her mother, who needed help to go to the bathroom. Now that she was awake, this woman, who was suffering from dementia, thought it was time to get up. Rather than confronting her or angrily telling her to go back to bed, her daughter instead reminisced with her about pleasant times they had spent together when the daughter was young. In a short while, the mother went back to sleep. Many caregivers do not have the patience or skill to take that approach, especially in the middle of the night, yet it undoubtedly calmed the woman and reduced the time her daughter was kept awake.

We expand on these approaches for coping with stressful behaviors later in the chapter. Our point here is that some factors associated with the stresses of caregiving are potentially modifiable. Strain on caregivers is in part due to the problems they are facing and in part to how they respond and the resources available to them for managing the problem.

Caregiving Involves Continuity and Change

The fifth point concerns continuity and change in the caregiving role. For many families, caregiving stretches over a period of several years. It is not uncommon, for example, for families to care for someone with dementia at home for a period of 10 years or more (Aneshensel et al., 1995). During this sustained effort, stressors emerge and recede in importance, and there are important transitions that alter a caregiver's involvement.

Three critical transitions in caregiving warrant examination: (1) transition to the caregiving role; (2) transition from community care to institutional placement; and (3) bereavement. We probably know the least about the transition to the caregiving role. Research and clinical interventions typically take place after families have been providing care for a while. Occasionally, however, clinicians treat families when they are considering becoming caregivers for a parent or at the outset of their relative's disability. There are opportunities for interventions in this early phase of caregiving that can prevent problems later on, which we will discuss, but unfortunately, most families do not get much help at this point.

A lot more is known about the transition from community to nursing home. The placement decision is often the most difficult thing families face during the course of caregiving. Rather than relieving stress on caregivers, placement simply alters the type of stresses they experience (S. Zarit & Whitlatch, 1992; Aneshensel et al., 1995). Caregivers do get relief from the stress of everyday care routines, but they encounter new stressors in the nursing home, including how to interact with their relative and with staff at the facility, concern about how to pay for care, and, frequently, guilt over having placed a spouse or parent. Not surprisingly, then, placement has been found not to lower emotional distress among family caregivers (S. Zarit & Whitlatch, 1992; Aneshensel et al., 1995).

We find similar results with the final transition, bereavement. Following the death of a relative suffering from dementia, caregivers continue to experience distress for some period of time (Aneshensel et al., 1995). Although depression and similar symptoms gradually decrease, some caregivers remain depressed for a sustained period of time.

There is, then, both continuity and change over the course of caregiving. It is important to view family care as a complex, ongoing process that is characterized both by considerable individual differences and by key transitions that require families to make new adaptations. There are no simple formulas for understanding caregiving or simple stages that reduce it to an uncomplicated pattern. Research on caregiving provides a framework for viewing the broad phenomenon, for conducting assessments to identify the particular strengths and problems within a given family, and for pinpointing potentially modifiable features of the stress process.

DEMENTIA AND FAMILY CAREGIVING: TREATMENT APPROACHES

Caregivers who are providing ongoing care of an older person face many stresses and problems, which can be addressed by a carefully planned clinical intervention. Over the years, we have developed a model for treatment of caregivers that emphasizes both the specific clinical techniques to be used and different forms that treatment can take (S. Zarit & Zarit, 1982; S. Zarit, Orr, & Zarit, 1985; S. Zarit, 1996). This approach (Figure 12.1) starts with assessment of the patient and caregiver. The model then emphasizes three treatment techniques—(1) providing information, (2) problem solving, and (3) support—and three treatment modalities—(1) counseling the caregiver, (2) family meetings, and (3) support groups. Though designed specifically for caregivers of dementia patients, many features of this approach have wider applications.

Empirical tests of this model have found it to be effective in reducing strain on the family caregiver and reducing inappropriate placement into nursing homes (Mittelman et al., 1995; Whitlatch, Zarit, & von Eye, 1991;

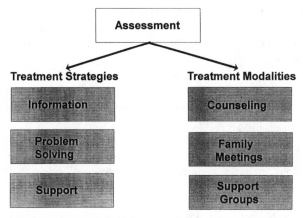

FIGURE 12.1. Model of intervention with caregivers.

Whitlatch, Zarit, Goodwin, & von Eye, 1995). From that perspective, it is a cost-effective intervention; the expense of the clinical intervention is offset by delaying more costly care in a nursing home.

Issues in Assessment of Caregivers

Caregivers may seek help for themselves, but the most typical situation is when they seek help for their relative. A family member other than the primary caregiver may sometimes bring the older person in for an evaluation. In these situations, clinicians begin with the designated patient, conducting an assessment of the patient's problems and the impact on the family. When the assessment reveals the need to involve the caregiver in treatment, the clinician then helps the family understand why that is needed and what it can accomplish.

An important part of the assessment is to find out about the older person's medical condition. In addition to the information the family provides, it is usually helpful to obtain the care recipient's medical records. Among the useful facts are (1) onset and course of symptoms, (2) physicians' diagnoses, (3) past and current treatments and their effects, and (4) other medical problems and medications. It is helpful to develop a collaborative relationship with the physician who is primarily involved in treatment of the patient's problems. The clinician may be able to provide information to the physician about ongoing behavioral or emotional problems that could lead to changes in medication or other medical intervention. In some cases, it may turn out that the medical evaluation has been inadequate, and then the therapist can discuss with the family the possibility of getting another opinion. We refer a client for another evaluation when a dementing illness has been diagnosed if the workup was not adequate or our observations of the patient do not support the diagnosis. We also refer patients who have unusual or atypical symptoms or diseases and so might benefit from an evaluation by a specialist.

Besides evaluating what has been done medically, the clinician should assess the family's understanding of the patient's illness, symptoms, treatment, and prognosis. As discussed later, providing information about these issues is often an important part of treatment.

A third part of the assessment is to identify stressors: the patient's disabilities, what type of help the patient needs on a regular basis, what portion of the help the caregiver provides, and the patient's cognitive functioning, behavior, and mood. As we emphasized earlier, it is important to determine which problems are present and which of those the caregiver experiences as stressful or problematic. The Memory and Behavior Problems Checklist can be used for this assessment (see Appendix 5.1). It is also useful to find out how caregivers manage these problems.

A similar approach should be taken in assessing secondary stressors, that is, the extent to which caregiving may affect other roles and activities. Caregiving undoubtedly affects these other roles, but caregivers may be able to tolerate or manage some of the strains. We should not assume that there is conflict with employment or in other family relationships but should determine which problems are actually present. A long-term goal is to prevent a buildup of stress in caregiving that would have adverse consequences for other areas of the caregiver's life.

In some instances, we may also have questions about the caregiver's cognitive functioning. We do not routinely recommend assessing the caregiver's cognitive functioning, since that is a distraction and may even upset the caregiver. We do conduct an evaluation, however, if the caregiver requests one (which usually then can be used to give reassurance that nothing is wrong) or if we observe evidence of forgetfulness that goes beyond everyday memory lapses.

Another focus of the assessment is the wider family network. The clinician should determine who the important family members are and what their current involvement and view of the situation is. Among the points to consider are how much help other family members provide, how much contact they have with the caregiver and the care recipient, what their understanding of the patient's condition and the caregiver's needs seems to be, and if there is conflict between the caregiver and other family members. Semple (1992) has suggested that there are three types of family conflict: (1) over the patient's diagnosis and treatment, (2) over the amount and type of care the caregiver is providing, and (3) over the amount of help provided by other family members. As in any family situation, the clinician must recognize that he or she is hearing one side of the story and that the perspective of the other family members may be quite different. In addition to family, friends, neighbors, and volunteers may be providing some help.

It is also important to determine what formal services the caregiver or care recipient have used, what has been helpful, and what has not worked out. Before clinicians suggest that caregivers use formal services, they should know what a caregiver has previously tried and if a particular service did not work out.

Finally, clinicians should evaluate caregivers' emotional distress. This assessment can be done clinically or by having the caregiver complete a rating scale or form, such as a depression inventory or caregiver strain measure. The advantage of obtaining this type of measure is that it provides a baseline against which subsequent treatment can be evaluated. The possibility of suicidal and homicidal thoughts should be evaluated as well. Although not common, instances occur in which a despondent, caregiving husband takes his wife's life and then his own. Clinicians can conduct a standard assessment of these issues and also follow up on any statements or behaviors by the caregiver indicating a possible risk of suicide or homicide.

Based on the initial evaluations, the clinician and caregiver can set goals for treatment. Goals include clarifying issues of diagnosis and treatment, finding out information about care resources, lowering stress on the caregiver, and treating behavior problems of the patient. Sometimes the goal is broader, such as when a family member is trying to decide about taking on the caregiving role. Usually, this situation involves sons or daughters, since spouses routinely assume this role for one another. Children may be asking about whether they should provide care themselves or find a setting in which their parent can be helped, or they may be trying to decide which of the children will take on the role. There are no right or pat answers to these questions. Families must make these decisions consistent with their own values and in light of the resources available to help them with caregiving. Clinicians should be nonjudgmental and make sure their own values do not color the decision. They can also provide families with information about care alternatives for their parent. Families often view the situation as a dichotomy between providing all the care themselves or putting a parent in a nursing home. Telling families about community and residential programs gives them options that might better suit their relative and themselves.

Treatment Techniques

Providing Information

The starting point of clinical intervention with caregivers is to provide the information they need about their relative's illness and the treatment and care options available so that they can make informed decision. We usually begin by finding out what they know about their relative's illness and answering their questions. Families typically report that they did not get much information from physicians at the time the diagnosis was made and that they would have liked more (Aneshensel et al., 1995). In some instances, physicians provided little or no information; in other cases, the family was not able to absorb the information or did not have time to formulate questions. In either case, the therapist can help families get the information they want. We typically discuss the illness with the family—and with patients who are not too impaired cognitively. We also give families books and pamphlets that explain the illness they are dealing with. If there are technical questions we cannot answer, we refer them to their physician or to an appropriate specialist.

When dealing with progressive disorders like dementia, the clinician needs to be honest but tactful in providing information. We give families a general idea about the likely progression and note that there are individual differences in symptoms and their rate of progression. We then answer their questions in an honest and direct manner.

Patients with chronic and incurable diseases and their families may seek out experimental or alternative treatments. These treatments provide hope in the face of a bleak prognosis. But experimental or unproven treatments outside research settings may be of questionable value. The clinician can help families weigh the potential advantages and disadvantages of unconventional approaches. The primary advantage, of course, is that the proposed treatment might help with the patient's symptoms. Common disadvantages are side effects of the treatment and its cost.

Beyond questions about the illness, families often misunderstand or misinterpret the patient's behavior. These misunderstandings increase stress on the caregiver and may also inadvertently contribute to the patient's problems. Misunderstandings are particularly common in dementia. When patients ask the same question over and over again, caregivers may conclude that patients are trying to annoy them or that they are too lazy to listen to the answer or that they could correct the problem by trying harder. In other words, families believe that patients should be aware of their memory problems and do something to control them, and they become impatient and angry with them for not doing so. Patients, however, usually have little or no insight into their condition and are not able to limit themselves. We help families view these problems as part of the disease, to understand that patients with dementing illnesses cannot remember and often cannot acknowledge that they cannot remember. By viewing the problems as symptoms of a disease and not as willful or under the patient's control, the family can make more adaptive responses.

This approach is extended to a variety of problems involving memory and interpretations of reality. Families often find themselves arguing with patients over issues such as whether an object was stolen or misplaced or whether the patient's mother is still alive or not. In arguing with dementia patients, families are falling into a logical trap. They are trying to reason with patients about the facts of a situation, but the patient's ability to understand the facts has been diminished by the disease. No matter how much families reason or argue with patients, they cannot win the argument. What is particularly frustrating for families is that their relative often can argue in a logical way while totally ignoring the evidence, as shown in the following example.

A wife caring for her husband recounted an argument she had had with him. He had always loved horses and had taken care of several horses after his retirement. Because of his progressive dementia, he could no longer continue doing so. One day he began to insist that there were two horses in the garage and that he had to give them food and water. No amount of arguing dissuaded him. He began taking water out to the horses and insisted that his wife buy feed for them. Finally exasperated with these continual arguments, she told him that she would go out to the garage with him where he could show her the horses. If she could see the horses, she would buy food for them. They went out to the garage, and she said she could not see the horses. He insisted they were there. When she asked if she could touch them, he put her hands on their two automobiles. In frustration, she asked, "If there are two horses here, wouldn't the garage be filled with manure?" to which he replied, "No, not with how little we're feeding them."

This example illustrates that the dementia patient's distortions are relatively resistant to reasoning and even to demonstrations that they are incorrect. Yet this patient responded to the caregiver's points in a logical way. This apparent logic engages caregivers, and they persist in trying to reason with patients who can no longer respond to a factual argument.

In these situations, it is important to help families see that their relative's ability to respond to the facts of a situation is limited and that they need to use other approaches. We encourage families to approach problems in two ways. First, we want them to think why someone with a memory-impairing disease behaves this way. Second, we want them to consider what someone behaving this way might be feeling. We can illustrate this approach with three common problems: paranoid accusations, wanting to see one's mother, and wanting to go home.

Paranoid accusations are common in dementia and usually have their basis in the patient's increasing memory loss (see Chapter 10). Typical accusations involve someone coming in and stealing money or stealing the patient's purse, wallet, or other valuable objects. Families see that the patient has misplaced the object and try to reason with the patient or persuade the patient that he probably hid it. Patients, however, typically deny that they misplaced the object and get upset when it is suggested they are incorrect.

Instead of arguing, families are encouraged to view the problem as due to memory loss, that patients have misplaced the object and cannot remember doing so, much less where the object is. Rather than responding to the facts of the situation, caregivers can ask themselves what the patient must be feeling and then respond to those feelings. Whatever the facts of the situation, the patient's emotional reaction is valid and real. Patients may be upset, frustrated, or fearful. Caregivers can address the patient's feelings by empathizing (e.g., "You're upset that you can't find your money") rather than arguing with the patient. They can also respond in ways that are calming (e.g., reassuring patients that they have plenty of money).

As dementia progresses, patients sometimes ask to see their mother. Often the first response by families, and by many professionals as well, is to tell patients that their mother is dead. Because of the patient's memory loss, this information often is experienced as new, and the patient becomes more upset and agitated. As their agitation increases, their requests to see their mother can become more frequent. We have known families who even showed patients their mother's obituary, but these attempts to orient patients to the facts of the situation make no difference whatsoever. Instead of arguing over whether the patient's mother is alive or not, the family should try to understand the behavior in light of the patient's memory problems. They can think about what their relative must be feeling when she says she wants to see her mother and respond to those feelings.

We once consulted in a special care unit for dementia patients on a case in which the patient wanted to see her mother. The staff believed their role was to reorient patients to reality, but no amount of telling the patient that her mother was dead had an effect. Staff then decided they would try to trick her. When she asked to see her mother, they had her dial a number on the phone, which rang in another part of the unit. A staff member answered and told her that her mother was in the bath and could not come to the phone. Although her memory deficits were pronounced, the patient remembered this conversation, and 5 minutes later she told the staff, "My mother is surely out of the bath by now. Can I call her again?" Finally frustrated with their inability to reason with the patient or to trick her, the staff tried responding to her feelings. When she asked to see her mother, the nurse asked her to sit down, have a cup of tea with her, and talk about her mother. That approach had a calming effect and reduced the frequency of her requests to see her mother. Families (or staff) can also look at old photographs or in other ways reminisce about the patient's mother.

Wanting to go home is a similar problem. Even patients who have lived in the same house for a long period of time may insist that they are not at home and that they want to go home. In our experience, no amount of arguing can change their mind. We have known families who take the patient back to the home he grew up in, only to find out that he does not recognize it. Just as with the other examples, the facts of the situation are not important. Sometimes families can distract patients by taking them out for a walk or a ride. When they come back to their house, the patient now recognizes it. A more general solution is to respond to the valid part of patients' communication, their feelings. In wanting to go home, patients may be expressing insecurity or bewilderment that the present is not making sense. A calm, reassuring response can lower the patient's anxiety. Reminiscing, looking at old photographs, or diverting patients to other activities can all be helpful.

Families facing extensive costs for long-term care should be encouraged to seek legal and financial advice. In particular, spouses need to be aware of how they can protect a portion of their assets and income if their husband or wife goes into a nursing home (see Chapter 9). If families do not have a lawyer to turn to, we refer them to someone who specializes in elder law.

Besides discussions with the clinician, families find it helpful to read pamphlets and books about caregiving. *The Thirty-Six Hour Day* (Mace & Rabins, 1991) is very popular among caregivers of dementia patients. The Alzheimer's Association and other organizations offer a variety of pamphlets and other helpful information.

Problem Solving

The heart of intervention with family caregivers is a behavioral technique called problem solving, which is used to manage problem behaviors. This approach was introduced in Chapter 11. Here we describe how we use problem solving in conjunction with caregivers and teach them how to use it themselves.

The steps we use in problem solving with caregivers are shown in Table 12.1. The starting point is to identify a problem and assess when it occurs. Most often the problem is a behavior, such as agitation or getting the caregiver up at night. In some instances, the caregiver may not be able to be specific about what behaviors or problems are most difficult or stressful, so the assessment can focus on identifying when the caregiver feels upset. Using a form to record problems (see Appendix 12.1), caregivers note when the targeted behavior occurs. Caregivers also record what happened right before

TABLE 12.1. Problem-Solving Process

1. Pinpoint a behavior and assess when it occurs and how often.
2. Identify antecedents and consequences.
3. Identify possible strategies for intervention (brainstorm).
4. Select a strategy (use pros and cons).
5. Plan and rehearse implementing the strategy.
6. Try out the strategy and evaluate it.

the problem (antecedents) and what occurred afterwards (consequences). The antecedent events may trigger or set off the problem behavior, and the events that follow, called consequences, may reinforce the problem behavior. We have found, for example, that inactivity or daytime naps frequently trigger agitation and restlessness. Another common antecedent of behavior problems is patient discomfort, such as pain or hunger. The consequences of problems are how caregivers respond. Caregivers may inadvertently reinforce problem behaviors. They may ignore patients when they are not causing any problems but give them attention when they act out.

We encourage caregivers to write down this information when it occurs, because it is difficult to remember the specific sequence of events leading up to and following a problem. This written record also provides a clear baseline of the frequency of the problem, which can be used to evaluate the effects of an intervention.

Once caregivers have clarified when and how often a problem occurs, it is possible to consider possible solutions. Solutions may emerge out of the pattern that has been observed. For example, if a patient becomes upset following a period of inactivity, a possible solution is to head off the problem by introducing activities. Caregiver and clinician talk about ways of doing that. Similarly, if the consequence of a behavior is that the patient gets attention, caregivers can identify ways of giving attention for positive behaviors instead.

Rather than suggesting a specific solution, we encourage caregivers to identify their own interventions. This approach builds on caregivers' own coping abilities, as well as teaching them how to use problem solving. Sometimes, however, caregivers feel too frustrated or hopeless to come up with solutions. They need to be encouraged to say anything that comes to mind. We ask them to brainstorm ideas and to avoid censoring any thoughts they might have.

Once the caregiver has identified possible solutions, a decision is made about which one to try. At this point, some caregivers express reservations about the solution and indicate a reluctance to try anything. Their anger and frustration may come out, that they have to make all this effort when they are getting so little in return. Other caregivers feel hopeless and believe that nothing can make a difference. It is important to empathize with these feelings—they are quite understandable given the circumstances in which caregivers find themselves. But the clinician should not dwell on these emotions. Instead, it is important to direct the caregiver back to the problem and to taking a more active role in controlling it. That can be done using the method of "pros and cons." This approach, developed as part of the cognitive-behavioral treatment of depression by Beck and his associates (Beck et al., 1979), involves evaluating the likely pros and cons of each solution. The caregiver writes down the advantages and disadvantages on a piece of paper. Writing down these responses serves to cut down on endless ruminations and to clarify which solution may actually be worth trying. For some caregivers, it may be necessary to try out any solution compared to doing nothing. The goal is to get the client to engage in some new behavior as a way of disrupting old patterns.

Once a solution has been identified, we encourage the caregiver to rehearse the steps involved in carrying it out. Rehearsing the behavior ensures that the caregiver can actually carry out the plan. A caregiver may, for example, decide to respond calmly when the patient asks the same question over and over and then distract the patient with an activity. Rehearsing this approach with us, it may become evident that the caregiver is too angry to answer the question in a patient manner. We then work on shaping a better response or taking a different approach.

When caregivers have a plan they are comfortable with, the next step is to try it out. As with other behavioral interventions, the time and place for the new response should be scheduled. The caregiver should continue monitoring the targeted problem to find out if the new response results in a change in frequency. If the intervention is successful, the targeted behavior will decrease. If not, caregiver and clinician can look at other possible solutions.

The goal is to eliminate or at least decrease how often a problem occurs. In situations where there is partial improvement, some caregivers dwell on the remaining incidents, not the improvement. For example, increasing a patient's activity during the day might reduce the number of nights that he wakes up the caregiver from six to two times a week. The caregiver, however, might complain that she has gotten no relief because she is still being awakened, thus ignoring the overall improvement. In that situation, the clinician uses the records the caregiver made of how frequently the problem occurs to demonstrate that there has actually been improvement and then discusses the significance of bringing the problem partly under control.

The following example demonstrates the use of problem solving. A woman was caring for her husband, who was suffering from Alzheimer's disease. Her biggest problem was that her husband became agitated between 4:00 and 6:00 P.M. every day. During this time, he would rearrange the furniture in the living room, throw things on the floor, and generally make a mess. While he was doing this, his wife was busy preparing dinner. On her therapist's prompting, the woman kept a record of her husband's agitated behavior for a week. Reviewing the records together, therapist and caregiver noted that the problem did not occur on one day during the previous week. They then explored what was different about that day. During the afternoon, the woman had taken her husband for a ride. They had done this other afternoons as well, but on this day her husband said he was hungry. Initially, she thought he would spoil his appetite for dinner if he ate then, but she decided that was not important, and they stopped for a sandwich. Based on this information, the clinician and the woman hypothesized that he might get hungry in the late afternoon. The caregiver decided to serve dinner at 5:00 P.M. rather than at 6:00 to see if that made a difference. The following week her records indicated that the amount of agitation in late afternoon was greatly reduced.

This example illustrates a number of important points about problem solving. Based on the initial information of agitation during late afternoon, several hypotheses could have been generated, for example, that this problem was part of the sundowner's syndrome and that better illumination might help. The hypothesis emerged in this case by focusing on the day the problem behavior did not occur and what was different about the sequence of events on that day. It was also built on an understanding of the effects of dementia. Patients sometimes do not report hunger, thirst, or even pain. We have even observed dementia patients who have fallen and fractured a bone but do not report discomfort. The discomfort from hunger, thirst, or pain can be a trigger for disturbed behavior. The solution, then, emerged from the observations the patient's wife made and drew on an understanding of how dementia affects behavior.

This type of approach has been found to work with many different kinds of problems, including agitation, not sleeping at night, and incontinence. Although solutions are often unique to the particular context in which a problem occurs, common solutions include increasing the amount of activity, eliminating daytime naps, modifying daily routines, giving patients more frequent snacks, identifying sources of discomfort or pain, and providing affection or other positive reinforcement for adaptive rather than maladaptive behavior. A variation of this approach, which was discussed in the previous chapter, involves increasing the rate of pleasant activities engaged in by dementia patients (Teri, 1994).

Another possible solution for problem behaviors is medications (see Chapter 11). By using medications within a problem-solving framework, it is possible to evaluate their effectiveness. Caregivers can obtain a baseline of how often targeted behavior is occurring prior to the introduction of a medication and then how the frequency changes after the patient has begun taking the medication. These records indicate clearly if the medication is having its intended effect. Medications that are not effective then can be discontinued. The judicious use of medications reduces the risk of adverse side effects and paradoxical reactions.

Solutions, including medications, can lose their effectiveness over time. At that point, it is important to reassess the situation to find out what has changed and to try a new approach. Caregivers, however, can react to changes catastrophically, feeling they have lost the little control they had or believing that the situation is now unmanageable. It is important to help them interpret a change as a normal setback. Before they give up, caregivers can try to find out if there is something different they can do to improve the situation.

Problem solving can be targeted to other concerns besides problem be-haviors. It can, for example, be used to pinpoint when a caregiver feels es-pecially stressed or emotionally drained and identify the specific event or sequence of events that gives the caregiver trouble. Solutions can include finding better ways to manage the triggering events or getting relief for the caregiver before the amount of stress builds up too high.

We have emphasized problem solving as a series of steps, with progress monitored through the use of written records. This framework can be used without formally going through each step. Clinicians who are not experienced with behavioral approaches or with dementia, however, should go through the whole sequence to make sure that the solutions that emerge are specific to the targeted problem and its context. Another advan-tage of formally going through the sequence is to teach caregivers how to use the approach themselves. Problem solving can complement the way caregivers deal with difficult situations. Caregivers learn new skills that re-place approaches that are not effective in managing a dementia patient.

Providing Support

The third treatment technique is providing support. Support emerges natu-rally from a therapeutic relationship that is empathic and nonjudgmental. Support from a therapist can help a caregiver explore difficult issues and gain confidence to try out new approaches.

In order to prepare for the long-term challenges they will face, care-givers must be able to get support from family, friends, and formal service agencies. Support includes both assistance with caregiving tasks and emo-tional support. The type of assistance a caregiver might benefit from usually emerges from discussions of what kinds of things are the most difficult to manage and when the caregiver feels the most stressed or exhausted.

The clinician helps caregivers identify potential sources of support and overcome barriers to their use. Barriers can be practical and emotional. It can be difficult, however, to differentiate between realistic reasons for not using a particular type of assistance and exaggerations of the possible nega-tive consequences.

Accepting help from family and friends is difficult for many caregivers. Some are reluctant to ask for help because they believe they should be able to manage on their own. Caregivers may feel embarrassed or ashamed of the care recipient's behavior or their own need for help. Parents sometimes do not want to burden their children by asking for help and may even try to protect their children from knowing how bad the situation has become. In other instances, the caregiver believes that he or she should not have to ask for help, that the family should offer it.

Caregivers erect similar barriers to accepting help from formal agen-cies. They may believe that no one else can do the job as well or that they should be able to manage everything by themselves. They may also say that the care recipient will not accept help or will become angry at the caregiver for getting help. Caregivers may be concerned that the helpers are not reliable or do not have adequate training.

When caregivers are reluctant to get help for situations that warrant it, clinicians should work with them in a collaborative way to identify the reasons for their reluctance. Using a cognitive-behavioral method of questioning (Beck et al., 1979; see Chapter 8), the clinician helps caregivers identify the thoughts that precede their feelings of reluctance to or anxiety about getting a particular type of help. It is then possible to find alternative ways of looking at a situation or arranging for help. For example, a caregiver may feel that asking her children for help with their father would place too big a burden on them, or that if they wanted to help, they would offer. Through examination of these assumptions and alternative ways of looking at the situation, the clinician may identify that the caregiver's children do not actually know what help she needs. It is also possible to suggest that by not helping, they are missing an opportunity to do something for and with their father while they still have the chance. Of course, the particular way of reframing the caregiver's thoughts about accepting help depend on the situation. Caregivers often fear the worst will happen if they get help. The clinician can point out that events will not necessarily turn out as they expected. Finding examples in caregivers' past experiences when they expected something bad to happen but it did not is also useful. Another objection that caregivers may raise is that they are the only ones who can provide help, that no one else can do it right. The clinician can suggest that it is important for the patient to see other people or to have a change of scenery. Identifying the potential benefits for the patient is helpful when caregivers believe that they are being selfish for seeking help. When caregivers are reluctant to get help, despite a high level of stress, the clinician can explore what their goals are and the consequences of not getting help. Most involved family caregivers want to provide help for as long as they can. By helping them look at the consequences of trying to do everything themselves, they can see that they will burn out quicker.

Again, we want to stress that these ways of reframing the acceptance of help are suggestions, not formulas. The particular way of reframing a situation must emerge from a collaborative and supportive discussion with the caregiver. This discussion should never become badgering or bullying, and clinicians need to be prepared to accept that caregivers choose to handle a situation in a less than optimal way. By building a supportive and accepting relationship, the clinician leaves open the door that the caregiver will become more willing to get help over time.

Caregivers are sometimes reluctant to use services because of practical and realistic barriers. Some service programs are not adequately prepared to handle difficult clients. When evaluating formal services, clinicians can be more helpful if they know how various agencies function. That way, they can assist caregivers to differentiate real barriers from the caregiver's own worries and fears. When there is a real barrier, it may be possible for the clinician to work with the caregiver to plan how to overcome it or to intervene directly with the agency. A typical problem is that home health agencies sometimes do not send the same person to the house for every visit. Sending a different person for each visit can be disruptive for both the family caregiver and the care recipient, especially when the latter has a memory disorder. The caregiver may be able to approach the agency about getting one person to come out or to find another agency that is be more cooperative.

Treatment Modalities

Counseling

Much of the work we have described takes place in one-to-one counseling sessions with the caregiver. An important part of these sessions is development of a therapeutic relationship that gives caregivers the security to examine the problems they are facing and to try out new approaches for managing them. A delicate balance needs to be established regarding expression of emotions. Caregivers often feel angry, depressed, worried, guilty, or frustrated and may have no one else to talk to about these emotions besides the therapist. These feelings are keys for identifying what problems are the most pressing and where clinicians should intervene. Some caregivers who are distressed may have trouble expressing their emotions or targeting what bothers them. More commonly, however, caregivers can readily express their feelings but find it hard to move beyond that point. The clinician needs to create an environment in which the caregiver feels safe in expressing strong emotions but is not encouraged to dwell on them.

The goal for treatment is to find ways of addressing modifiable features of the situation that contribute to the caregiver's distress. Of course, some things cannot be changed, such as their relative's illness and the sense of loss they be feeling. It may seem to many caregivers that the only way of dealing with these feelings is to leave the situation, which can be a frightening thought. The clinician must be able to show caregivers how taking specific steps can make their situation better, even though the patient's illness has not been cured. Starting with small steps, clinicians can provide information, use problem solving, and give support as ways of demonstrating that some things can be changed.

Treatment can address a variety of other issues, including ambivalence over assuming the caregiving role, long-standing problems in the relationship between the caregiver and care recipient, and feelings of guilt. Many caregivers need the opportunity to clarify what their role should be and to set limits to their involvement. If caregivers can articulate what they believe is the right thing for them to do, then it is possible to work with them to develop a plan to do that and to let go when it is the right time. It is important that clinicians convey that there is no right way to be a caregiver, that caregivers must decide what is best for them. Counseling can also involve the care recipient, as described in Chapter 11.

The duration of counseling can be brief and problem focused or long term. Some caregivers need a framework for managing their problems and make considerable progress in five to 10 sessions. These caregivers often have good coping strategies and other resources that can quickly be focused on the situation. When treatment is brief, the door should be left open for caregivers to return if the situation changes and they feel they are no longer managing well.

Other cases are more complicated. Caregivers may be feeling high levels of distress or have inadequate coping strategies for managing the situation. The family situation may be especially difficult or complicated. We have found that in these instances weekly sessions for a sustained period of time are useful. When the situation is stabilized, the time between sessions can be lengthened, though regular sessions can be resumed during a crisis.

Family Meetings

Families are the most important source of support and assistance to caregivers. Unlike formal agencies, which operate within a bureaucratic framework, family members can help in flexible ways and outside business hours. But families may not provide help when the caregiver thinks it is needed or may disagree with the primary caregiver about the care their relative should get. These nonsupportive interactions can be especially debilitating to caregivers already under a great deal of pressure.

Because of how central other family members are to the caregiver's well-being, we have found that direct interventions are useful. A carefully orchestrated family meeting can reduce misunderstandings and conflict over care while building support for the primary caregiver. A single family meeting with telephone follow-up usually suffices (S. Zarit, Orr, & Zarit, 1985), though some treatment protocols use two family sessions (Mittelman et al., 1995).

Planning for the family meeting begins with the primary caregiver. The clinician needs to learn about the family structure and relationships before the family meeting, though recognizing that the perspective of the caregiver is limited. From a family systems perspective, it is useful to get a sense of how a family functions, for example, who is influential and who is not, who is close to and distant from whom, and what the roles of the caregiver and care recipient have been in the family. It is also important to identify conflict over caregiving issues, as well as disagreements over other issues that might interfere with the family's pulling together to support the caregiver. Finally, the clinician and caregiver should explore what kind of help the caregiver would like to get and what is realistic to expect the family to provide. Issues concerning the patient's diagnosis should be clarified before the family meeting, because that will often be a topic of discussion.

The caregiver decides who to invite to the family meeting and when and where to hold it. Family meetings can be held in a clinician's office, though we have had more success when they are held in a family member's home. Families are less likely to respond defensively at home than when called to a mental health professional's office. By going to their home, the clinician demonstrates a commitment to the family that engenders trust.

In the family meeting, the clinician recapitulates the process the caregiver has been going through, moving from providing information to problem solving and support. As a first step, it is important that everyone has the same information about the diagnosis and the possibilities for treatment. Family members may have partial, distorted or incorrect information. In cases of dementia, the primary caregiver usually accepts that the illness is irreversible before other family members, who may continue to question the diagnosis or bombard the caregiver with suggestions about possible treatments they have heard or read about. Although meant to be helpful, this kind of suggestion is frequently experienced by the caregiver as an added stressor (MaloneBeach & Zarit, 1995). Clinicians can address these issues in a gently authoritative and nondogmatic manner. Especially in cases of irreversible disorders like Alzheimer's disease, it is important to assure everyone that everything that can be done is being done. Because the media frequently report the results of new research on possible treatments for Alzheimer's and similar diseases, families may want to continue a search for a cure. As was done earlier with the caregiver, the clinician needs to provide honest answers about the prospects of treatment without dashing all hope that something can be done. The goal is to reframe people's wish to do something from searching for a medical cure to providing support and assistance.

When the family understands the care recipient's condition, the meeting can turn to the caregiver. The clinician can ask the caregiver what is stressful and what kinds of things can help. In some cases, it is the first time the family has thought about the caregiver's situation in that way. When the caregiver's needs are expressed, the family's problem-solving ability comes into play. Usually, there is someone in the family who is an organizer and problem solver and who takes over at that point to develop a plan. The plan can include having family members provide emotional or instrumental support or helping arrange for or pay for formal help. The tasks that the family agrees to do should be scheduled. It should be clear what each person will do and when. The clinician makes sure that no one has overcommitted and that all the tasks are achievable within the proposed time frame.

The best kind of plan involves giving everyone some responsibility. It is important that people do not argue over whether someone is doing too much or too little. The clinician should emphasize that each person can contribute in a different way and that every kind of help is important.

The following example illustrates giving everyone a task and emphasizing that each task is important. This family sought help because the daughter-in-law of a woman suffering from dementia decided to go back to work. She had been providing most of the care for her mother-in-law but could no longer do so. Her husband, the patient's son, was too angry with his mother to spend more time with her because of long-standing problems in their relationship. The patient's daughter wanted to do more for her mother, but she was ill and lived some distance away. She felt guilty that she could not spend more time with her mother. In this situation, the clinician worked with the family to construct tasks for each person. The daughter-in-law said she could continue to visit the mother (who lived in a retirement home) but would go less frequently. The son was willing to talk to the manager of the retirement home about his mother's condition in order to see what additional support the home might provide. He would also talk with his uncle, who lived in the same retirement home, encouraging him to spend more time with the patient. This was something he thought his uncle would be willing to do. Although the daughter could not visit, she could talk with her mother on the phone. When she expressed guilt over not doing more, the therapist stressed to her that this was an important and valuable activity. Follow-up indicated that the plan worked: the family was satisfied with the arrangements they made for their mother and with each other.

The clinician's role in a family meeting is to be neutral and supportive. Already having a relationship with the primary caregiver, the clinician should be sure to note other people's perspectives and observe how the family functions and makes decisions. Caregivers who are strong may be perceived as not needing help and may even have alienated potential helpers. On the other hand, when caregivers are perceived as weak, other family members may deprecate what they have done or blame them for some of the current problems. In these situations, the therapist must keep the focus on how to stabilize the care situation without getting into discussions of the caregiver's or anyone else's personality.

The therapist should use but not try to change family process. Family meetings are not family therapy and should not be used to treat long-standing problems or to redress the balance of power within a family. That is not what the family asked for help with, and it is not necessary for addressing the problems at hand. Rather, the clinician should focus on caregiving issues, identifying common family goals (e.g., providing more support) and developing a plan to reach the goals.

We have been able to work with families who have long-standing conflicts yet can reach an agreement on care-related issues. In one case, a family was so divided that it seemed at first that the family meeting could not be held, because no one could be identified to host the meeting who would be considered neutral by everyone else. Finally, a more distant relative was identified to whom both sides of the feuding family talked, and the meeting was held at that relative's home. The outcome was positive, with the family learning for the first time how severe their mother's disabilities were and rallying around their stepfather to provide help. After discussing their mother's diagnosis, the stress their stepfather was under, and his need for occasional respite, one daughter pulled out her calendar and said that the five children could each take a weekend a month to care for their mother. They agreed on a schedule and also planned to hire help with cooking and cleaning for their stepfather. Follow-up indicated that everyone fulfilled his or her obligations.

This example shows that it is possible to conduct a family meeting when there is conflict around other, long-standing issues. It also shows how families can be creative in generating their own solutions. There are situations, however, where family meetings are not helpful. It is probably not advisable to conduct a family meeting with severely disturbed families who have poor boundaries, disordered communications, and little history of success in dealing with common tasks and problems. In some families the conflict over care may be too intense for a family meeting. As an example, a son who was the primary caregiver for his mother, who was in a nursing home, had made the decision to maintain her old home, at considerable expense, because he felt it was good for her to be able to visit it. His brothers were furious with him and believed that he was squandering the inheritance that was due to them. They had not provided any help with caregiving and, according to the caregiver and his wife, were concerned only about their inheritance. We arranged a family meeting, but the brothers declined to attend. Their refusal to come actually had a positive effect, confirming for the caregiver and his wife that his brothers were not interested in their mother's well-being. He and his wife now felt more comfortable with the decisions they had made and validated in their belief that they were doing the right thing for the mother.

The size of family meetings depends on how many relevant people there are who should be invited. We have had meetings with just one other person and meetings with as many as 25 people. We have even held family meetings in which some of the participants came from overseas. In one such case, the key person providing emotional support to the caregiver was her sister, who lived in Europe, but was visiting when the family meeting took place. During the meeting this sister expressed how badly she felt that should could not help more. The caregiver was able to assure her that her letters and phone calls were very special to her and provided her with help that no one else could provide. This face-to-face meeting allowed for expressions of support that probably could not have taken place otherwise.

Despite the planning the therapist does before the family meeting, he or should be prepared for surprises. Some family members use the forum to reveal information that greatly changes the situation. In one family, two daughters were overseeing the care of their mother, who had severe Alzheimer's disease and was being assisted by a live-in housekeeper. The daughters were close to one another, but both had secrets that they revealed during the meeting. One daughter revealed that she and her husband were trying to have a baby, and that if she got pregnant, she would be able to do much less for her mother. Her sister revealed that she was about to change jobs and could also do less for their mother. They each felt they were letting the other person down and had been reluctant to talk openly about the changes in their lives. By bringing out what they had been hiding from each other, they realized that they had reached the limit of what they could do for their mother, and they decided it was necessary to plan for nursing home care. Though they felt sad that they could not continue to keep their mother at home, they believed they had made the right decision. At follow-up, the sisters had remained close and supportive of each other, placement had gone smoothly, and the first sister was pregnant.

We have also made interventions short of a full-scale meeting that accomplished the same goals. Included are phone conversations with key family members, for example, a child of the caregiver, or joint office sessions that involve one or two other family members. For some families, these more informal arrangements are preferable. The gains that can be made from face-to-face family meetings, however, should not be overlooked, especially the benefit of having everyone in the room together hearing the same information and being given the opportunity to contribute to a plan for support.

Support Groups

Support groups for caregivers, particularly those assisting someone with Alzheimer's disease or another dementing illness, have become immensely popular. Part of a grass-roots movement that began in the late 1970s to assist caregivers and build support among the general public for treatment of Alzheimer's disease, support groups have flourished and led to the development of advocacy organizations such as the Alzheimer's Association. Research on support groups suggests that they are not as effective as one-to-one counseling or a combination of counseling and family meetings in reducing stress on caregivers (Toseland, Rossiter, Peak, & Smith, 1990; Whitlatch, Zarit, & von Eye, 1991). Support groups should not be the first line of help or only source of help for caregivers. But their enduring popularity indicates that they are helpful in important ways.

The special properties of support groups enhance the three treatment techniques, information, problem solving, and support. Groups are an effective way of disseminating information among caregivers. Caregivers share their first-hand experience with various community helpers and resources; they discuss which physicians are helpful, which attorneys to consult, and how to find good home helpers to assist the patient. They also share information about treatments, such as which drugs help patients, something that should be closely monitored by the group leader but that can be productive.

Groups also provide a special kind of support that is not available elsewhere, that of sharing experiences with people who are in the same situation. Caregivers feel less isolated after attending groups. Hearing how other people respond to similar situations can be a normalizing experience. It helps caregivers understand that the strong emotions they feel are an expected part of the stress of caregiving, not something that is wrong with them. In one group of caregivers who did not know each other well, one man burst out that he had gotten so angry at his wife (who had dementia) that he had put his fist through the wall. The group sat for a minute in stunned silence, and then everyone began saying that how they felt angry and frustrated, too, but had been ashamed of those feelings. By acknowledging their anger to one another, group members felt less isolated and could now identify their anger as something to work on rather than hide.

In a similar way, caregivers are able to draw on one another's experiences to overcome their reluctance to accept help. They learn first-hand about the benefits of getting help and realize that it is not shameful or a sign of weakness to accept help. By giving as well as receiving support, group members gain a sense of their own competence and feel more positive about their involvement.

Problem solving takes on a new dimension in support groups. Caregivers often come up with original solutions that we would not have imagined. They also are more willing to try solutions when a peer suggests them. Many years ago one caregiver told a story in a group about how she had been trying to cross a busy intersection with her husband, who was suffering from dementia. Her husband had become frightened and would not cross the street when the light was green. The caregiver caught her breath and realized that forcing him to cross would not work. Instead, when the light turned green, she took his arm gently and in her softest voice said, "Honey, it's time to cross." He walked readily with her. The other group members were struck by this example of using affection rather than confrontation, and several tried this approach during the next week, with considerable success. Over the years, we have suggested using affection to deal with many different kinds of problem behaviors, a solution that first emerged from caregivers themselves.

One thing that groups may be able to do particularly well is to encourage caregivers to take better care of themselves. The group can promote using respite services such as adult day care or taking breaks from caregiving. In one group, for example, a man agonized for several weeks about whether it was appropriate for him to take a vacation. He was currently visiting his wife every day in a nursing home. He finally was able to go off on a brief vacation and found that it replenished him and that his wife did not notice let alone suffer from his absence. A few weeks later another member of the group announced that she was taking a vacation and thanked the caregiver who had done so first for showing her that it was possible to go away without causing one's spouse any distress.

Probably the most dramatic example of caregivers encouraging one another to take better care of themselves occurred when one long-standing member of a group complained that he had been having chest pains and that his doctor wanted him to have a thorough examination. He was ambivalent about going to the hospital because he was concerned about what would happen to his wife in the meantime. He had actually made arrangements for his daughter to care for his wife, but he told the group that he had changed his mind and was going to go home rather than keep his doctor's appointment. The group insisted that he go to the doctor, and so he kept the visit. After examining him, his doctor hospitalized him immediately and he had heart bypass surgery, which was successful. Without the intervention of the group, this man would not have had the immediate treatment he needed.

Groups, of course, are not inherently helpful. Therapeutic processes emerge or fail to emerge from the interactions in the group. A group that is dominated by an opinionated, self-centered person will not be helpful and under some circumstances can be harmful. A major role of the support group leader is to create a therapeutic environment in which everyone's opinion is heard and respected, no one dominates the group, and no one is ignored. There needs to be both a sense of universality, that everyone is in the same boat, and a sense of differences, that it is all right to have different responses and feelings. In some mature groups (that is, groups with long-standing members), participants often create this therapeutic environment themselves, telling new members how much they have gained from the group and stressing that everyone's experience is different and that there is no single best way to do things.

As an example, one group member struggled for a long time over whether or not to place her husband in a nursing home. She wanted to know when the right time was, a question that caregivers often ask. The leader suggested that the right time was when she was ready. In other words, she needed to make the decision herself, not base it on what anyone else might think. This perspective helped her through the placement and the period afterwards when she sometimes felt guilty or regretful. Later on, she frequently shared this philosophy with other participants in the group as a way of stressing both their shared experience and that each person has to make the decision in his or her own way.

Support groups are organized in many different ways. Some are led by clinicians and others have lay leaders. While a lay person can be an effective leader, we believe that any leader should have training in group process so that the leader can step in to maintain a therapeutic or supportive environment. The frequency with which groups meet also varies. Most community groups meet monthly. Research protocols have sometimes used weekly meetings, which may be especially helpful when caregivers first seek help. Finally, groups differ in terms of how they operate. Some groups emphasize information almost exclusively; they invite speakers and focus on specific topics. Other groups focus more on sharing feelings and experiences. As we have stressed throughout, we believe it is important to create an atmosphere in which caregivers feel they can express their feelings but are not encouraged to dwell upon them. They should be encouraged to identify the features of the situation they can change and not remain stuck on the things they cannot change.

Nursing Home Placement

There is probably no decision more difficult or stressful to families than that of placing a relative in a nursing home. We want to give this decision special attention and examine the role clinicians play.

As we have emphasized, this decision should be the family's, not the clinician's. Each family has a different commitment and resources for providing care in the home. Some families may be willing to make great sacrifices while others are unwilling or unable to do so. The clinician should not dogmatically state that a family ought to place an elder in a home or that there is a right time to do so. Instead, clinicians should make sure families feel comfortable talking about the issue and viewing it an option. If a family has not brought up placement, the clinician can make a ubiquitous statement to introduce the topic, such as, "Many people in your situation have thought about placing their relative in a nursing home. Have you thought about that?" When families bring the topic up themselves, the clinician should assure them that it is an appropriate option and that there is no shame in placing someone in a nursing home.

As discussed earlier, placement changes but does not relieve stress on caregivers. A particular challenge is how families will pay for long-term care. It is irresponsible to encourage a precipitous placement before the family has worked out the finances.

Finally, the clinician's involvement should not end with placement. Caregivers often need a variety of help following nursing home placement. Spouse caregivers, in particular, feel guilty and lonely. Caregivers also need to work out how often they will visit and how to interact with staff in productive ways.

CONCLUSIONS

Caring for a disabled older relative can be a stressful experience. Family caregivers may find themselves providing around-the-clock help, with few breaks and little assistance from anyone else. Although an older person's disabilities may be irreversible, there may be features of the situation that can be changed to lower stress on the caregiver. We have developed a model of intervention composed of three treatment techniques—information, problem solving and support—and three treatment methods—one-to-one counseling, family meetings, and support groups. Each technique and method provides a different resource for families and can be useful in lowering stress. In the end, the goal is to help families clarify their preferences and assist them as much as possible in providing care in a way consistent with their values and beliefs. Clinicians can provide technical expertise and support that helps families do the best they can and minimize the physical and emotional costs to themselves.

APPENDIX 12.1. DAILY RECORD OF PROBLEM BEHAVIORS

Time of day	Behavior	What happened before	What happened after

13

Consultation in Institutional Settings

One of the most important roles for mental health professionals is providing consultation and treatment in institutional settings. The consultant role requires specialized skills and knowledge that are not typically part of general clinical training. In nursing homes, hospitals, adult day care programs and other such settings, staff are confronted with a wide range of behavioral, emotional, and cognitive problems of older clients that they do not have the time or training to manage effectively. A mental health consultant can assess the possible causes of the problems and intervene with patients, staff, and family members to maximize the patient's functioning and reduce strain on an already overburdened staff.

In this chapter we emphasize consultation in nursing homes because nursing homes are the most important institutional setting for older adults and, compared to hospitals, one in which mental health professionals are likely to have little prior experience or training. Our approach combines basic consultation principles with an understanding of the tenets of geriatric mental health practice and the unique features of the nursing home setting. This approach can be applied to the other important institutional settings for mental health consultation, such as hospitals, by incorporating a similar understanding of how those settings function and of the role and opportunities for the mental health consultant within them (see Haley, 1996).

MENTAL HEALTH CONSULTATION IN NURSING HOMES

With the extension of Medicare coverage to include mental health services in nursing homes, mental health professionals have moved extensively into these settings. Unfortunately, many of these providers have no background

320

in psychogeriatric care and are not able to give pertinent and helpful consultations. Companies sometimes contract with nursing homes to provide mental health services, sending in clinicians who have had little or no prior training to provide clinical services of dubious value. Their emphasis is more on how to produce billable hours than on giving high-quality care. This situation wastes money and deprives patients, staff, and family of proper treatment. Good care costs no more to the facility or family than inadequate care, but it requires clinicians with the appropriate competencies.

The need for mental health services in nursing homes is considerable. As Michael Smyer and his colleagues (Smyer 1989; Smyer, Cohn, & Brannon, 1988) have emphasized, nursing homes have become the mental hospitals of our era. Estimates of the prevalence of residents with significant mental disorders in nursing homes have ranged from 50% to over 90% (e.g., German, Shapiro, & Kramer, 1986; Rovner, Kafonek, Filipp, Lucas, & Folstein, 1986). Despite these high rates, most patients do not receive treatment for their mental health problems (Burns et al., 1993; Shea, Streit, & Smyer, 1994).

The most frequent disorders are those which are prevalent in the general population of elderly—dementia, delirium, and depression. The clinician may, however, encounter the full range of psychiatric diagnoses in these settings. Consultations involve diagnostic questions, but usually the most important work is development and implementation of a multifaceted treatment plan that addresses the pertinent medical, psychological, interpersonal and environmental dimensions of functioning.

The mental health professional has an important role to play in nursing homes. Besides bringing expertise on geropsychiatric problems, the consultant has the time to spend with patients to figure out what is going on. Staff are busily caught up in daily routines and do not have enough time to get to the root of complex problems. Therapeutic staff such as occupational, physical, or speech therapists also spend a lot of time with patients, but they are task oriented and do not have the opportunity to see the bigger picture. Patients often recognize this role and say to us, "You're the first person to take time to listen to me."

Another important consideration is that regulations in nursing homes emphasize the use of behavioral and other nonpharmacological interventions as the first choice for management of behavior problems. As part of the Omnibus Budget Reconciliation Act of 1987, nursing homes have been restricted in their use of antipsychotic medications and physical restraints to control behavior. Use of these approaches must be now be carefully justified. This regulation grew out of recognition that antipsychotic medications are not consistently effective with agitated behavior (Schneider, Pollock, & Lyness, 1990) and that medications and restraints were frequently used when more positive approaches were available. A consultant can help staff with patients who are agitated or have other behavioral problems to develop interventions to control those problems. Solutions may in some cases involve the use of psychotropic medications or restraints, but these approaches are used as part of an overall treatment plan; they are not a reflexive response to behavior problems.

Consultations can be intellectually challenging because of the variety and complexity of problems presented. Like solving a puzzle or mystery, the clinician must sort through several levels of data to identify likely contributing factors and possible avenues for intervention. Consultations are also satisfying because results can generally be seen immediately. Despite the age and disability of patients in nursing homes, interventions can often be successful in alleviating the presenting problem and making the situation better for patients, their families, and staff.

Another challenging feature of consultations is that successful interventions focus on both the patient and the care system. In his classic text, Caplan (1970) differentiated between four primary types of mental health consultation: (1) client-centered case consultation, (2) consultee-centered case consultation, (3) program-centered administrative consultation, and (4) consultee-centered administrative consultation. Because of the nature of the nursing home setting and the population of residents and staff, the consultation may involve elements of each of these approaches. Although the consultation is often client centered, the optimal solution may involve working with the consultee and, in some cases, with program or administrative systems. Nursing homes are not resource rich, and staff may have little training or experience in handling mental health problems. Thus, a lot of what we do is building the capability of the staff to manage mental health problems. Because many residents are limited in their ability to change by their physical impairments, interventions with staff may be the best avenue for approaching a problem. When a consultant encounters repeated similar problems related to administrative or program policies, then intervention at that level may be appropriate. These opportunities for intervention at different levels of the nursing home community is another reason we find this work satisfying.

Mental health services in nursing homes can be organized in different ways. The clinician can be a salaried employee of a facility, an arrangement found in some larger nursing homes. The more common arrangement is for clinicians to be consultants who are called in as needed. One value of the clinician being a consultant rather than a member of the staff is reassurance to patients and sometimes to staff about the confidentiality of the conversation. As a consultant, the clinician can represent the patient's interests, not the institution's. Many patients, especially those on Medicaid, may feel vulnerable or that they have no choice about where they are living. A mental health professional who is a caring outsider can be a better advocate for patients.

Related to the issue of the focus of consultation is the question of goals.

In particular, consultants are often confronted with questions about the extent to which residents might be able to function independently in some areas. Parmalee and Lawton (1990) have described care in nursing homes as organized around the autonomy–security dialectic. Autonomy represents the patient's preferences for independence and control over his or her personal environment, while the institution, sometimes in conjunction with the family, stresses the need for keeping patients safe and secure. There are many threats to autonomy in nursing homes, including the lack of privacy due to shared rooms and the tendency for nursing and medical staff to make decisions for patients about their care or to provide too much care. A series of compelling studies by Margaret Baltes and her colleagues (M. Baltes, 1994; M. Baltes, Kindermann, Reisenzein, & Schmid, 1987) have documented that staff reinforce dependent behavior and ignore or punish independent behavior. At the same time, there are legitimate needs for safety, especially for patients who are not competent to evaluate the risks of their own actions. We emphasize supporting autonomy when possible, that is, when it does not compromise the resident's safety or that of other residents or staff. When patients or their families indicate their preference for autonomy, whether in making decisions about the type of care provided or regarding use of safety measures to prevent falls or other accidents, we believe it is important to find ways to support this preference. Often minor modifications in the usual way of doing things in the nursing home can set a balance between autonomy and security that is acceptable to everyone. Several of the examples later in the chapter address this issue.

DIVERSITY OF NURSING HOME SETTINGS

The organization of long-term care in the United States and in other countries is changing rapidly as providers recognize the limitations of traditional nursing home care and try new ways of arranging services. Traditional nursing homes are only one type of long-term residential facility. There are other, newer types of care facilities for disabled elders as well as increasing variability within institutions licensed as nursing homes.

Two recent developments in nursing homes have considerable impact on how care is provided. The first involves creation of subacute medical care units in many nursing homes. Since the early 1980s, Medicare has provided incentives to hospitals to limit the length of inpatient stays. The result is that many older patients are discharged "sicker and quicker" and may require ongoing medical and nursing care. Sometimes care can be provided at home, with visits from home nursing personnel or by coordinating home care with outpatient services such as physical therapy. In other instances, patients are discharged from the hospital to a nursing home subacute unit. These units have a higher level of medical services and more skilled personnel than chronic care units. Subacute programs are often located in a wing of a traditional nursing home that offers chronic care in other parts of the building. The emphasis in subacute units is on providing rehabilitation services so that the patient can return to the community. In contrast to chronic care, subacute care that follows a hospitalization is covered by Medicare for up to 120 days.

There is little information to date on how many hospitalized older people go to nursing homes on discharge from hospitals or what proportion are able subsequently to return home. Nursing homes have always included a small proportion of short-term patients, but this group of residents is now growing rapidly. Because of the stable and high reimbursement provided by Medicare, subacute units have become a very important part of a nursing home's financial foundation. (One of the ironies of shorter hospital stays is that they appear to lead to greater use of nursing homes. Thus, it is not clear whether shorter stays are actually producing cost savings in Medicare or merely shifting costs from one part of the program to another).

For the consultant, the main implication of subacute care is that some nursing home consultations involve issues of transition back to the community. In contrast to hospital settings, where the patient's stay is increasingly brief, the subacute unit provides consultants with the opportunity to implement treatment for issues such as depression or family conflict that can improve rehabilitation and ease the move back home.

While the number of subacute units is increasing rapidly, nursing homes predominantly provide chronic care. It is within chronic care that we see the second major development in nursing homes, the formation of separate units for care of people with dementia. These programs are typically identified as Alzheimer's or special care units. The number of Alzheimer's programs has grown rapidly in the last decade, but there is no consensus as to what constitutes special care (Holmes et al., 1994; Maslow, 1994). The one consistent feature that marks most programs is that the unit is locked. Other than that, facilities may offer a variety of special environmental features, such as indoor and outdoor areas where residents can wander, orienting information to help residents identify their own rooms or other facilities on the unit, and more homelike furnishings and decorations. Activities are geared for dementia patients who benefit from a high level of activity.

Part of the impetus for development of Alzheimer's units has been the recognition that the traditional medical model of nursing homes is not appropriate for these patients, who primarily require supervision and structured activities (e.g., Sloane & Matthew, 1991). Special programs for dementia have also been developed outside nursing homes. These programs emphasize social models of care for dementia patients and for people with other chronic physical disabilities. In the United States, these facilities are typically called "assisted living" residences, though in some states they are licensed as "board and care" homes. Like nursing homes, board and care or assisted living facilities can vary widely (see Kane & Wilson, 1993). Some assisted living facilities serve only older people, including those with dementia. Others serve old and young with physical disabilities. Board and care is a designation that has historically served the chronically medically ill, and some facilities mix younger mentally ill or substance abusers with older patients. That type of program is often very frightening to older residents. Finally, units may be licensed or unlicensed. Small, unlicensed facilities are often hidden from public view but sometimes provide a high quality of care (Morgan, Eckert, & Lyon, 1995). In Europe, similar developments are shifting dementia care from a medical to a social setting (Malmberg & Zarit, 1993).

For the consultant, it is important to recognize that there are many different and changing arrangements in long-term care. Nursing homes differ in many important ways from assisted living programs, but they also vary among themselves. As we emphasize in the following section, one of the first tasks in consulting is to understand the structure and organization of the facility.

PRINCIPLES OF CONSULTATION IN NURSING HOMES

Consultation in nursing homes involves applying principles that have been shaped for the setting and population. In this section, we describe how we approach consultation and the specific issues mental health professionals must address in nursing homes.

Understand the Setting

The consultant needs to understand the nursing home setting and how it is organized. We describe a general framework, but the particular organization within a home should be determined by the consultant.

Nursing home staff are organized in a hierarchy. It is important to understand how this hierarchy works and to learn at what levels effective interventions can be made. The consultant must also learn how to work with the different shifts. Information given to one shift needs to be conveyed to the other two shifts.

Smyer and his colleagues (1988) describe the hierarchy as a pyramid, with a few administrative and supervisory personnel at the top and nursing assistants at the bottom. Supervisors have the most influence over the program and policy but the least impact on day-to-day care. Although they have the least training and influence in the hierarchy, nursing assistants have the most contact with residents.

The director of nursing (DON) is usually the most influential person on patient care in the hierarchy. The DON oversees the clinical operation of the facility and is in charge of whatever happens clinically. The consultant should develop a good working relationship with the DON, establishing procedures for conducting consultations and getting support for the types of interventions the consultant makes. A helpful way of working with the DON is to set up regular (e.g., monthly) meetings to review the cases the consultant has seen.

The nursing home administrator (NHA) is less critical for mental health consultation. Although technically in charge of all aspects of the facility, administrators are usually involved in paperwork and details related to business practices and regulations. While there are exceptions, administrators usually do not get involved in clinical activities and may not even have a clinical background. In contrast to the DON, consultants spend little time with administrators.

The next level of the hierarchy is the nursing supervisors. Nursing supervisors are registered nurses (RNs) who oversee clinical operations. Depending on the size of the facility, only one or two nursing supervisors may be on duty per shift. They are often the key people in making referrals to the consultant and in implementing changes.

Licensed practical nurses (LPNs) head units of the home. They oversee provision of regular nursing services to patients. Despite limited training, they have considerable responsibility for management of patients, and their work can be very stressful.

Finally, nursing aides or nursing assistants provide most of the ongoing care and spend the most time with patients. They may have little formal training or preparation for their work except for a small amount of federally mandated inservice training. The extent and depth of this training varies, as do opportunities for continuing education. Some aides have many years of experience and are highly skilled. Others have little or no background and may simply go through the motions of doing their job.

Another dimension of how nursing homes are organized is specialized units or levels of care that serve different patients and functions. As we noted earlier, nursing homes may offer subacute care or special Alzheimer's care, in addition to traditional long-term chronic care. The consultant needs to be familiar with the levels of care offered in a particular nursing home. Solutions may sometimes involve moving patients from one unit to another, where a particular kind of care is more likely to be provided or to be appropriate.

Medical staff are an important part of the hierarchy. The medical staff can be organized in different ways. Some nursing homes have a physician on staff who sees all residents. Other nursing homes have a few physicians who regularly see patients at the facility. In most homes, residents can see their own physicians if the doctor is willing to come to the facility or the patient can get transportation to the doctor's office. Physicians who regularly visit the home have varying degrees of involvement; some do little more than reviewing charts, others spend considerable time with patients and staff.

A critical step for the mental health consultant is to develop a relationship with staff physicians or other physicians who regularly see patients in the facility. This can be done by establishing credibility with the physicians when consulting on cases. Credibility can be gained by how the consultant presents information. Both written reports and verbal communications need to be succinct and free of psychological jargon. Physicians tend to dismiss jargon as "psychobabble," even if the recommendations are sound. A report that speculates at length about the psychodynamics of a patient might be appropriate in a mental health facility but will not be helpful in a nursing home. Instead, the consultant needs to get to the point, summarizing the results of an assessment or providing a recommendation in a clear, succinct way.

Another important way to establish credibility is to become knowledgeable about the common medical problems and medications used in nursing homes. Not only does this knowledge facilitate communication with physicians, but it is critical in determining whether current medications or illnesses are contributing to the resident's behavior, emotions, or cognitive status.

The following example illustrates the value of medical knowledge when working with physicians. We were asked by the physician at a nursing home to consult in the case of an 80-year-old woman. The physician was someone we had previously not worked with much. She wanted to know if the patient, who was suffering from Parkinson's disease, had a normal end-of-life depression or if her depressive symptoms warranted more aggressive treatment. In evaluating the patient, we noted (as we usually do) the current medications. The medications included the antidepressant Sinequan, which has anticholinergic effects and is not the best choice for someone suffering from Parkinson's disease, as it tends to worsen the movement disorder. When we provided feedback to the physician, she said she did not recognize the name of the antidepressant and asked what the generic name is. We told her it is doxepin. She recognized it as a tricylcic antidepressant and decided to change it. By being able to provide the physician with the generic name as well as other pertinent information as part of the consultation, we established our credibility with her and have collaborated successfully on several cases since.

Credibility with physicians and nurses also depends on familiarity with the common illnesses encountered in nursing homes. The consultant should have a good background in dementia, Parkinson's disease, stroke, chronic obstructive pulmonary disease (COPD), and diabetes. It is important to be able to make a differential diagnosis between dementia and stroke or other conditions, as well as to understand the behavioral and cognitive implications of these disorders. A useful resource is Morrison's (1997) *When Psychological Problems Mask Medical Disorders.*

A common referral is any patient who cries a lot. The first question to determine is whether the patient has suffered a stroke. If the patient has had a stroke, crying can be part of a depressive reaction, but in some instances it is not meaning-based crying (i.e., there is no depressive content). Whether related to depression or not, crying can be treated with SSRIs, with behavioral approaches (providing attention when the patient is not crying), and by increasing activity levels.

Besides a familiarity with common illnesses and their features, clinicians should also be able to recognize the terminal phases of disease. Terminal decline is frequently accompanied by anxiety and depression, which should be treated differently from typical affective disorders. Care in the terminal phase of an illness should emphasize making the patient comfortable and addressing any specific concerns or unfinished business. It may be useful to help family, and sometimes also staff, to let go of the dying patient, that is, to stop trying to intervene actively or to talk about recovery. In turn, families and staff may need support prior to and after the patient's death. Again, by having the time to talk with everyone involved, the mental health professional can play a very important role in the care of dying patients. The consultant, of course, needs to be comfortable dealing with the dying process and able to separate his or her own beliefs from the preferences of the patient and family.

Start with the Person Who Requested the Consultation

The second principle of consultation is to talk first with the person who requested the consultation. This point may seem elementary, but in a busy nursing home with its focus on patient problems, the easiest course is to see the patient first. We think it is beneficial to start with the staff member who requested the consultation to get an idea about the reasons for the consultation. A brief note or verbal request may not contain all the relevant information. A face-to-face discussion (or a telephone call, if the consultant has a good relationship with the person making the referral) can provide valuable information that will guide the consultation and may also contribute to the solution. By going to this person first, the consultant also supports the hierarchy in the nursing home. Changes that will benefit the patient need to be made within that structure, so the consultant needs the support of the people who can effect change.

Another reason to start with the person who made the request is that consultation addresses an interaction between staff and patient, staff and family, or sometimes all three. Solutions often involve changing the interaction, not the patient. The real issue sometimes turns out to be the staff's well-being, not the patient's. Starting the consultation with the person who requested it recognizes that person's role and engages him or her in the process. That person may turn out to be peripherally involved, such as when a DON or nursing supervisor requests help with a patient on behalf of staff nurses or nursing assistants but is not involved in care. By going to the supervisor first, the consultant can gain support for the interventions that will be made.

Read the Whole Nursing Chart

Another basic issue, but one we find inexperienced consultants omit, is to read the whole nursing chart. The chart contains useful information about the typical functioning of the patient and about ongoing medical and nursing care and medications. There are two key points for the consultant when reading the chart. The first is to look for discrepancies. Do the observations of the patient's behavior, mood, or functional capacities seem to vary? Do these variations follow any pattern, such as changing with different shifts? Do different staff have varying impressions of the patient's behavior or capabilities? Another type of discrepancy is between how medications are supposed to be given and how they are actually administered. We have seen instances, for example, where antidepressants are given as needed, rather than on a regular basis. That pattern of administration is not adequate to build up to a therapeutic level of the medication.

The second point about chart information is that consultants should retain their objectivity. It is possible that some of the data in the chart are inaccurate or outdated, especially when the patient's condition has changed. This is often the case where the first person making a note in the chart writes that the patient is disoriented or confused. Everyone who follows may make a similar note but not really evaluate specifically what the patient's cognitive problems are or if the patient's functioning has changed. On occasion, it may turn out that there is a different problem than dementia or delirium, as indicated in the following example.

We consulted on a woman who had suffered anoxia during surgery to repair a hip fracture. In an initial note in her chart, someone wrote that the patient was pleasantly confused. Then everyone repeated that statement in each subsequent note. It appeared that they had stopped evaluating her and merely repeated the initial impression. She had, in fact, begun to improve as her post-surgical delirium receded. Our examination identified areas where she had improved and now functioned at a better level.

Gather Information from All Relevant Sources

The fourth principle is to gather information from all relevant sources, including the staff who actually spend time with the patient. A nursing supervisor may not have all the relevant information about the problem or how staff have tried to deal with it.

Another valuable source of information is the patient's family or other involved caregivers. The consultant needs to identify the main family members involved in the patient's care. Because many family members visit their relatives frequently, the consultant may meet them in the course of talking to staff and patients. Or it may be necessary to telephone them, particularly adult children who are employed and do not come to the nursing home during daytime hours. In any case, it is important to have a conversation with the family early in the consultation process in order to obtain a history of the patient and the family's view of current problems.

When patients are competent, it is necessary to get their permission before talking with the family. That is important legally and because it establishes the confidentiality of the relationship between clinician and patient (see Chapter 14). When patients are not competent, the family should be involved because they have legal and financial responsibility. At one home where we work, Social Services informs the family that a consultation has been arranged. That way it is not a surprise when we call them. If competence has not been established (and establishment of competence may, in fact, be the reason for the consultation), the consultant should assume that the patient is competent until evidence suggests differently.

Respond in a Rapid and Relevant Way

The consultant needs to respond in a rapid and relevant way. The pace in nursing homes is quick and decisions about problem patients need to be made in a timely way. Staff become impatient with a consultant who dallies before conducting the consult or who is slow in reporting the result. The sluggish consultant may find that recommendations have become irrelevant and that staff have taken steps on their own to manage the situation.

The consultant makes a response at several levels. One important response is a note in the medical chart. This is a necessary and legally required step. The note should be clear and brief and should provide the necessary information for the physician and staff to understand the problem and take steps to correct it. As we have stressed previously, it is important to use jargon-free language. The note should not go through all the steps in the consultant's reasoning. Rather, it should briefly summarize conclusions and recommendations.

One of the most important considerations is to write the note at a level that is comprehensible to anyone reading it. Many of the nursing assistants and even some of the RNs have limited educational backgrounds, yet these are the staff who will implement the consultant's recommendations. The note should be written so that they can easily understand what the consultant is proposing. As an example, a consultant may discover that a patient has a vision impairment, and that some of his difficult behaviors are caused by staff who start talking to this man before he can see them. The consultant notes in the chart: "Be in the patient's line of vision when you speak to him."

The consultant should be aware that a note in the patient's chart can be read by any staff member. For that reason, the note should not contain any confidential information that the patient or anyone else reveals. That information should be kept in a separate, locked case file, which the consultant maintains with the confidentiality of a therapy file.

The note in the chart can clarify how staff can respond to an ongoing, difficult situation. We are often asked to consult when staff have difficulty involving patients in activities. Sometimes we find that a person is reluctant to participate but can be encouraged. In these situations, our note in the chart reads something like "When trying to get Mrs. Q. involved in activities, don't take an initial 'no' for an answer." Another patient may be competent to choose not to get out of bed or become involved in activities. As an example, we were asked to consult in the case of a woman who had been an artist and had always led a somewhat reclusive life. She was in the nursing home because of a hip fracture. She already suffered from painful arthritis and never regained the ability to bear weight on her hip. In the nursing home, she refused to do more for herself or to get involved in more therapy. The staff of nursing homes often have difficulty dealing with patients like this one who could function at a higher level but refuse to do so. They asked for a consultation to determine whether the patient was competent to make this decision or her refusal reflected depression. The evaluation revealed that the patient was competent and fully understood the decisions she made and their implications. She was also not depressed. The note we made in her chart reinforced the idea that she was competent to refuse to do more for herself and that staff should not bother her about it.

We stress the chart note because we find that many consultants in nursing homes do not know how to convey information effectively that way. In addition to the note, it is important to respond to all the relevant people involved in the case: the referral source, physician, nurses, nursing assistants, family, and patient. In some cases, the intervention is developed with key people on the staff or even with the patient. In other cases, the consultant explains the recommendations and enlists support in implementing them.

Follow Through

An important part of a consultation in a nursing home is follow-through. There typically needs to be follow-through with all the involved parties—patient, staff, family—to see how the proposed actions have worked out. Mental health professionals who consult in settings such as rehabilitation or psychiatric hospitals are accustomed to conducting their evaluation and then writing a detailed report. A psychologist, for example, may test the patient and then write a report on the results that addresses the reason for consultation. The psychologist is unlikely to have any further contact with the patient or any follow-up with the staff. The difference between that kind of consultation and a consultation in a nursing home is that the problems in nursing homes typically involve long-term adjustment to the facility. Patients in other in-patient settings typically leave quickly, so consultations involve diagnostic questions or address a short-term problem. The nursing home patient is usually not going anywhere else. Although the consultation may involve diagnostic questions, there is almost always a component dealing with management of behavior. In order to be most effective, the consultant should follow up to see how well the recommendations have been implemented and to provide additional support or make changes if the plan is not working. Some problems require a longer-term involvement just to figure out what may be triggering or reinforcing problem behaviors.

Another important reason for follow-up is that the staff of nursing homes do not have much background in mental health problems or behavioral management. The consultant provides that expertise in a tactful and respectful way. But it is usually not sufficient to lay out a plan, even in clear and concise language, and expect that staff will carry it out as planned. The staff may not fully understand the plan or may be too preoccupied with other problems to give it their full attention.

PUTTING THE PIECES OF THE PUZZLE TOGETHER: EFFECTIVE CONSULTING

The recommendations the consultant makes usually focus on improving the care or living situation of a patient, but the concerns of the family and staff are also important. Family and staff usually must be involved in treatment recommendations to some degree. At minimum, they must consent to the recommendations and not disagree or actively subvert them. More typically, the consultant recommends ways they can change their interactions with the patient. Another important focus is to alter the communications family and staff have with each other. In a way, the consultant is often being asked to consider the well-being of the family and staff, as well as that of the patient. In doing so, the consultant must make sure that each person's interests are balanced. It is important not to lose sight of the patient or the patient's interests, but at the same time, many consultations concern problems that staff or family are having with the patient or with each other. Although the patient may be the overt reason for the consultation, solutions often lie in interventions with family and staff.

Helping Families Get What They Want

An important role for consultants is to empower families. They need to feel that they can have an impact on the care their relative is receiving, while appreciating the limitations of the situation and the fact that the care will not be as consistent or as personal as they would like or as they might give themselves. A starting point in forming a relationship with the family is to empathize with their complaints. The consultant should not become defensive or move too quickly to propose solutions but should instead listen and reflect the family's feelings.

Concerns Families Have

Families are most likely to raise concerns about the kind of care the patient receives. They wonder if their relative is receiving appropriate and sufficient care. They may be feeling guilty about placement and may even be wondering if they should move their relative back home. The family may also be having difficulty communicating with staff. The most frequent concerns, however, are the personal care the home provides the patient—whether the patient is bathed carefully enough or taken to the toilet frequently enough and whether the staff speak respectfully to the patient and family or make the family feel guilty.

Sometimes the staff and family have different goals that lead to misunderstandings, as illustrated in the following example. We were asked to consult on a man who had suffered a severe stroke and was moved to the nursing home after a stay in an acute hospital. He had rallied somewhat in the nursing home and wanted to go home. The staff was telling him that when he got better, he could go home. This made his wife feel terrible. Despite his recovery, he was still was too disabled for her to manage. In addition to the disabilities from his stroke, he weighed more than 200 pounds and was cognitively impaired, both of which contributed to her reluctance to take him home again. Because she felt badly about not wanting to take him home, she did not indicate her wishes directly to the staff. Compounding the situation was the fact that one of the nurses was caring at home for her own husband, who had suffered a stroke. We suggested that the patient's wife tell the staff that she could never give her husband the kind of care they did. This intervention helped the staff understand that he could not go home, and it helped his wife feel better about her decision. We also took the opportunity of a care planning meeting to change the focus of his care from short term to long term. During the meeting, his wife did not say directly that she did not want to take him home, so we brought the issue up and worked with her and the staff to develop a new plan for the patient to stay in the facility.

We should note that the nursing homes where we have been consulting are better than average in quality of care. Families are likely to have other issues if the care is really substandard. A consultant in a nursing home that is substandard needs to take an activist role with the administrator and director of nursing. The bottom line is that it does not cost more to do care right.

Teaching the Family How the System Works

Nursing homes are complex organizations with their own rules and procedures for how things get done. Families usually do not have any idea how this system works, and their frustrations often result from their not knowing who to approach about a problem or how to phrase a request.

One of the most important things for families to learn is whom to talk to about which problems. When they see something they do not like about the care their relative is receiving, they may walk up to the first staff person they see and mention it. They are then surprised and angry when no changes are made in the patient's care. The consultant should be familiar with how the nursing home typically organizes care and who is likely to incorporate the family's suggestions into daily routines so that the consultant can guide the family to the best source of help. Typically, the family can work with the LPN who consistently cares for the patient. In some nursing homes, it is better to ask the nursing supervisor who the best person is to talk to about the patient. The family should then go to that person with their suggestions about the patient's care. When visiting, families notice the staff who are kind or go out of their way to help patients, and they often develop a relationship with them as a way of assuring better care for their relative.

Nursing homes sometimes designate a spokesperson to talk with the family, a good solution for channeling the complaints of a particularly demanding family or when the medical and nursing care problems are complex. Most nursing homes do not routinely designate a contact person for the family.

It is important that the family feel that the staff care about the patient. When the patient has a pleasant personality, staff often become attached to the patient and go out of their way to do extra things. (When one of these patients dies, the staff grieve and may need extra support.) By contrast, when the patient is a difficult person, the family may mainly hear complaints from the staff. In part, these complaints are a function of the regulations in nursing homes. The staff are obligated to report all incidents to the family, such as if a patient injures himself or touches someone else. If the family is only hearing about these incidents, they may feel depressed or criticized by the staff because their relative is so difficult. Hearing about these complaints adds to their guilt. We try to get the staff to be more balanced in their communications with families. When staff report an incident about a problem patient, they should also make sure to mention the good days the patient is having or any other positive behaviors.

In a parallel way, some families need to learn how to soften their complaints and give the staff complements as well as suggestions. We have known caregivers who voice a lot of complaints about the staff to us but maintain easy and friendly relationships with them. In the end, their relatives get better care because the staff like the family and want to do more for them. When the family complains excessively or does not show respect for the staff, the care their relative receives suffers. The consultant needs to work with complaining families to use better strategies to get what they want, which is better care for their relative.

Are Groups for Families or Patients in the Nursing Home a Good Idea?

We prefer family groups that are run outside the facility. Families can talk more freely about the problems and concerns they have in a group not connected with the facility. Just as a consultant who is not employed by the facility can give the family an independent perspective on their concerns, so can groups that are run in the community, not the nursing home. Families can also learn about other facilities from the people attending the group. That information is often valuable, because it helps families put their own situation into a broader perspective.

Groups for patients that focus on reminiscence or socializing can have positive benefits (Woods, 1996). These groups can usually be run by recreational therapists (RTs) or other staff. They do not need a mental health professional and usually do not have an explicit mental health focus. The mental health consultant can work with the RT to decide what kind of group is appropriate. The RT should not try to conduct a therapy group but should be given guidelines on identifying problems (e.g., someone who is depressed) for referral to the consultant.

Spayd and Smyer (1996) provide a concise description of the uses of therapy groups in nursing homes. We do not, however, think that therapy groups for patients are generally a good idea. There are several factors that we feel make therapy groups inappropriate in this setting. First, patients live with each other on a 24-hour basis, and that is a deterrent to their talking about personal issues. There is so little privacy already in a nursing home that groups would be perceived as another privacy threat. Second, patients are often hesitant about getting attached to one another or find it hard to reach out and form friendships. They are all old and ill, so there is not a lot of socialization among residents even at meals or social events. This is in contrast to personal care homes or retirement homes where residents pair off and form friendships. In those facilities, the residents function better and are able to form social relationships. The main social relationships patients in nursing homes have are with family or old friends. We should facilitate those relationships as much as possible. The goal that patients should socialize more with one another or form friendships usually comes from staff and sometimes families, not from patients themselves.

Individual Therapy with Patients

In contrast to groups, we find that individual therapy is appropriate and helpful with some patients. People who are depressed or who are dealing with the implications of their illness or placement can sometimes benefit from therapy. We have briefer sessions (e.g., 30 minutes) with nursing home patients if they do not have the stamina for a longer session. These sessions can reduce feelings of depression and isolation. Sessions can also identify ways the resident can get more needs met by the nursing home staff or by family and friends. Interventions are usually short term, though in rare instances we have treated a patient for a sustained period of time, usually for chronic depression. Spayd and Smyer (1996) describe other uses of individual psychotherapy in nursing homes.

Confidentiality is an important condition for psychotherapy in any setting and more so in nursing homes. It is essential that the therapist and client be able to meet in private. Residents usually share double rooms and so do not have their own private place to go. The therapist needs to assure them that they will have privacy and that they will not be interrupted. Nursing homes usually have examining rooms or other rooms that can be used for this purpose. It is also critical to maintain the confidentiality of what the patient says. The therapist should make a note in the chart that the session took place but should never put in the chart any information that was revealed during the session. The therapist should keep detailed notes and summaries in his or her own locked files, preferably outside the nursing facility. Being able to assure a resident of complete confidentiality is often a prerequisite to developing a therapeutic relationship.

Empowering and Training Staff

Much of the work of the consultant is to enhance the capability of staff to manage problems. In overt and subtle ways, the clinician can help staff learn how to deal more effectively with patients and their families and to manage the many pressures placed on themselves. When trying to help patients with chronic physical or psychological problems, it is often easier and quicker to get staff to take a new approach than to focus solely on the patient.

One effective approach for dealing with a problem patient is to identify the staff who are working with that patient and then do a mini-inservice around that problem. The inservice should focus on practical issues for managing that problem. The clinician should model problem solving (see Chapter 11) and give the staff solutions. Solutions should be concrete and behavioral; that is, they should direct the staff to respond in a specific way.

The following example illustrates the use of a problem-focused inservice. The patient was a narcissistic woman who was heavy and required two people to assist her with transfers. She would periodically go limp during the transfers, which led to injuries to the staff. The nursing supervisor was furious with the patient because she was injuring her staff, and the staff did not particularly like the patient.

The intervention developed in the inservice was complex. The first step was to help the staff think about solutions, rather than focusing on their anger. We started by reframing the nursing supervisor's presentation of the problem, from "I can't let the patient continue to do this to my staff" to "How can we solve the problem?" Doing that led to two solutions. One solution was to have a third person stand by during transfers to help out if the patient went limp. That took staff time but also prevented injuries. Another solution was proposed by a social worker on the team. The patient was poorly socialized, so no roommate had been able to stand her. She had little contact with anyone and was very angry, which in part was reflected in her going limp. In the past, she had been placed with roommates who had poor functioning because of her own bad behavior. The social worker proposed moving her in with a psychologically healthy patient. This move was made with good results. The new roommate told the woman she needed to get up, get dressed, and go to the dining room. She responded to this challenge and started doing more for herself. Her going limp during transfers disappeared.

This solution is contrary to the usual procedures, which are to put problem people together. It is, of course, not something that works every time, and it can be unfair to the high-functioning individual to be paired with someone with pronounced social and emotional problems. In this instance, however, the psychologically healthy resident had a positive effect on the problem resident without suffering from having to share a room with her.

We want to stress that a mini-inservice is just that, a small working group focused on a specific problem. This type of approach should not try to serve the function of providing ongoing inservice training to the whole staff. When a number of common problems emerge from different patients and units, however, then the consultant can organize an inservice on that topic for the whole staff.

Another important role the consultant can play is to validate the staff's feelings in dealing with difficult families. Families can place excessive or unrealistic demands on staff or treat them disrespectfully. The consultant should empathize with the staff's distress over being treated this way and then help them develop strategies to deal more effectively with these families. The particular solution depends on the family and type of problem. As we noted earlier, one approach is to balance positive and negative comments about the patient. Helping staff be more assertive about what they can and cannot do is also useful. In extreme instances, one staff person may be appointed to deal with a very demanding or complaining family.

One of the dilemmas a consultant faces is that the complaints made by families usually have some basis in reality. Even in the best nursing homes, staff have too many demands and too little time to respond to them. Patients sometimes have to wait too long for someone to assist them, and staff may not always do the best job bathing or dressing a difficult patient. The consultant must walk the difficult path of encouraging staff to do the best they can within the constraints put on them and helping families learn to make more realistic and appropriate demands.

ENVIRONMENTAL AND PROGRAMMATIC INTERVENTIONS WITH DEMENTIA PATIENTS

An important dimension in nursing homes is the environmental characteristics of the setting. It has long been recognized that features of the setting influence behavior and that modifications in the environment can be used to enhance an individual's capabilities. The work of M. Powell Lawton (e.g., Lawton, 1986; Lawton & Nahemow, 1973) has provided a framework for understanding the influences of the setting on individual behavior and competence. Central to this framework is the concept of the person–environment fit. In an optimal situation, the demands of the environment in a setting do not exceed the individual's capability for responding. People with higher levels of competence function best in settings that provide adequate challenges, while individuals with more limited abilities need appropriate amounts of support and assistance. Settings that provide more challenges than an individual can manage are experienced as frustrating and overwhelming and sometimes lead to catastrophic responses. In turn, settings that are understimulating are experienced as boring and may lead to a deterioration in adaptive behavior, as the individual no longer has opportunities to engage in certain skills or activities.

Probably the most important use of environmental design in nursing homes and other residential care settings has been the creation of special units for dementia patients. There is as yet no consensus on what constitutes a special care unit or what the essential features should be (Holmes et al., 1994). In some places, special care for dementia represents little more than a locked door, with no additional programming or staff capabilities than found in a traditional nursing home unit. In other places, however, special care has resulted in significant improvements in the quality of residential life for both dementia patients within the unit and for cognitively intact residents in other units of the facility.

The mental health consultant can be instrumental in helping staff implement a sound program of special care that maximizes the abilities and quality of life of dementia patients, and, in some instances, the consultant may even have the opportunity to be involved in the initial design of a facility. We present several key components that are fundamental to special care for dementia patients.

Locked Unit and Freedom of Movement

When the dementia unit is locked, staff do not have to worry about residents leaving the facility. Residents can wander freely within the unit. This freedom enhances their autonomy and avoids power struggles with staff. Some dementia patients walk a great deal during the day. Encouraging this activity is helpful, because it gives patients something to do and also tires them out, reducing behavior problems during the day and sleep problems at night.

Even with a locked unit, there can be a struggle around the entrance, with residents trying to force the door or waiting for someone to come in so they can scoot out. Some units have been designed so that the main entrance is hidden from view. Other units use the floor plan to divert residents away from the entrance. Facilities can be designed to reduce residents' feelings of confinement in other ways. Many special units have a secured outdoor walking area that patients can freely access. In our experience, only a few residents use these outdoor areas consistently, but knowing they can go out on their own may be important to some residents. The design of other units includes indoor walking areas. One such design is construction of the unit in a circle so that residents can walk inside continually without coming to a barrier or exit. Other designs can offer interesting indoor walking paths. The main goal is to offer residents freedom of movement with little need for ongoing staff supervision.

There are some risks associated with free movement. Residents can fall and suffer serious injuries, such as a fractured hip. Some special care units inform families of this risk at the outset (e.g., S. Zarit, Zarit, & Rosenberg-Thompson, 1990). The alternative is to restrain patients, which reduces quality of life and also can lead to other complications, such as a more rapid decline in functional competence. Another risk of unrestricted movement is that residents can get into altercations with one another or with staff. Using a behavior management framework, the consultant may be able to identify the triggering events for these altercations and work with staff to prevent or reduce their occurrence.

Environmental Cues

Special care facilities typically use environmental cues to help residents. Most nursing homes, whether they provide special dementia care or not, provide basic orienting information, such as the date and the weather. Some facilities still provide orientation classes, which drill patients in this information. We believe orientation classes are not valuable and that staff efforts are better directed to other activities that are more likely to be rewarding for residents. Some orienting information posted in the unit is probably helpful to some patients. But staying oriented is not possible for dementia patients. The issue is to find ways to enhance functioning despite intellectual deficits.

Environmental cues can help residents identify their own rooms. Special units have used a variety of solutions to this problem. Sometimes rooms or doors to rooms are painted different colors. Placing residents' names on the doors is not usually effective because some residents no longer read. A more effective strategy is to place a photograph of the resident outside the room, especially a picture taken several years earlier. Residents may not recognize their current appearance but remember how they looked in the past. Another strategy is to have a window box at each door that contains objects residents associate with themselves. In a facility that used this approach, one resident who had been a hunter had a bow in his window box while another resident who was an avid bingo player had a bingo card in hers.

Some facilities allow residents to bring in their own furniture or other possessions. Having their own furniture may help residents recognize their own room and also feel more comfortable in the setting. The main risk is that valuables might be taken by another resident or by staff. This vulnerability is at the heart of the dilemma facing institutions that want to provide a homelike atmosphere but cannot guarantee enough security to make it feasible.

Signs and cues are frequently used to denote other facilities on the unit, such as dining and social areas. It is probably useful to use visual cues when possible, but there is no consensus on what type of approach works best.

Sensory Stimulation

One of the most important but often neglected design issues is the amount of sensory stimulation, in particular, light and noise. Exposure to light can contribute to maintaining good sleep patterns (Dowling, 1996). In a typical nursing home unit, there is little exposure to daylight, while at night lights in the corridor and other locations in the unit remain on. Because exposure to light regulates biorhythms and the sleep–wake cycle, it should not be surprising that some residents of nursing homes mix up day and night. Dementia may predispose people to sleep problems (e.g., Bliwise, 1994), but environmental factors potentiate them.

Some research on dementia patients suggests that regular exposure to daylight reduces sleep problems at night, as well as increased confusion in late afternoon and early evening (sundowner's sydrome) (see Dowling, 1996, for a review). We observed this relation between exposure to light and sleep patterns in a specially designed assisted living residence for dementia. This facility has a sitting area with large windows where residents typically gather during the daytime. Initially, staff were concerned that residents would be upset by looking out the windows, so they darkened the windows with shades. Staff then observed a marked increase in disturbed behavior in early evening. When the windows were opened again so that residents were fully exposed to daylight, the amount of sundowning decreased.

In the same manner, exposure to bright lights in the middle of the night can alter residents' sleep–wake cycle, making it more difficult for them to go back to sleep. When it is necessary to assist a resident at night, staff should keep lights as dim as possible, providing the resident (and any others who are wakeful) with the cue that it is, indeed, nighttime.

Noise levels are an important irritant in nursing home environments. Restricting noise levels is considered an important part of overall sleep hygiene (practices that promote good sleeping patterns) (National Institutes of Health, 1990). The role of noise, however, has received little attention in studies of sleep disturbances of the elderly in nursing homes. In our visits to facilities in other countries, particularly Sweden, we have been struck by how much less agitated dementia patients are. Certainly many factors are involved, including cultural differences and greater autonomy for residents. But one of the most striking differences is how much quieter Swedish nursing homes and group homes for dementia are compared to facilities in the United States. In the United States, there is typically an intercom system paging people throughout the facility. Television sets may be blaring, staff talking loudly, dishes on food carts rattling, and so on. Noise levels can remain high even at night. In contrast, Swedish facilities do not have intercoms and greatly limit noise from other sources. Although we do not know the effect of this type of random noise on dementia patients, it certainly does not improve behavior and may be a contributing factor to increased agitation and problems sleeping at night.

A recent study by Burgio and his associates (1996) suggests that the type of noise in a residential setting may be related to agitation. Using the observation that residents' agitation decreased when they were exposed to white noise (while sitting under a hair dryer in the beauty salon of the facility), the researchers designed a trial in which agitated residents wore earphones that played pleasant environmental sounds (mountain stream or ocean sounds). Reductions in verbal agitation were found both in a laboratory trial and in the nursing home unit. The researchers speculate that white noise may reduce agitation by presenting calming audio input. An alternative explanation is that the headphones block out the typical random clatter in nursing homes. In any case, level and type of noise may be an important and potentially modifiable environmental feature associated with agitated behavior.

The amount and type of visual stimulation is also an important consideration. Issues such as whether there should be a lot of variety or limited amounts of visual stimulation and the role of familiar objects remain to be resolved. Our recommendation is an overall design that is calm and orderly and emphasizes familiar furnishings, rather than looking like a clinic or hospital.

Structured Activities

An important feature of special care is to engage residents in activities that allow them to use their remaining abilities. Traditional nursing homes have provided programs in arts and crafts as well as social programs. With dementia, it may be better to build on past abilities to the extent possible rather than try to teach a new skill. Swedish group homes, for example, structure the day around familiar household activities. Some U.S. nursing homes have tried exercise equipment, which benefits some dementia patients (Fisher, Pendergast, & Calkins, 1991). Walking has been found to improve communication (Friedman & Tappen, 1991). Some facilities have made use of videotapes recorded by the resident's family (Lund, Hill, Caserta, & Wright, 1995). In many facilities, activities are available only during the daytime, but structured programs during the evening and on weekends may be helpful. An activities specialist who is familiar with the emerging literature on working with dementia patients is a key part of the program. Zgola (1987) presents a useful framework for involving dementia patients in activities.

Behavioral Management

Behavioral management can play a central role in special care. We use the problem-solving approach described in Chapter 11 to identify antecedents (triggers) and consequences (reinforcers) of behaviors and for designing and implementing interventions in nursing homes. As with situations in the home, each problem involves a unique set of triggering or reinforcing events. Based on observations of these events, we develop a hypothesis about how the behavior is functioning in that setting and an intervention designed to disrupt the current pattern of triggering events and reinforcers.

Staff often have difficulty managing the activities of daily living, such as dressing or bathing a patient. Again, each situation is unique, and it is important to examine the unique causes for each case. The best choice is to allow residents as much autonomy as possible, letting them do activities their own way as long as that is feasible. It is better to have a resident who dresses in a somewhat idiosyncratic manner than a struggle over dressing. Staff may, however, have to work with family on this issue so that family do not assume that the patient is being neglected.

Bathing is often a difficult problem. Dementia patients frequently become agitated when staff try to bathe or shower them. In some cases, their fear seems to come from being undressed. Both the attitude and the gender of the staff may be issues. With some difficult patients, the struggle over bathing can be solved by allowing them to keep their underwear on, changing it after the bath or shower. The temperature in the bathroom can also be an issue. Dementia patients appear to have difficulty regulating body temperature and chill easily. A bathroom that is too cold can be unpleasant to them. Finally, a lot of verbal reassurance as well as making bathrooms more homelike can reduce problems.

One area where there has been considerable research is management of incontinence. The method of prompted voiding—in effect, placing patients on a schedule and reminding them to go to the bathroom—has been found to be very effective in reducing incontinence in nursing home residents, including that of dementia patients (e.g., Burgio et al., 1990; Schnelle et al., 1989; Schnelle, Newman, & Fogarty, 1990).

Activities play an important role in preventing or reducing behavior problems. Sleeping in the daytime and inactivity are frequent antecedents of sleep problems at night. While the literature is not conclusive, at least some evidence suggests that increasing daytime activities improves sleep at night in dementia patients (see Dowling, 1996, for a review). In a similar way, inactivity and napping are frequent antecedents of agitation or other problem behavior in the daytime. An effective strategy is to involve patients in activities in advance of periods of agitation or other problems. Activities can head off agitation as well as avoid the reinforcement of inappropriate behaviors that occurs when staff respond mainly to problems.

Autonomy

An overriding issue in interventions is striking the right balance between autonomy and security. Autonomy is at the heart of so much that is involved in special Alzheimer's care, as well as care of residents who do not have cognitive deficits (Hofland, 1995).

Care of dementia patients is so challenging because they often try to maintain control without recognizing their limitations. It is easy to fall into struggles with them over bathing, dressing, following routines, and a whole host of safety issues. As we noted earlier, a locked unit removes one source of struggle, but there are many other ways staff try to limit a resident's autonomy. The key is to do as little limiting as necessary, consistent with the safety of residents.

Group homes for dementia in Sweden offer residents much more autonomy than typical facilities in the United States or in many other countries for that matter (Malmberg & Zarit, 1993). Residents sign a lease to an apartment when they enter the group home. Their apartment, which contains a kitchenette and private bathroom, belongs to them. They have a key to the apartment and do not share it with anyone else. They are, in fact, encouraged to lock the door so that other residents do not wander in. Apartments are furnished with their own possessions and are homelike, not institutional, in appearance. The risk that someone might steal valued possessions is minimized because residents do not share their rooms with anyone and they can keep their doors locked.

Group homes have been found to be a viable living environment for all but the most agitated dementia patients (Malmberg & Zarit, 1993). They are remarkable for their low rates of behavioral disturbance, compared to U.S. facilities. Many factors undoubtedly contribute to their success, such as the low level of noise in them and the amount of training staff receive. But residents' autonomy may be the crucial dimension. Having one's own apartment automatically eliminates the problems that come with having a roommate, which are endemic in U.S. facilities. Double rooms are an anachronism based on a medical model of care. While they make sense in a hospital, where people stay for only a few days, shared rooms are not appropriate in a long-term residence. Beyond shared rooms, however, the attitude conveyed in group homes by allowing residents keys and locks supports their autonomy and may reduce fears and struggles that are commonplace in more typical care facilities.

CASE EXAMPLES

We end this chapter with two case examples that illustrate the consultation process and the principles we have presented.

Case 1. An Issue of Competence

During a hospitalization, a woman's condition deteriorated rapidly and it was assumed she was terminally ill. Hospice was ordered and she was moved to a nursing home. She had probably suffered from a bad reaction to a cardiac medication, and in the nursing home she actually began to clear up mentally and improve physically. When she began insisting on going home, the staff asked for a consultation.

Normally, the woman's improvement would not have posed a problem. The complicating factor was that the patient's daughter was a physician, and she was the person who ordered hospice in the first place. The attending physician approached us about doing a consultation, stating that she "felt" that the patient was probably competent to make the decision to go home. We replied that it would be important to carry out a careful evaluation of competence, given the circumstances and the need to deal with the patient's daughter in a tactful way.

In a competence evaluation, it is important to decide first what question is being asked. In this case, the question was "Does the patient understand how to make decisions?" Answering this question required two steps. First, we determined the quality of her thinking using the comprehension and similarities subtests of the WAIS-III (Wechsler, 1997a). The comprehension subtest evaluates a patient's ability to understand common situations, and the similarities subtest assesses abstracting ability. We also administered a global cognitive screening test, the Mini-Mental State Examination (Folstein, Folstein, & McHugh, 1975). We then talked with the resident about the decision she was making, asking practical questions such as "Where would you go if you left the nursing home?" "What kind of care would you need?" and "What do you think would happen if you left?" We evaluated the quality of her thinking and the degree to which she indicated an awareness of the risks and problems she might encounter.

In this case, the resident was found to be competent. The challenge, then, was to approach her daughter carefully and to help the daughter reevaluate her view of her mother's situation. With the daughter now aware of the changed circumstances, she agreed to moving her mother back home.

Case 2. Don't Fix What Isn't Broken

When a patient is functioning adequately, it is important to avoid destabilizing the situation with unnecessary change. The following case was referred to us by a new and relatively inexperienced physician. The patient was an older woman who had been taking a major tranquilizer. Concerned about the amount of sedation and mild Parkinsonian side effects, the physician decided to switch her to another medication with potentially fewer side effects but also less sedation. In the process of being withdrawn from the first medication and put on the second, the patient became extremely agitated and difficult to deal with, using profane language and occasionally acting abusively. A consultation was called for. We reviewed the available information on the woman, which indicated that she had been a long-term psychiatric patient at a state hospital with a diagnosis of chronic schizophrenia. The original medication was, in fact, controlling her symptoms despite the side effects. We decided to talk with the doctor about the medication change. It turned out that he did not know why the woman had been placed on a powerful antipsychotic medication in the first place. Now that he had a better understanding of the patient's history, he put her back on the original medication and took steps to control its side effects.

CONCLUSIONS

Working in nursing homes and other institutional settings can be one of the most rewarding activities for a mental health professional. The consultation process offers a variety of challenges, ranging from interesting diagnostic issues to complex interventions that involve staff, resident, and family alike. The consultant sometimes provides treatment and in other cases serves as a resource for staff and families to learn new approaches to what is a very stressful situation for everyone involved. Problems arise when family and staff see their interests as diverging, but the consultant can reframe and redirect their viewpoints so that everyone agrees on the best approach to a problem.

A successful consultant needs a strong foundation in geropsychological knowledge and skills as well as an appreciation of how to function within a complex system. The ability to work with people from many different social backgrounds—from physicians to nursing assistants—is another important component. Nursing homes do not have the resources they need to manage all the complex problems of residents and their families. The consultant brings expertise on the behavioral, emotional, and interpersonal problems of residents and their families and helps to increase the staff's competence in dealing with these problems.

14

Ethical Issues
in Geriatric Psychology

Ethical issues are always a part of clinical practice, but they can take on new variations with older clients. As they do when working with younger clients, clinicians need to place practice with older people within the framework of ethical principles and the code of conduct that has been developed to guide their profession. In this chapter, we examine how established ethical standards can be applied to practice with older clients. As psychologists, we draw on a set of principles developed by the American Psychological Association (1992), "Ethical Principles of Psychologists and Code of Conduct." These standards are built on a foundation of six general principles: (1) competence, (2) integrity, (3) professional and scientific responsibility, (4) respect for people's rights and dignity, (5) concern for others' welfare, and (6) social responsibility. We encourage readers who are not psychologists to become familiar with the ethical guidelines developed by their professions.

A theme of this book has been the similarities and differences in clinical practice with older and younger adults. In many situations, clinicians need specialized knowledge and training to be able to address the problems of an older adult. The situation is similar with respect to ethical issues in practice. All the varied ethical dilemmas that arise with younger clients also arise with older clients, but some concerns are more frequently encountered or require special deliberation that goes beyond standard training in ethical conduct. For the purposes of this chapter, we have chosen the three most frequently encountered ethical dilemmas in a geriatric practice: competence of the clinician, confidentiality, and end-of-life issues.

Parts of this chapter were published previously in J. Zarit and Zarit (1996). Copyright 1996 by the American Psychological Association. Reprinted by permission.

COMPETENCE OF THE CLINICIAN

A basic tenet of ethical conduct is not to practice beyond one's competence and training. The need for mental health professionals to work with the elderly has always been greater than the number of trained people who could potentially provide services. With the expansion of coverage under Medicare in the late 1980s, many people who do not meet minimum requirements for training and experience in geropsychology have been pressed into providing services.

The problem of undertrained professionals seems greatest in nursing home settings. Although hard data are difficult to come by, reports by clinicians across the country suggest that many mental health professionals have been practicing in nursing homes without much understanding or knowledge of clinical issues in later life. The greatest abuse seems associated with corporations that recruit but do not necessarily train professionals adequately to go into nursing homes. In nursing homes, we have reviewed case notes and other documents prepared by clinicians who had little or no background in geriatrics, and have found the lack of competence in assessment and treatment to be startling. Given how poor the quality of services were, they should not have been billed to Medicare, but of course they were. As we noted earlier, contracting with a company to provide services as opposed to identifying a clinician with appropriate training is not advantageous to nursing homes.

As a result of the growing evidence of practice in nursing homes of dubious value, Medicare carriers in some states have placed restrictions on provision of mental health treatment in nursing homes. In other words, practice by people without adequate competence is calling into question the ability of everyone who practices.

One response to this growing concern is the development of standards for training in geriatric mental health. The American Psychiatric Association has had a formal specialization in geriatric psychiatry for several years. Work groups associated with the American Psychological Association have developed guidelines for training and experience (Knight, Teri, Wohlford, & Santos, 1995). Not everyone who works with older people needs to be a specialist. However, a minimum requirement should be some prior exposure and training. Part of the ongoing problem is that very few graduate and professional programs include geriatrics as part of their curriculum or clinical experiences. Most professionals (including physicians) emerge from training without a sufficient foundation in geriatrics to practice effectively.

Competence and qualifications of professionals to practice with the elderly will continue to be an important issue. If Medicare and managed care providers try to limit practice to professionals with appropriate credentials, there are likely to be considerable disputes in professional groups in defining competence for practice with older people. Regulation, however, is a blunt instrument that will only partly resolve the problem while certainly introducing new paperwork and other difficulties for people who practice responsibly.

We expect that readers of this volume are familiar with this problem and that many of you have already had professional training and supervised experience in geriatrics. For those of you for whom this is your first exposure, we want to stress the importance of obtaining more training through course work, through continuing education, and by working with clinicians experienced in geriatric practice. All of us concerned about the well-being of older people must be advocates for training and specialization in geriatrics. There is a very difficult line to walk with insurance carriers. They need to recognize the value of competent psychological care so that they do not throw the good practitioners out with the bad. It is also important to work with nursing homes and with the general public to understand the potential benefits of psychological assessment and treatment and having trained people provide those services.

CONFIDENTIALITY

Confidentiality is a basic ethical principle in practice with people of any age, but it takes on different patterns in a geriatric practice. There are many potential threats to confidentiality. Confidentiality can be differentially affected by the client's living situation (independently community dwelling, assisted living, nursing home, hospital), by the nature of the psychological problem (functional vs. organic), and by whether or not family members are involved in the therapy. Furthermore, there is a much higher incidence of concurrent medical treatment with older than with younger clients, which requires frequent consultation between the mental health specialist and a variety of physicians. Because there are such important differences in the kind of confidentiality issues that arise, depending on the setting in which the older person lives, we have organized our discussion according to place of residence. We end the section by examining situations where professionals must break confidentiality.

Community Living

For older adults who live independently in the community and do not suffer from dementia or similar problems, confidentiality issues are generally the same as they would be for a younger client. In other words, an older person is entitled to the same confidentiality as any other client. For example, if a concerned son or daughter calls about their mother who is in treatment, a release must be obtained from the client before a conversation with her children can take place. The therapist and the client should also discuss whether to allow unlimited consultation with family members or to confine the communication to specific domains.

Family members are much more likely to contact therapists about elderly clients than younger ones, as are neighbors and other interested community members, so a well-thought out response to calls is essential. When an unexpected call occurs, the best response is to listen to the information being given without divulging whether or not the person is in your care, then advise the caller that he or she may wish to raise this concern with the person and that any professional who is involved with that person will need a signed release to communicate with the caller directly. This tactic allows the clinician to assess whether there is a dangerous situation without compromising the client's confidentiality.

The dilemma then becomes how to use the caller's information. Of course, if the situation involves imminent danger to a client or other people, confidentiality is no longer an issue. In other situations, it may be in the client's best interest to have the therapist talk with the caller. The therapist must then find a way to steer the client toward the information, hopefully resulting in a signed release. "Ethical Principles of Psychologists and Code of Conduct" (American Psychological Association, 1992) contains specific tenets regarding confidentiality that can be used to guide decision making.

The situation is slightly different when the client has been referred for evaluation of an organic impairment or where a dementing illness (Alzheimer's disease, vascular dementia, or some other memory impairment) is known to be present. It is usually critical to coordinate this kind of assessment with the client's physician and to exchange information that can clarify the diagnosis. If a power of attorney (POA) for health care is in effect, releases to obtain information from or to send reports to physicians or other professionals must be signed by that person. This is one of the most troubling of situations for therapists, particularly because many dementia patients retain some awareness of their intellectual deficits. If the clinician's observations in the initial interview lead to the opinion that the patient retains some capacity for decision making, it is advisable to obtain signed releases from the patient as well, even though they may not be considered legally binding in the face of the POA. (Guardianship is used rarely as a legal device for older people with compromised intellectual functioning; a POA is the most typical way this situation is handled, but clinicians need to be aware of the specific legal mechanisms available in the state in which they practice. Usually, a POA must be specific for health care. Someone with POA to manage finances can take over management of health affairs only if another POA for that purpose is signed.)

A common dilemma for clinicians arises when a client has been referred for an initial evaluation of memory impairment and competency has been found to be significantly compromised, yet no POA exists. Some clients in those circumstances will quite willingly sign releases to allow the psychologist to talk with their physician when their specific purpose is explained to them. Others may not be willing to sign releases at all. If a client is reluctant to sign a release to his or her primary physician on an initial visit, it may be possible to reintroduce the issue in a subsequent session after some trust has been established.

One way to circumvent this problem is to include a form for release of information at intake. Medicare, in fact, requires that psychologists offer to consult with the primary physician at the onset of treatment. Often this physician has referred the client, but a signed release is still mandated. An example of this type of release is shown in Figure 14.1. This release, of course, does not resolve the problem of sharing information with the family, which can be done only with the client's consent. In almost all cases, however, that is not a problem, for clients give permission to talk with their family. Information should be shared with the family only when it is relevant and in the client's best interests, for example, when the family is providing care for the client and the results of the assessment will help them plan more effective care.

A difficult ethical dilemma is whether a release signed by someone who is believed to be incompetent is valid. From a legal perspective, until an individual has been declared legally incompetent, which requires a court appearance, they are considered competent. That does not, however, relieve clinicians of their obligation to weigh conflicting ethical concerns. The deci-

---

Medicare Consultation Release

It may be beneficial to you for me to contact your primary care physician regarding your psychological treatment or regarding any medical problems for which you are receiving treatment. In addition, Medicare requires that I notify your physician, by telephone or in writing, concerning services I provide unless you request that notification not be made.

Please check one of the following.

____ I authorize you to contact my primary care physician, whose name and address are shown below, to discuss the treatment I am receiving under your care and to obtain information concerning my medical diagnosis and treatment.

____ I do not authorize you to contact my primary care physician about the treatment I am receiving under your care or to obtain information concerning my medical diagnosis and treatment. I am providing you with the name and address of my primary care physician only for your records.

Signature and date

FIGURE 14.1. Sample release of information form.

sion to obtain a consent to release information from a client with questionable competence must be based on the evaluation that doing so is in the client's best interest. This problem fortunately occurs only rarely in practice. Instead, individuals usually have been encouraged to sign POAs by physicians and attorneys while they are still (sometimes marginally) competent. We should also add that a finding of dementia or other type of cognitive deficit does not necessarily mean an individual is no longer legally competent (see Chapter 6). Rather, competence depends on understanding the specific issues involved, in this case, giving consent for release of information (Grisso, 1994).

The following example indicates the kind of complications that can arise regarding confidentiality when several members of a family are involved. The initial contact was made by John, a 48-year-old attorney who had power of attorney for his father, Harry, who had developed clear organic impairment following open-heart surgery. While the main focus was on his father, John requested help for both his parents. He had observed that his mother, Mary, was not coping well with his father's impairments. The initial evaluation was made on the father. The mother (who also had POA for her husband) was present. Mary did not consider herself in need of any help but simply wanted her husband restored to his former self. From a practical perspective, beginning with an assessment of Harry would clarify the extent of his deficits and the kinds of problems his wife had to cope with. As often happens in caregiving situations, Mary could then be brought into treatment as the focus shifted from finding out what was wrong with the father to identifying what the family could do to manage the problems effectively. Mary signed consent forms for information about her husband to be freely communicated with her son and all the physicians involved in her husband's care.

After a few visits, John called, wanting a summary of the treatment. Since his mother had signed a release to discuss his father, John was given a summary. In the course of the conversation, it became clear that John wanted to talk as much about his mother's functioning as about his father's. He expressed concern that she was becoming overwhelmed by having to care for her husband and that she was behaving oddly, for example, kicking her husband under the table if he said something she objected to. As it became apparent that the focus of the discussion was shifting from the father to the mother, it was necessary to obtain a release from her. Through the process of assessment of her husband, Mary had become engaged in trying to understand his difficulties and her reactions to them. At this point, she was eager for open communication among everyone and gave the release for the therapist to talk with her son. This step became important later when the decision was being made to place Harry in a nursing facility, which required many conversations with John about what would be in both Harry's and Mary's best interest.

In general, if a clinician anticipates the need to speak with family members, it is wise to obtain releases early in treatment. When dealing with a frail older person, questions about moving the person to a more protective setting are very common, and families naturally want to be involved in the decision making. The therapist can be helpful in this situation, because the family often turns to him or her for an expert opinion in choosing among the available options. The therapist can also assure that the client's best interests are taken into account rather than those of the most forceful person in the family.

This example raises another issue. It is generally preferable that a therapist treat only one person in a family, except when explicitly conducting marital or family therapy. With older clients, however, special circumstances involve one therapist seeing two or more family members. These situations typically involve dementia and other chronic disabilities. Issues that may be discussed include arranging and coordinating care for the disabled person, making long-term plans for care, and the impact the disability has on the primary caregiver and other family members. The use of multiple therapists in such a situation would unnecessarily complicate the treatment process for the family.

The therapist who is seeing several family members must take steps to avoid the pitfalls inherent in this type of situation. The therapist must consider if he or she can take a position that is in everyone's best interests. That may require being able to reconcile very different viewpoints about issues such as placement. The therapist must also be sure not to reveal anything said to him or her in confidence by one family member to anyone else in the family. In general, tactfulness and respect for each person's opinions are critical. While communications can become complicated, it remains preferable to channel everything through a single therapist than to add more specialists to a situation in which the family is already overburdened with doctors. Of course, the usual constraints about seeing more than one person in a family would apply when treating an older person who functions independently.

Assisted Living Facilities

When a client lives in an assisted living facility, confidentiality issues can be rather tricky. Assisted living implies that the person has relinquished control over certain aspects of daily living, such as meals, housekeeping, bathing, and/or the administration of medication. Assisted living may include a "board and care" residence or "boarding home." In some states, retirement hotels and residences that previously catered to the well elderly are adding services so that people can remain in the facility despite declining functioning. In a more formalized "personal care residence," nursing care is available though not routinely provided. These facilities differ, however, from nursing homes, which are licensed and regulated as medical facilities (see Chapter 8).

Residents of assisted living facilities vary considerably in their functioning. Some are fully competent and seek out a therapist as any other adult might do. Others are physically or intellectually compromised. The referral may come from the client, their family, or their physician, or from a community agency or the facility.

Consistent with maintaining the confidentiality of the client's communications, it is best to limit the transmission of information to the least number of people who need to know. While some facilities keep a chart that resembles a nursing home or hospital chart, the clinician should not write in the chart. In a nonmedical setting, the fact that a client is even seeing a mental health professional is confidential information. With an appropriate release, however, the clinician can consult with staff on care issues. All confidential records should be kept in the therapist's office, as would be done with any other client. A self-referred client should be asked if he or she wants the primary physician kept informed, and a release should be either signed or denied. Beyond that, the only time the facility needs to know about therapy is in a situation involving danger for the client or other people or if competence becomes an issue.

When the family requests treatment, an assessment should be made concerning the extent to which they should be involved in treatment and whether it is in the client's best interest for the therapist to stay in communication with them. Releases must be signed to allow free exchanges of information. Occasionally a physician refers a client who does not have any identified family members. Again, if the client is competent, the only release necessary is for the physician. But if the client is not competent, then it may be necessary to communicate with the facility to determine whether the client has or needs the involvement of a geriatric case manager or if an appropriate public agency should assume guardianship to insure that the person's best interests are being protected. In this case, a release from the patient to communicate freely with the facility would still be necessary.

Sometimes the clinician would like to share the findings of the evaluation with the facility, but the resident refuses to give consent. This problem can be especially troubling when the resident is demented and having obvious difficulties in the facility. We have often encountered older clients who are early in the dementia process and aware of some of their deficits. Out of their anxiety and fear over what is happening to them, they refuse to allow any communication to occur between the therapist and the facility. Their right to confidentiality must be respected unless the situation is or becomes dangerous. Usually, if the relationship continues, it is possible to obtain the release at a later time in such a way that clients agree to at least a limited communication with the facility that would be in their own best interest.

Nursing Home or Hospital

In these settings, Medicare requires that each visit be documented with the date, type of service provided, length of service, some indication of the content of the service, and a signature. Because these records are open to all medical and ancillary personnel who have access to records, and because security of the records is light, it is preferable to make only the necessary entries to ensure continuity of care in the facility and to keep extended notes in more secure confidential files in the clinician's own office. For example, if a client is depressed, that would be the notation in the chart in the facility, along with any suggestions for how staff might assist the client or recommendations that the patient be evaluated for antidepressant medication. In the clinician's own files would be the documentation of what the client said, what tests were used, and so on.

Usually patients in nursing homes and hospitals have signed a blanket release from confidentiality that pertains to all who treat them, allowing free communication among professional staff. It still is important to consider the client's privacy and best interests. Just because it is permissible to communicate with staff members does not mean that it is in the client's best interest to communicate everything. Care should be taken to communicate only what is necessary for the staff to know about a client without violating the client's privacy. Bear in mind that residents in nursing facilities and patients in hospitals feel intruded on and powerless, and the mental health professional may be the only person they can confide those feelings to.

One of the most useful roles of a mental health professional in the nursing home is consultant to staff about behavior problems of patients, particularly cognitively impaired patients, but also those with other problems that put undue stress on the staff (see Chapter 13). The best way to protect client confidentiality in these situations is to make positive suggestions to staff in very general terms, rather than discussing a particular patient. When the consultant talks about a class of patients, rather than an individual, it allows the staff member to think about applying suggestions across a variety of patients, which helps them stay oriented to the suggestions in a professional rather than a personal way.

Even if the patient or the person holding POA has authorized communication within the nursing home or hospital, it is still necessary to obtain a specific release before communicating with family members other than the person with POA. While this step sounds obvious, it is not always possible to anticipate the particular family structure (or dysfunctions) that will be encountered. So a certain amount of vigilance is necessary when responding to family members who inquire about their relative.

Confidentiality issues, then, can arise in a variety of different ways for older people, depending on the setting in which they live, the client's competence to give consent, the involvement of family, and the need to exchange information with other health care providers. Situations arise where clinicians must weigh the competing demands of different ethical principles. The clinician's responsibilities to clients, particularly in protecting confidentiality, should guide all decisions about treatment and release of information.

Exceptions to Confidentiality

For certain types of communications, clinicians are obligated to break confidentiality. Although state laws vary somewhat, mental health professionals are generally required to take steps to prevent clients from committing suicide or from harming other people. This responsibility includes the duty to inform an intended victim of violence. Reporting child abuse is mandatory, especially abuse involving sexual activity. These statutes apply whether one's client is old or not.

The issue of suicide in late life is complex. Even though a client is old, state laws requiring clinicians to intervene to prevent suicide still apply. When clients talk about suicide, we discuss with them our responsibilities, letting them know that we must intervene if we see an imminent risk. Of course, we also work with the client on the issues that are leading to the suicidal ideation.

A clinician might in principle support rational suicide, for instance, to forestall intolerable pain or inevitable deterioration, but encouraging a suicide or neglecting to intervene is a violation of professional ethics and state law. Whether or not clients have the right to end their lives, especially in extreme circumstances that cannot be remedied, is an important ethical issue. Many people do not agree with the way those issues are currently addressed by the legal system, but professionals must to work within that framework. We continue discussion of this issue later, when we turn to decisions to refuse treatment.

The other issue involving exceptions to confidentiality that is different in geriatric practice is elder abuse. Elder abuse laws are not as widespread as child abuse laws, and in some states, the duty to report elder abuse is voluntary. Elder abuse statutes also vary in their definitions, particularly of psychological abuse and neglect.

When clinicians have a choice about reporting, they can take into consideration how serious and chronic the abuse has been and whether psychological interventions are likely to be sufficient to prevent further abuse. We would not report, for example, a family caregiver who got so frustrated with a dementia patient that she pushed him once in anger, even though it might be covered under some interpretations of the legal statute. Instead, we would work with the caregiver to understand her anger and head off future outbursts. On the other hand, we would not hesitate in reporting a nursing aid who was consistently abusing patients. Whatever the clinician's specific course of action in an abusive situation, it must be an effective intervention.

END-OF-LIFE ISSUES

We begin with an example that illustrates the complexity of end-of-life decisions. The clients are Bess, a 70-year-old woman with Alzheimer's disease, and her 72-year-old husband of 45 years, Frank. Bess was referred by a neurologist, who requested a neuropsychological evaluation after diagnosing her dementia. In the course of the evaluation, it became apparent that Bess was acutely and painfully aware of her deficits and clinically depressed as a result. She began psychotherapy and continued until her memory deficits became sufficient to contraindicate talking therapy. As she declined, treatment shifted to Frank, who had become increasingly depressed and angry about the hopeless deterioration he saw taking place in his wife. They were seen together and separately over a 5-year period, both in the office and later at home, when Bess was no longer able to leave the home because of degenerative arthritis and increased fear of falling outside the home. Eventually, she started falling helplessly to the floor at night, and Frank had to call the police and neighbors to help get her up. When he realized that he could no longer take care of her, he placed her in a nursing home. Three months after she went to the facility, and on the urging of his son-in-law who was a physician, Frank asked that Bess be coded as DNR (do not resuscitate) and also that no extraordinary means be used to prolong her life.

Bess was severely aphasic but was able to communicate her unhappiness about her situation both through an anguished expression and very occasionally by asking plaintively, "Why me?" During the therapy we previously had conducted with Bess, we established that her first choice was to be cared for at home but she would accept a nursing home if it became necessary. She also talked at great length about how unhappy she was with what had become of her. She did not want to be a burden to Frank and worried about his depression. While she was still able to, she granted Frank power of attorney, including responsibility for health care decisions.

About 6 months after she entered the nursing home, Bess suddenly became ill. Tests showed that she had been bleeding internally, probably secondary to the nonsteroidal anti-inflammatory medication she had been taking for her arthritis. What followed was a series of ethical dilemmas about whether the situation should be defined as "end of life," which would then trigger the prohibition on using extraordinary means, and about the hidden implications of decisions that physicians ask families to make about treatment.

The physician, Dr. Smith, explained the situation to Frank and very gingerly asked him if he wanted Bess to have a transfusion. Frank responded by asking Dr. Smith what he would normally do. The physician interpreted Frank's response as an indication that he wanted treatment started, so Bess was transferred to the hospital for the transfusion. Once the transfusion was started, she immediately had an allergic reaction, which is very rare. The physician stopped the transfusion. Bess was running a temperature of 102, and the physician asked Frank if he wanted an IV started to hydrate her. He replied, "Yes," so that Bess would not be dehydrated. She was then returned to the nursing home.

At the nursing home, some of the staff were upset that the IV had been started in light of Bess's "no extraordinary measures" status. Given her physical situation, they felt she was clearly in decline and would die soon. Without the IV, the process would take anywhere from 5 to 14 days, but with the IV, she could linger for much longer. Dr. Smith had not explained that to Frank. The nursing staff asked us to discuss the dilemma with Frank, given the length and nature of our relationship. Frank was distraught by the turn of events, so the options were delicately explained to him. Then we called the physician and asked what his intentions were. (It was helpful that we had already worked with Dr. Smith on several cases and had developed a good collaborative relationship.) Dr. Smith explained that when he started the IV in the hospital he explained to Frank that it would only be in place for 4 days, just to rehydrate Bess after the transfusion reaction. Once her physical status was stabilized, it would be removed. And, indeed, on the fourth day, when the IV came loose, the nurses were instructed not to replace it. At that point, Bess was in a coma, nonresponsive, and dying. She lingered for another 5 days, being kept as comfortable as possible, and then expired peacefully.

Our role in this situation was complex. Because of the nature and longevity of our relationship with Frank, we were thrust into the role of the person who could best lay out the choices that could be made. The physician was prepared to abide by Frank's wishes not to prolong Bess's life needlessly, but he did not make explicit exactly what each choice meant. Frank was relying on the physician to make the decisions for him, including determining the point at which no further treatment should be given, but the physician was bouncing the decision making back to Frank. The choice had already been made not to resuscitate nor to take extraordinary steps to prolong life, but Frank was put in the position of determining whether or not the transfusion and then the IV were extraordinary steps. After we intervened, Frank was able to defer to the physician, who followed the original plan of removing the IV after 4 days. Frank felt that a medical protocol had been followed, rather than that he had made a decision that might shorten his wife's life.

In this example, we found ourselves in the situation of advising the caregiver on the decisions. We had to remain neutral, not indicating a personal preference for one decision over another. The clinician's own personal biases must not enter into such a decision. As mental health professionals, we have tremendous power to influence our clients, and in a situation like this one, we have to continuously assess whether our own values and biases are influencing the decision-making process.

A major question is whether that is a role therapists ought to assume. Because of the nature of the psychotherapeutic relationship, which involves talking extensively to clients and getting to know their beliefs, attitudes, and values, mental health professionals may be in a unique position to address end-of-life issues. Physicians rarely have the time to spend with their patients or the patients' families to explore these issues in depth. Consequently, many geriatricians and family practice physicians are eager for help in this kind of decision making and even to defer some of the explanation of alternatives to the mental health professional. Occasionally, the physician may make a referral to a therapist specifically to determine what the individual's wishes are, particularly if there is a question about competence or if depression or anxiety might be clouding the patient's decision-making abilities. As in the example, the intervention with a patient can gradually include a widening circle of concerned family members, who can be involved individually or in a family session. On the other hand, mental health professionals have not been prepared specifically for this role, which can be emotionally demanding and includes knowing the explicit and implicit medical, legal, and ethical considerations for addressing end-of-life situations.

A growing body of legal and ethical writing bears on end-of-life issues. Most writers on these issues make a distinction between active euthanasia and passive approaches that involve withholding procedures that might prolong life (Thomasma, 1992). Active approaches, such as that of Jack Kervorkian, are clearly more controversial. As we stressed earlier, whatever one's personal opinion of euthanasia, there is a legal and ethical obligation to prevent suicides, assisted or otherwise.

Legal and ethical issues concerning the decision to cease or withhold active treatment of terminally ill individuals are complex and evolving. There has been considerable debate over whether decisions should be made according to the principle of beneficence—appropriate people choose what is in the patient's best interest—or the principle of autonomy—the patient or his or her proxy makes the decision. The Cruzan case has had a large influence on legal standards for cessation of treatment (see White, 1992). Nancy Cruzan was a young woman who fell into a persistent vegetative state as a result of injuries suffered in a serious automobile accident and was kept alive on life supports. Her family sued to have her life supports removed. The courts eventually ruled in favor of the family, largely on the basis of testimony that the patient had stated in conversations before the accident that she preferred not to be kept alive in that kind of condition. In deciding for the family, the court endorsed the principle of autonomy.

The principle of autonomy in end-of-life decisions is supported by passage of the Patient Self-Determination Act, which was part of the Omnibus Budget Reconciliation Act of 1990 (Sections 4206 and 4751 of OBRA, 1990, Public Law 101-508). Under the provisions of this act, all Medicare and Medicaid provider organizations, including hospitals and nursing homes, must obtain at the time of admission advance directives that indicate the patient's preferences about terminating treatment. When the patient is not able to respond, the closest family member indicates a preference, as in the DNR order in the previous example. A concurrent trend that has grown out of the publicity received by the Cruzan case and similar situations is for people to execute advance directives (sometimes called living wills) that indicate their preferences concerning medical treatment in extreme situations.

Though these approaches offer people some degree of control over end-of-life decisions, there remain many problems and questions. From a practical perspective, most people do not have advance directives (Moore et al., 1994). Complicating the situation is the fact that health care providers often do what they believe to be appropriate, regardless of an advance directive or power of attorney. That happens especially if the family is divided over what the appropriate treatment should be (Moody, 1992). Some ethicists raise serious objections to the principle of autonomy. Dresser (1992), for example, argues that the patient's prior choices should not influence current decisions, because the person may not have foreseen this particular situation and might now make a different choice. Proxy decisions by family members are criticized even more strongly, because, in the absence of an advance directive, the family cannot truly know what the patient wanted (Rhoden, 1988).

The importance and complexity of these issues have grown out of a long-standing trend in medicine, whereby what were previously considered heroic or extraordinary measures are becoming standard procedures for care. An obvious example is the use of hydration and feeding tubes for late-stage dementia patients. Are these kinds of procedures heroic measures, or have they become routine and expected care? Does hydration or a feeding tube contribute to the comfort of an end-stage patient, or do these procedures needlessly prolong suffering? As Sherwin Nuland (1993) has observed in his powerful book, *How We Die*, we have the medical technology to do all sorts of amazing things, but at the end of life, do we merely make people uncomfortable rather than helping them die peacefully? Thomasma (1992) made a powerful critique of this trend in medicine, arguing that we need to reverse current premises in end-of-life situations. Rather than assuming that everything must be done to prolong life, he proposes that the "default mode" of modern medicine should be to do nothing to extend life in a hopeless situation, except if requested by the patient, by the family, or by an advance directive. While the debate among medical ethicists continues, medical technology is extending the boundaries of life-and-death decisions in new and unexpected ways, placing families in situations for which they are not prepared.

Beyond the ethical dimensions involved in these situations, clinicians need to be aware of the practical implications of medical decisions in life-threatening situations so that they can help patients and their families obtain the kind of care they prefer. As illustrated in the case example, medical personnel have developed a set of implicit rules in end-of-life situations, where each decision has certain consequences. Families are asked to make decisions but often without being aware of the long-term implications. Once procedures to manage an acute situation are started, physicians will usually feel obligated to continue them. It is very difficult to discontinue some procedures, such as feeding tubes and respirators, after they have been started, if the patient cannot survive independently without them. In the example, the physician could have argued for the need for continued hydration or might have encouraged the use of a feeding tube. Indeed, the decision to cease hydration would have been controversial in many medical settings. In some nursing homes or hospitals, staff actively oppose removing these treatments and have gone to court to prevent it. The result is that families who do not want to prolong suffering sometimes find themselves on an irreversible course of doing just that because they have made decisions without fully understanding what their choice meant.

A related consideration is that physicians, hospitals, and nursing homes need to support the decisions reached by patients and their families. Some physicians do not agree to follow specific advance directives or to implement the treatment plan proposed by the family; some facilities have their own guidelines. Once a terminal phase of care has begun, it may be impossible to reconcile these differences in beliefs. Families caring for someone with a predictable course of decline, such as dementia, should be encouraged to talk about terminal-stage care ahead of time with the patient's physicians to make sure that the patient's preferences are likely to be implemented.

One of the more problematic aspects of these situations is determining whether a patient has entered a terminal phase. Physicians may be reluctant to make this determination and, as in the example above, turn to the family for guidance about whether or not to continue treatment. In other instances, physicians insist on initiating treatment in situations the family regards as terminal. As physicians' skills in prolonging life continue to improve, the decision that a situation is terminal may become increasingly social, not medical.

One further consideration is that older people and their families need to understand the implications of their decisions concerning use of different types of medical facilities. Specifically, the patient's preferences as indicated by do-not-resuscitate orders, no-extraordinary-measures orders, or advanced directives are all invalid in an emergency room and in situations in which paramedics have been called. In emergency situations, emergency medical technicians and physicians need to be able to respond to the crisis immediately before them, and they do not honor advance directives or DNR orders. As a result, a severely impaired dementia patient who has a significant medical event, such as a myocardial infarction or cardiovascular accident, may be taken to the emergency room and resuscitated, contrary to the wishes of the patient and family. The only physician who can honor advance directives is the primary care physician, so it is advisable for family members to consult with this doctor before making a trip to the emergency room. When the older person resides in a nursing home, the family should make similar arrangements with the staff. Some nonmedical programs, such as adult day care or assisted living facilities, may feel obligated to call for emergency help, despite the presence of a DNR order. It may fall on the mental health professional to make explicit to the family what the consequences will be of using emergency services and to help them discuss these issues with nursing home staff or other people involved in the patient's care.

The mental health professional should not decide what is best for the patient or family but should instead help families understand the implications of their decisions and help them make decisions that reflect their preferences and those of the patient. To be effective and helpful in the decision-making process, we need to be able to present the various choices in a nonjudgmental and clear manner, and to do so we must understand our own values and clearly differentiate them from our clients' values. As an example, we may believe that patients deserve a natural death, unencumbered by technology, except to keep them as comfortable and free from pain as possible. Some patients and families may value prolonging life as long as possible. Each family must find its own answer to the dilemma of doing everything they feel should be done without needlessly prolonging suffering. Whatever the situation, our role is to help people articulate their values and then to make decisions in a manner consistent with those values.

CONCLUSIONS

Beyond the basic issues of becoming competent and comfortable in treating older people, clinicians need to develop an understanding of the complex legal and ethical issues involved. Foremost among these are confidentiality and end-of-life issues. The "Ethical Principles and Code of Conduct of Psychologists" provides a framework and set of principles for addressing the dilemmas that are encountered. But because the principles are broad and abstract, clinicians often find themselves having to apply and extend the basic tenets in situations for which there are no specific precedents. It is important for clinicians to approach these decisions very carefully, getting input from colleagues, and examining their own biases and values so that they are able to differentiate what they would want for themselves from their clients' best interests. There is clearly a need for more education in this area and for development of forums for discussion of ethical dilemmas in the care of older people.

References

Abas, M. A., Sahakian, B. J., & Levy, R. (1990). Neuropsychological deficits and CT scan changes in elderly depressives. *Psychological Medicine, 20,* 507–520.

Adams, W. L. (1995). Potential for adverse drug–alcohol interactions in elderly retirement community residents. *Journal of the American Geriatrics Society, 43,* 1021–1025.

Adams, W. L. (1997). Interactions between alcohol and other drugs. In A. M. Gurnack (Ed.), *Older adults' misuse of alcohol, medicines, and other drugs* (pp. 185–205). New York: Springer.

Adams, W. L., Magruder-Habib, K., Trued, S., & Broome, H. L. (1992). Alcohol abuse in elderly emergency department patients. *Journal of the American Geriatrics Society, 40,* 1236–1240.

Akiskal, H. S., & McKinney, W. T. (1973). Depressive disorders: Toward a unified hypothesis. *Science, 5,* 20–29.

Albert, M. S. (1988). Assessment of cognitive function. In M. S. Albert & M. B. Moss (Eds.), *Geriatric neuropsychology* (pp. 57–81). New York: Guilford Press.

Albert, M. S., Duffy, F. H., & Naeser, M. (1987). Nonlinear changes in cognition with age and their neuropsychologic correlates. *Canadian Journal of Psychology, 41,* 141–157.

Albert, M. S., & Moss, M. B. (Eds.). (1988). *Geriatric neuropsychology.* New York: Guilford Press.

Albert, M. S., Wolfe, J., & Lafleche, G. (1990). Differences in abstraction ability with age. *Psychology and Aging, 5,* 94–100.

Alexopoulos, G. S. (1994). Biological correlates of late-life depression. In L. S. Schneider, C. F. Reynolds, B. D. Lebowitz, & A. J. Friedhoff (Eds.), *Diagnosis and treatment of depression in late life* (pp. 99–116). Washington, DC: American Psychiatric Press.

Alexopoulos, G. S., Meyers, B. S., Young, R. C., Mattis, S., & Kakuma, T. (1993). The course of geriatric depression with "reversible dementia": A controlled study. *American Journal of Psychiatry, 150,* 1693–1699.

Alexopoulos, G. S., Young, R. C., Abrams, R. C., Meyers, B., & Shamoian, C. A. (1989). Chronicity and relapse in geriatric depression. *Biological Psychiatry, 26,* 551–564.

Alexopoulos, G. S., Young, R. C., & Shindledecker, R. D. (1992). Brain computed to-mography findings in geriatric depression and primary degenerative dementia. *Biological Psychiatry, 31,* 591–599.

American Psychiatric Association. (1990). *The practice of electroconvulsive therapy: Recommendations for treatment, training, and privileging.* Washington, DC: Author.

American Psychiatric Association. (1994). *Diagnostic and statistical manual of mental disorders* (4th ed.). Washington, DC: Author.

American Psychiatric Association. (1997). *Practice guidelines for the treatment of patients with Alzheimer's disease and other dementias of late life.* Washington, DC: Author.

American Psychological Association. (1992). Ethical principles of psychologists and codes of conduct. *American Psychologist, 47,* 1597–1611.

Ancill, R. J., Embury, G. D., MacEwan, G. W., & Kennedy, J. S. (1987). Lorazepam in the elderly: A retrospective study of the side-effects in 20 patients. *Journal of Psychopharmacology, 2,* 126–127.

Aneshensel, C. S., Pearlin, L. I., Mullan, J. T., Zarit, S. H., & Whitlatch, C. J. (1995). *Profiles in caregiving: The unexpected career.* New York: Academic Press.

Anthony, J. C., & Aboraya, A. (1992). The epidemiology of selected mental disorders in later life. In J. E. Birren, R. B. Sloane, & G. D. Cohen (Eds.), *Handbook of mental health and aging* (2nd ed., pp. 27–72). San Diego: Academic Press.

Anthony, J. C., LeResche, L., Niaz, U., Von Korff, M. R., & Folstein, M. F. (1982). Limits of the Mini-Mental State as a screening test for dementia and delirium among hospital patients. *Psychological Medicine, 12,* 397–408.

Anthony-Bergstone, C. R., Zarit, S. H., & Gatz, M. (1988). Symptoms of psychological distress among caregivers of dementia patients. *Psychology and Aging, 3,* 245–248.

Atkinson, R. M. (1990). Aging and alcohol use disorders: Diagnostic issues in the elderly. *International Psychogeriatrics, 2,* 55–72.

Atkinson, R. M., Ganzini, L., & Bernstein, M. J. (1992). Alcohol and substance-use disorders in the elderly. In J. E. Birren, R. B. Sloane, & G. D. Cohen (Eds.), *Handbook of mental health and aging* (2nd ed., pp. 516–556). San Diego: Academic Press.

Atkinson, R. M., & Kofoed, L. L. (1982). Alcohol and drug abuse in old age: A clinical perspective. *Substance and Alcohol Actions/Misuse, 3,* 353–368.

Atkinson, R. F., Tolson, R. L., & Turner, J. A. (1990). Late versus early onset problem drinking in older men. *Alcoholism: Clinical and Experimental Research, 14,* 574–579.

Atkinson, R. M., Turner, J. A., Kofoed, L. L., & Tolson, R. L. (1985). Early versus late onset alcoholism in older persons: Preliminary findings. *Alcoholism: Clinical and Experimental Research, 9,* 513–515.

Bacellar, H., Muñoz, A., Miller, E. N., Cohen, B. A., Besley, D., Selnes, O. A., Becker, J. T., & McArthur, J. C. (1994). Temporal trends in the incidence of HIV-1-related neurologic diseases: Multicenter AIDS Cohort Study, 1985–1992. *Neurology, 44,* 1892–1900.

Bachman, D. L., Wolf, P. A., Linn, R. T., Knoefel, J. E., Cobb, J. L., Belanger, A. J., White, L. R., & D'Agostino, R. B. (1993). Incidence of dementia and probable Alzheimer's disease in a general population: The Framingham Study. *Neurology, 43,* 515–519.

Baddeley, A. (1992). Working memory. *Science, 255,* 556–559.

Baldwin, R. C., & Jolley, D. J. (1986). The prognosis of depression in old age. *British Journal of Psychiatry, 149*,574–583.

Baltes, M. M. (1994). Aging well and institutional living: A paradox? In R. P. Abeles, H. C. Gift, & M. G. Ory (Eds.), *Aging and quality of life* (pp. 185–201). New York: Springer.

Baltes, M. M., Kindermann, T., Reisenzein, R., & Schmid, U. (1987). Further observational data on the behavioral and social world of institutions for the aged. *Psychology and Aging 2*, 390–403.

Baltes, M. M., Neumann, E. M., & Zank, S. (1994). Maintenance and rehabilitation of independence in old age: An intervention program for staff. *Psychology and Aging, 9*, 179–188.

Baltes, M. M., & Wahl, H. W. (1992). The dependency–support script in institutions: Generalization to community settings. *Psychology and Aging, 7*, 409–418.

Baltes, P. B. (1987). Theoretical propositions of life-span developmental psychology: On the dynamics between growth and decline. *Developmental Psychology, 23*, 611–626.

Baltes, P. B. (1997). On the incomplete architecture of human ontogeny: Selection, optimization, and compensation as foundation of developmental theory. *American Psychologist, 52*, 366–380.

Baltes, P. B., & Kliegl, R. (1992). Further testing of limits of cognitive plasticity: Negative age differences in a mnemonic skill are robust. *Developmental Psychology, 28*, 121–125.

Baltes, P. B. & Lindenberger, U. (1997). Emergence of a powerful connection between sensory and cognitive functions across the adult life span: A new window to the study of cognitive aging? *Psychology and Aging, 12*, 12–21.

Barclay, L. L., Zemcov, A., Blass, J. P., & Sansone, J. (1985). Survival in Alzheimer's disease and vascular dementias. *Neurology, 35*, 834–840.

Barrett, L. I. (1997). Reagan's long goodbye. *Time, 149*(12), 82.

Beck, A. T. (1976). *Cognitive therapy and the emotional disorders*. New York: International Universities Press.

Beck, A. T., Freeman, A., & Associates. (1990). *Cognitive therapy of personality disorders*. New York: Guilford Press.

Beck A. T., & Greenberg, R. L. (1974). *Coping with depression*. New York: Institute for Rational Living.

Beck A. T., Rush, A. J., Shaw, B. F., & Emery, G. (1979). *Cognitive therapy of depression*. New York: Guilford Press.

Becker, J. T., Huff, J., Nebes, R. D., Holland, A., & Boller, F. (1988). Neuropsychological function in Alzheimer's Disease. *Archives of Neurology, 45*, 263–268.

Beizer, J. L. (1994). Medications and the aging body: Alteration as a function of age. *Generations, 18*, 13–17.

Bem, D., & Allen, A. (1974). On predicting some of the people some of the time: The search for cross-situational consistencies in behavior. *Psychological Review, 81*, 506–520.

Bender, M. B. (1952). *Disorders in perception, with particular reference to the phenomena of extinction and displacement*. Springfield, IL: Thomas.

Benton, A. L. (1974). *Revised Visual Retention Test*. New York: Psychological Corporation.

Benton, A. L. & Hamsher, K. deS. (1976). *Multilingual Aphasia Examination*. Iowa City: University of Iowa.

Berg, S., Nilsson, L., & Svanborg, A. (1988). Behavioral and clinical aspects—Longitudinal studies. In J. P. Wattis & I. Hindmarch (Eds.), *Psychological assessment of the elderly* (pp. 47–60). London: Churchill Livingstone.

Beutler, L. E., Scogin, F., Kirkish, P., Schretlen, D., Corbishley, A., Hamblin, D., Meredith, K., Potter, R., Bamford, C. R., & Levenson, A. I. (1987). Group cognitive therapy and alprazolam in the treatment of depression in older adults. *Journal of Consulting and Clinical Psychology, 55*, 550–556.

Bigler, E. D., Rosa, L., Schultz, F., Hall, S. & Harris, J. (1989). Rey–Auditory Verbal Learning and Rey–Osterrieth Complex Figure Design performance in Alzheimer's disease and closed head injury. *Journal of Clinical Psychology, 45*, 277–280.

Bille-Brahe, U. (1993). The role of sex and age in suicidal behavior. *Acta Psychiatrica Scandinavica, 371*, 21–27.

Birkhill, W. R., & Schaie, K. W. (1975). The effect of differential reinforcement of cautiousness in intellectual performance among the elderly. *Journal of Gerontology, 30*, 578–583.

Blau, E. & Ober, B. A. (1988). The effect of depression on verbal memory in older adults. *Journal of Clinical and Experimental Neuropsychology, 10*, 81.

Blazer, D. (1993). *Depression in late life* (2nd ed.). St. Louis: Mosby.

Blazer, D. (1994). Epidemiology of late-life depression. In L. S. Schneider, C. F. Reynolds, B. D. Lebowitz, & A. J. Friedhoff (Eds.), *Diagnosis and treatment of depression in late life* (pp. 9–20). Washington, DC: American Psychiatric Press.

Blazer, D., George, L. K., Hughes, D. (1991). The epidemiology of anxiety disorders: An age comparison. In C. Salzman & B. Lebowitz (Eds.), *Anxiety in the elderly* (pp. 17–30). New York: Springer.

Blazer, D., Hughes, D. C., & George, L. K. (1987). The epidemiology of depression in an elderly community population. *Gerontologist, 27*, 281–287.

Blessed, G., Tomlinson, B. E., & Roth, M. (1968). The association between quantitative measures of dementia and of senile change in the cerebral grey matter of elderly subjects. *British Journal of Psychiatry, 114*, 797–811.

Bliwise, D. L. (1994). Dementia. In M. Kryger, T. Roth, & W. Dement (Eds.), *Principles and practice of sleep medicine* (2nd ed., pp. 790–800). Philadelphia: Saunders.

Bohnen, N., Warner, M., Kokmen, E., Beard, M., & Kurland, L. (1994). Alzheimer's disease and cumulative exposure to anesthesia: A case–control study. *Journal of the American Geriatrics Society, 42*, 198–201.

Boller, F., Mizutani, T., Roessmann, V., & Gambetti, P. (1980). Parkinson disease, dementia, and Alzheimer's disease: Clinicopathological correlations. *Annals of Neurology, 7*, 329–335.

Bondi, M. W., Monsch, A. U., Galasko, D., Butters, N., Salmon, D. P., & Delis, D. C. (1994). Preclinical cognitive markers of dementia of the Alzheimer type. *Neuropsychology, 8*, 374–384.

Bonner, D., & Howard, R. (1995). Treatment-resistant depression in the elderly. *International Psychogeriatrics, 7*, 83–94.

Bootzin, R. R., Engle-Friedman, M., & Hazelwood, L. (1983). Insomnia. In P. M. Lewinsohn & L. Teri (Eds.), *Clinical geropsychology: New directions in assessment and treatment* (pp. 81–115). Elmsford, NY: Pergamon Press.

Botwinick, J. (1966). Cautiousness in advanced age. *Journal of Gerontology, 21,* 347–353.

Botwinick, J. (1969). Disinclination to venture response versus cautiousness in responding: Age differences. *Journal of Genetic Psychology, 115,* 55–62.

Botwinick, J. (1984). *Aging and behavior* (3rd ed.). New York: Springer.

Botwinick, J., & Storandt, M. (1974). *Memory, related functions and age.* Springfield, IL: Thomas.

Bourgeois, M. S. (1990). Enhancing conversation skills in patients with Alzheimer's disease using a prosthetic memory aid. *Journal of Applied Behavior Analysis, 23,* 29–42.

Branconnier, R. J., Cole, J. O., Ghazvinian, S., Spera, K. F., Oxenkrug, G. F., & Bass, J. L. (1983). Clinical pharmacology of bupropion and imipramine in elderly depressives. *Journal of Clinical Psychiatry, 55* (5, Pt. 2), 130–133.

Breitner, J. (1996). Inflammatory processes and antiinflammatory drugs in Alzheimer's disease: A current appraisal. *Neurobiology of Aging, 17,* 789–794.

Breitner, J., Gau, B., Welsh, K., Plassman, B., McDonald, W., Helms, M., & Anthony, J. (1994). Inverse association of anti-inflammatory treatments and Alzheimer's disease: Initial results of a co-twin control study. *Neurology, 44,* 227–232.

Brenner, D. E., Kukull, W. A., van Belle, G., Bowen, J. D., McCormick, W. C., Teri, L., & Larson, E. B. (1993). Relationship between cigarette smoking and Alzheimer's disease in a population-based case–control study. *Neurology, 43,* 293–300.

Brody, E. M., Kleban, M. H., Johnsen, P. T., Hoffman, C., & Schoonover, C. B. (1987). Work status and parent care: A comparison of four groups of women. *Gerontologist, 27,* 201–208.

Brown, G. W., Bifulco, A., & Harris, T. O. (1987). Life events, vulnerability and onset of depression: Some refinements. *British Journal of Psychiatry, 150,* 30–42.

Brown, R., Sweeney, J., Loutsch, E., Kocsis, J., & Frances, A. (1984). Involutional melancholia revisited. *American Journal of Psychiatry, 141,* 24–28.

Brown, R. G., & Marsden, C. D. (1984). How common is dementia in Parkinson's disease? *Lancet, 2,* 1262–1265.

Brun, A. (1987). Frontal lobe degeneration of the non-Alzheimer type: I. Neuropathology. *Archives of Gerontology and Geriatrics, 6,* 193–208.

Burgio, K. L., & Burgio, L. D. (1991). The problem of urinary incontinence. In P. A. Wisocki (Ed.), *Handbook of clinical behavior therapy with the elderly client* (pp. 317–336). New York: Plenum Press.

Burgio, L. D. (1996). Interventions for the behavioral complications of Alzheimer's disease: Behavioral approaches. *International Psychogeriatrics, 8,* 45–52.

Burgio, L. D., Engel, B. T., Hawkins, A., McCormick, K., Scheve, A. S., & Jones, L. T. (1990). A staff management system for maintaining improvements in incontinence with elderly nursing home residents. *Journal of Applied Behavior Analysis, 23,* 111–118.

Burgio, L. D., Schilley, K., Hardin, J. M., Hsu, C., & Yancey, J. (1996). Environmental "White Noise": An intervention for verbally agitated nursing home residents. *Journal of Gerontology: Psychological Sciences, 51B,* P364–P373.

Burns, B. J., Wagner, H. R., Taube, J. E., Magaziner, J., Permutt, T., & Landerman, L. R. (1993). Mental health service use by the elderly in nursing homes. *American Journal of Public Health,83,* 331–337.

Buschke, H. & Fuld, P. A. (1974). Evaluating storage, retention and retrieval in disordered memory and learning. *Neurology, 11*, 1019–1025.

Butters, N., Granholm, E., Salmon, D. P., Grant, I., & Wolfe, J. (1987). Episodic and semantic memory: A comparison of amnesic and demented patients. *Journal of Clinical and Experimental Neuropsychology, 9*, 479–497.

Butters, M. A., Salmon, D. P., & Butters, N. (1994). Neuropsychological assessment of dementia. In M. Storandt & G. R. VandenBos (Eds.), *Neuropsychological assessment of dementia and depression in older adults: A clinician's guide* (pp. 33–60). Washington, DC: Amercan Psychological Association.

Butters, N., Salmon, D. P., Cullum, C. M., Cairns, P., Troster, A. I., Jacobs, D., Moss, M. B., & Cermak, L. S. (1988). Differentiation of amnesic and demented patients with the Wechsler Memory Scale—Revised. *Clinical Neuropsychologist, 2*, 133–144.

Caine, E. D. (1981). Pseudodementia: Current concepts and future directions. *Archives of General Psychiatry, 38*, 1359–1364.

Caine, E. D., Lyness, J. M., King, D. A., & Connors, L. (1994). Clinical and etiological heterogeneity of mood disorders in elderly patients. In L. S. Schneider, C. F. Reynolds, B. D. Lebowitz, & A. J. Friedhoff (Eds.), *Diagnosis and treatment of depression in late life* (pp. 21–54). Washington, DC: American Psychiatric Press.

Camp, C. J., Foss, J. W., O'Hanlon, A. M., & Stevens, A. B. (1996). Memory interventions for persons with dementia. *Applied Cognitive Psychology, 10*, 193–210.

Camp, C. J., Foss, J. W., Stevens, A. B., Reichard, C. C., McKitrick, L. A., & O'Hanlon, A. M. (1993). Memory training in normal and demented elderly populations: The E-I-E-I-O model. *Experimental Aging Research, 19*, 277–290.

Camp, C. J., & Schaller, J. R. (1989). Epilogue: Spaced-retrieval memory training in an adult day-care center. *Educational Gerontology, 15* , 641–648.

Camp, C. J., & Stevens, A. B. (1990). Spaced-retrieval: A memory intervention for dementia of the Alzheimer's type. *Clinical Gerontologist, 10*, 58–61.

Canadian Study of Health and Aging Working Group. (1994). Canadian Study of Health and Aging: Study methods and prevalence of dementia. *Canadian Medical Association Journal, 150*, 899–913.

Caplan, G. (1970). *The theory and practice of mental health consultation.* New York: Basic Books.

Carlen, P. L., McAndrews, M. P., Weiss, R. T., Doniger, M., Hill, J. M., Menzano, B., Farchik, K., Abarbanei, J., & Eastwood, M. R. (1994). Alcohol-related dementia in the institutionalized elderly. *Alcoholism: Clinical Experimental Research, 18*, 1330–1334.

Carney, S. S., Rich, C. L., Burke, P. A., & Fowler, R. C. (1994). Suicide over 60: The San Diego study. *Journal of the American Geriatrics Society, 42*, 174–180.

Carr, D., Schmader, K., Bergman, C., Simon, T. C., Jackson, T. W., Haviland, S., & O'Brien, J. (1991). A multidisciplinary approach in the evaluation of demented drivers referred to geriatric assessment centers. *Journal of the American Geriatrics Society, 39*, 1132–1136.

Carstensen, L. L., & Fisher, J. E. (1991). Treatment applications for psychological and behavioral problems of the elderly in nursing homes. In P. A. Wisocki (Ed.), *Handbook of clinical behavior therapy with the elderly client* (pp. 337–362). New York: Plenum Press.

Cassel, C. K., Rudberg, M. A., & Olshansky, S. J. (1992, Summer). The price of success: Health care in an aging society. *Health Affairs, 11*, 87–99.

Cattan, R. A., Barry, P. P., Mead, G., Reefe, W. E., Gay, A. & Silverman, M. (1990). Electroconvulsive therapy in octogenaraians. *Journal of the American Geriatrics Society, 38,* 753–758.

Cercy, S. P., & Bylsma, F. W. (1997). Lewy bodies and progressive dementia: A critical review and meta-analysis. *Journal of the International Neuropsychological Society, 3,* 179–194.

Chambless, D. L., Sanderson, W. C., Shoham, V., Johnson, S. B., Pope, K. S., Crits-Christoph, P., Baker, M., Johnson, B., Woody, S. R., Sue, S., Beutler, L. Williams, D. A., & McCurry, S. (1996). An update on empirically validated therapies. *Clinical Psychologist, 49,* 5–18.

Ciompi, L. (1987). Review of follow-up studies on long-term evolution and aging in schizophrenia. In N. E. Miller & G. D. Cohen (Eds.), *Schizophrenia and aging: Schizophrenia, paranoia, and schizophreniform disorders in later life* (pp. 37–51). New York: Guilford Press.

Clausen, J. A. (1986). A 15 to 20 year follow-up of married adult psychiatric patients. In L. Erlenmeyer-Kimling & N. E. Miller (Eds.), *Life-span research on the prediction of psychopathology* (pp. 175–194). Hillsdale, NJ: Erlbaum.

Cohen, C. I. (1990). Outcome of schizophrenia into later life: An overview. *Gerontologist, 30,* 790–797.

Cohen, G. D. (1992). The future of mental health and aging. In J. E. Birren, R. B. Sloane, G. D. Cohen, N. R. Hooyman, B. D. Lebowitz, M. Wykle, & D. E. Deutchman (Eds.), *Handbook of mental health and aging* (2nd ed., pp. 894–912). New York: Academic Press.

Cohen, B. J., Nestadt, G., Samuels, J. F., Romanoski, A. J., McHugh, P. R., & Rabins, P. V. (1994). Personality disorders in later life: A community study. *British Journal of Psychiatry, 165,* 493–499.

Cole, M. G. (1983). Age, age of onset, and course of primary depressive illness in the elderly. *Canadian Journal of Psychiatry, 28,* 102–104.

Cole, S. A., Woodard, J. L., Juncos, J. L., Kogos, J. L., Youngstrom, E. A., & Watts, R. L. (1996). Depression and disability in Parkinson's disease. *Journal of Neuropsychiatry and Clinical Neurosciences, 8,* 20–25.

Collins, M. W., & Abeles, N. (1996). Subjective memory complaints and depression in the able elderly. *Clinical Gerontologist, 16,* 29–54.

Committee on Aging, Group for the the Advancement of Psychiatry (1994). Impact of tacrine in the care of patients with Alzheimer's disease: What we know one year after FDA approval. *American Journal of Geriatric Psychiatry, 2,* 285–289.

Conwell, Y. (1994). Suicide in elderly patients. In L. S. Schneider, C. F. Reynolds, B. D. Lebowitz, & A. J. Friedhoff (Eds.), *Diagnosis and treatment of depression in late life* (pp. 397–418). Washington, DC: American Psychiatric Press.

Conwell, Y., & Brent, D. (1995). Suicide and aging. I: Patterns of psychiatric diagnosis. *International Psychogeriatrics, 7,* 149–164.

Conwell, Y., Olsen, K., Caine, E. D., & Flannery, C. (1991). Suicide in later life: Psychological autopsy findings. *International Psychogeriatrics, 3,* 59–66.

Cooper, A. F., Garside, R. F., & Kay, D. W. K. (1976). A comparison of deaf and non-deaf patients with paranoid and affective psychoses. *British Journal of Psychiatry, 129,* 532–538.

Cooper, A. F., & Porter, R. (1976). Visual acuity and ocular pathology in the paranoid and affective psychoses of later life. *Journal of Psychosomatic Research, 20,* 107–114.

Cooper, J. W. (1994). Drug-related problems in the elderly patient. *Generations, 18,* 19–26.

Corder, E., Saunders, A., Strittmatter, W., Schmechel, D., Gaskell, P., Small, G., Roses, A., Haines, J., & Pericak-Vance, M. (1993). Gene dose of apolipoprotein E type 4 allele and the risk of Alzheimer's disease in late onset families. *Science, 261,* 921–923.

Corsellis, J. A. N., Bruton, C. J., & Freeman-Browne, D. (1973). The aftermath of boxing. *Psychological Medicine, 3,* 270–303.

Costa, P. T., Jr., & McCrae, R. R. (1988). From catalog to classification: Murray's needs and the five-factor model. *Journal of Personality and Social Psychology, 55,* 258–265.

Craik, F. I. M. (1994) Memory changes in normal aging. *Current Directions in Psychological Science, 3,* 155–158.

Crimmins, E. M. (1984). Life expectancy and the older population: Demographic implications of recent and prospective trends in old age mortality. *Research on Aging, 6,* 490–514.

Crook, T., Bartus, R. T., Ferris, S. H., Whitehouse, P., Cohen, G. D., & Gershon, S. (1986) Age-associated memory impairment: Proposed diagnostic criteria and measures of clinical change. Report of a National Institute of Mental Health Work Group. *Developmental Neuropsychology, 2,* 261–276.

Crum, R. M., Anthony, J. C., Bassett, S. S., & Folstein, M. (1993). Population-based norms for the Mini-Mental State Examination by age and educational level. *Journal of the American Medical Association, 269,* 2386–2391.

Cummings, J. L. (1985). Organic delusions: Phenomenology, anatomical correlations, and review. *British Journal of Psychiatry, 146,* 184–197.

Cummings, J. L. (1987a). Multi-infarct dementia: Diagnosis and management. *Psychosomatics, 28,* 117–126.

Cummings, J. L. (1987b). Dementia syndromes: Neurobehavioral and neuropsychiatric features. *Journal of Clinical Psychiatry, 48*(5, Suppl.), 3–8.

Cummings, J. L., & Benson, D. F. (1992). *Dementia: A clinical approach* (2nd ed.). Stoneham, MA: Butterworth–Heinemann.

Cummings, J. L., Miller, B., Hill, M. A., & Neshkes, R. (1987). Neuropsychiatric aspects of multi-infarct dementia and dementia of the Alzheimer type. *Archives of Neurology, 44,* 389–393.

Cunningham, W. R., & Owens, W. A., Jr. (1983). The Iowa State Study of the Adult Development of Intellectual Abilities. In K. W. Schaie (Ed.), *Longitudinal studies of adult psychological development* (pp. 20–39). New York: Guilford Press.

Curtis, J. R., Geller, G., Stokes, E. J., Levine, D. M., & Moore, R. D. (1989). Characteristics, diagnosis, and treatment of alcoholism in elderly patients. *Journal of the American Geriatrics Society, 37,* 310–316.

Davison, A. M., Walker, G. S., Oli, H., & Lewins, A. M. (1982). Water supply aluminum concentration, dialysis dementia, and effect of reverse-osmosis water treatment. *Lancet, 2,* 785–787.

DeArmond, S. J., & Prusiner, S. B. (1995). Prion protein transgenes and the neuropathology in prion diseases. *Brain Pathology, 5,* 77–89.

D'Elia, L. F., Boone, K. B., & Mitrushina, M. (1995). *Handbook of normative data for neuropsychological assessment*. New York: Oxford University Press.

DeHart, S. S., & Hoffmann, N. G. (1997). Screening and diagnosis: Alcohol use disorders in older adults. In A. M. Gurnack (Ed.), *Older adults' misuse of alcohol, medicines, and other drugs*. (pp. 25–53). New York: Springer.

De Leo, D., & Diekstra, R. F. (1990). *Depression and suicide in late life*. Toronto: Hogrefe & Huber.

Delis, D. C., Kramer, J. H., Kaplan, E., & Ober, B. A. (1987). *The California Verbal Learning Test*. New York: Psychological Corporation.

Delis, D. C., Massman, P. J., Butters, N., Salmon, D. P., Kramer, J. H., & Cermak, L. (1991). Profiles of demented and amnesic patients on the California Verbal Learning Test: Implications for the assessment of memory disorders. *Psychological Assessment: A Journal of Clinical and Consulting Psychology, 3,* 19–26.

Dennis, M. S., & Lindesay, J. (1995). Suicide in the elderly: The United Kingdom perspective. *International Psychogeriatrics, 7,* 263–274.

Ditter, S. M., & Mirra, S. S. (1987). Neuropathologic and clinical features of Parkinson's disease in Alzheimer's disease patients. *Neurology, 37,* 754–760.

Double, K. L., Halliday, G. M., McRitchie, D. A., Reid, W. G., Hely, M. A., & Morris, J. G. (1996). Regional brain atrophy in idiopathic Parkinson's disease and diffuse Lewy body disease. *Dementia, 7,* 304–313.

Dowling, G. A. (1996). Specific interventions: Behavioral intervention strategies for sleep-activity disruption. *International Psychogeriatrics, 8,* 77–86.

Drebing, C. E., Van Gorp, W. G., Stuck, A. E., Mitrushina, M., & Beck, J. (1994). Early detection of cognitive decline in higher cognitively functioning older adults: Sensitivity and specificity of a neuropsychological screening battery. *Neuropsychology, 8,* 31–43.

Dresser, R. S. (1992). Autonomy revisited: The limits of anticipatory choices. In R. H. Binstock, S. G. Post, & P. J. Whitehouse (Eds.), *Dementia and aging: Ethics, values and policy choices* (pp. 71–85). Baltimore: Johns Hopkins University Press.

Egbert, A. M. (1993). Clinical clues to active alcoholism in the older patient. *Geriatrics, 48*(7), 63–69.

Elder, G. H., Jr., Shanahan, M. J., & Clipp, E. C. (1994). When war comes to men's lives: Life-course patterns in family, work, and health. *Psychology and Aging, 9,* 5–16.

Elkin, J., Shea, M. T., Watkins, J. T., Imber, S. D., Sotsky, S. M., Collins, J. R., Glass, D. R., Pilkonis, P. A., Leber, W. R., Docherty, J. P., Fiester, S. J., & Parloff, M. B. (1989). National Institute of Mental Health Treatment of Depression Collaborative Research Program: General effectiveness of treatment. *Archives of General Psychiatry, 46,* 971–983.

Engle-Friedman, M., Bootzin, R. R., Hazlewood, L., & Tsao, C. (1992). An evaluation of behavioral treatments for insomnia in the older adult. *Journal of Clinical Psychology, 48,* 77–90.

Erikson, E. H. (1950). *Childhood and society*. New York: Norton.

Erikson, E. H., Erikson, J. M., & Kivnick, H. Q. (1986). *Vital involvement in old age*. New York: Norton.

Erker, G. J., Searight, R., & Peterson, P. (1995). Patterns of neuropsychological functioning among patients with multi-infarct and Alzheimer's dementia: A comparative analysis. *International Psychogeriatrics, 7,* 393–406.

Evans, D. A., Funkenstein, H., Albert, M. S., Scherr, P. A., Cook, N. R., Chown, M. J., Hebert, L. E., Hennekens, C. H., & Taylor, J. O. (1989). Prevalence of Alzheimer's disease in a community population of older persons. *Journal of the American Medical Association, 262,* 2551–2556.

Evans, L. K. (1987). Sundown syndrome in institutionalized elderly. *Journal of the American Geriatrics Society, 35,* 101–108.

Farberow, N. L., Gallagher-Thompson, D., Gilewski, M., & Thompson, L. (1992). The role of social supports in the bereavement process of surviving spouses of suicide and natural deaths. *Suicide and Life-Threatening Behavior, 22,* 107–124.

Farrell, K. R., & Ganzini, L. (1995). Misdiagnosing delirium as depression in medically ill elderly patients. *Archives of Internal Medicine, 155,* 2459–2464.

Feinberg, L. F., & Kelly, K. (1995). A well-deserved break: Respite programs offered by California's statewide system of caregiver resource centers. *Gerontologist, 35,* 701–705.

Ferrier, I. N., & McKeith, I. G. (1991). Neuroanatomical and neurochemical changes in affective disorders in old age. *International Journal of Geriatric Psychiatry, 6,* 445–451.

Ferster, C. B. (1973). A functional analysis of depression. *American Psychologist, 28,* 857–870.

Filipp, S. H. (1996). Motivation and emotion. In J. E. Birren & K. W. Schaie (Eds.), *Handbook of the psychology of aging* (4th ed., pp. 218–235). San Diego: Academic Press.

Fillenbaum, G. G. (1987a). Activities of daily living. In G. L. Maddox (Ed.), *The encyclopedia of aging* (pp. 3–4). New York: Springer.

Fillenbaum, G. G. (1987b). Multidimensional functional assessment. In G. L. Maddox (Ed.), *The encyclopedia of aging* (pp. 460–464). New York: Springer.

Finkel, S. I., & Rosman, M. (1995). Six elderly suicides in a 1-year period in a rural midwestern community. *International Psychogeriatrics, 7,* 221–230.

Finlayson, R. D. (1997). Misuse of prescription drugs. In A. M. Gurnack (Ed.), *Older adults' misuse of alcohol, medicines, and other drugs* (pp. 158–184). New York: Springer.

Finlayson, R. D., & Davis, L. J. (1994). Prescription drug dependence in the elderly population: Demographic and clinical features of 100 inpatients. *Mayo Clinic Proceedings, 69,* 1137–1145.

Fisher, N. M., Pendergast, D. R., & Calkins, E. (1991). Muscle rehabilitation in impaired elderly nursing home residents. *Archives of Physical Medicine and Rehabilitation, 72,* 181–185.

Flicker, C. (1988). Neuropsychological evaluation of treatment effects in the elderly: A critique of tests in current use. *Psychopharmacology Bulletin, 24,* 535–556.

Flicker, C., Ferris, S. H., Crook, T., Bartus, R. T., & Reisberg, B. (1986). Cognitive decline in advanced age: Future directions for psychometric differentiation of normal and pathological age changes in cognitive function. *Developmental Neuropsychology, 2,* 309–322.

Flicker, C., Ferris, S. H., & Reisberg, B. (1993). A longitudinal study of cognitive function in elderly persons with subjective memory complaints. *Journal of the American Geriatrics Society, 41,* 1029–1032.

Floyd, M.,& Scogin, F. (1996). Effects of memory training on the subjective memory functioning and mental health of older adults: A meta-analysis. *Psychology and Aging, 12,* 150–161.

Folstein, M. F., Anthony, J. C., Parhad, I., Duffy, B., & Gruenberg, E. M. (1985). The meaning of cognitive impairment in the elderly. *Journal of the American Geriatrics Society, 33,* 228–235.

Folstein, M. F., Bassett, S. S., Romanoski, A. J., & Nestadt, G. (1991). The epidemiology of delirium in the community: The Eastern Baltimore Mental Health Survey. *International Psychogeriatrics, 3,* 169–176.

Folstein, M. F., Folstein, S. E., & McHugh, P. R. (1975). "Mini-Mental State": A practical method for grading the cognitive state of patients for the clinician. *Journal of Psychiatric Research, 12,* 189–198.

Frank, E. (1994). Long-term prevention of recurrences in elderly patients. In L. S. Schneider, C. F. Reynolds, B. D. Lebowitz, & A. J. Friedhoff (Eds.), *Diagnosis and treatment of depression in late life* (pp. 317–329). Washington, DC: American Psychiatric Press.

Frank, E., Kupfer, D. J., Perel, J. M., Cornes, C., Jarrett, D. B., Mallinger, A. G., Thase, M. E., McEachran, A. B., & Grochocinski, V. J. (1990). Three-year outcomes for maintenance therapies in recurrent depression. *Archives of General Psychiatry, 47,* 1093–1099.

Friedman, R., & Tappen, R. M. (1991). The effect of planned walking on communication in Alzheimer's disease. *Journal of the American Geriatrics Society, 39,* 650–654.

Fries, J. F. (1983). The compression of morbidity. *Milbank Memorial Fund Quarterly, 61,* 397–419

Friss, L. R., & Whitlatch, C. J. (1991). Who's taking care? A statewide study of family caregivers. *American Journal of Alzheimer's Care and Related Disorders and Research, 6,* 16–26.

Fuld, P. A. (1978). Psychological testing in the differential diagnosis of the dementias. In R. Katzman, R. D. Terry, & K. L. Bick (Eds.), *Alzheimer's disease, senile dementia and related disorders* (pp. 185–193). New York: Raven Press.

Funkenstein, H. H. (1988). Cerebrovascular disorders. In M. S. Albert & M. B. Moss (Eds.), *Geriatric neuropsychology* (pp. 179–210). New York: Guilford Press.

Gallagher, D., Rose, J., Rivera, P., Lovett, S., & Thompson, L. W. (1989). Prevalence of depression in family caregivers. *Gerontologist, 29,* 449–456.

Gallagher, D., Thompson, L. W., Baffa, G., Piatt, C., Ringering, L., & Stone, V. (1981). *Depression in the elderly: A behavioral treatment manual.* Unpublished manuscript, Andrus Gerontology Center, University of Southern California, Los Angeles, CA.

Gallagher-Thompson, D., & Thompson, L. W. (1995). Psychotherapy with older adults in theory and practice. In B. Bonger & L. Beutler (Eds.), *Comprehensive textbook of psychotherapy* (pp. 357–379). New York: Oxford University Press.

Gallagher-Thompson, D., & Thompson, L. W. (1996). Applying cognitive-behavioral therapy to the common psychological problems of later life. In S. H. Zarit & B. G. Knight (Eds.), *A guide to psychotherapy and aging* (pp. 61–82). Washington, DC: American Psychological Association.

Gatz, M. (1994). Application of assessment to therapy and intervention with older adults. In M. Storandt & G. R. VandenBos (Eds.), *Neuropsychological assessment of dementia and depression in older adults: A clinician's guide* (pp. 155–176). Washington, DC: Amercan Psycholgical Association.

Gatz, M., Fiske, A., Fox, L. S., Kaskie, B., Kasl-Godley, J. E., McCallum, T. J., & Wetherell, J. L. (in press). Empirically-validated psychological treatments for older adults. *Journal of Mental Health and Aging*.

Gatz, M., & Hurwicz, M. L. (1990). Are old people more depressed? Cross-sectional data on center for epidemiological studies depression scale factors. *Psychology and Aging, 5,* 284–290.

Gatz, M., Lowe, B., Berg, S., Mortimer, J., & Pedersen, N. (1994). Dementia: Not just a search for the gene. *Gerontologist, 34,* 251–255.

Gatz, M., Pedersen, N. L., Berg, S., Johansson, B., Johansson, K., Mortimer, J. A., Posner, S. F., Viitanen, M., Winblad, B., & Ahlbom, A. (1997). Heritability for Alzheimer's disease: The study of dementia in Swedish twins. *Journals of Gerontology: Medical Sciences, 52A,* M117–M125.

Gatz, M., & Warren C. (1989, November). *Pathways to electroconvulsive therapy: Depressed elders and distressed families.* Paper presented at the annual meeting of the Gerontological Society of America, Minneapolis, MI.

Genensky, S., Zarit, S. H., & Amaral, P. (1992). Visual care and rehabilitation of the elderly patient. In A. A. Rosenblum, Jr., & M. W. Morgan (Eds.), *Vision and aging: General and clinical perspectives* (2nd ed., pp. 424–444). New York: Professional Press.

George, L. K. (1994). Social factors and depression in late life. In L. S. Schneider, C. F. Reynolds, B. D. Lebowitz, & A. J. Friedhoff (Eds.), *Diagnosis and treatment of depression in late life* (pp. 131–154). Washington, DC: American Psychiatric Press.

German, P. S., Shapiro, S., & Kramer, M. (1986). Nursing home study of the Eastern Baltimore Epdemiological Catchment Area Study. In M. S. Harper & B. D. Lebowitz (Eds.), *Mental illness in nursing homes: Agenda for research* (pp. 27–40). Rockville, MD: National Institute of Mental Health.

Girolamo, G., & Reich, J. H. (1993). *Personality disorders.* Geneva: World Health Organization.

Glasscote, R. M., Gudemen, J. E., & Miles, D. G. (1977). *Creative mental health services for the elderly.* Washington, DC: American Psychiatric Association

Golden, C. J., Ariel, R. N., McKay, S. E., Wilkening, G. N., Wolf, B. A., & MacInnes, W. D. (1982). The Luria–Nebraska Neuropsychological Battery: Theoretical orientation and comment. *Journal of Consulting and Clinical Psychology, 50,* 291–300.

Goldstein, G., Zubin, J., & Pogue-Geile, M. (1991). Hospitalization and the cognitive deficits of schizophrenia: The influences of age and education. *Journal of Nervous and Mental Disease, 179,* 202–206.

Goodman, C. R., & Zarit, S. H. (1994). Effects of education on assessment of age-associated memory impairment. *American Journal of Geriatric Psychiatry, 2,* 118–123.

Goodwin, F. K., & Bunney, W. E., Jr. (1973). Psychobiological aspects of stress and affective illness. In J. P. Scott & E. C. Senay (Eds.), *Separation and depression: Clinical and research aspects* (pp. 91–112). Washington, DC: American Association for the Advancement of Science.

Gorham, D. R. (1956). A proverbs test for clinical and experimental use. *Psychological Reports, 1,* 1–12.

Grant, R. W., & Casey, D. A. (1995). Adapting cognitive behavioral therapy for the frail elderly. *International Psychogeriatrics, 7,* 561–571.

Graves, A. B., White, E., Koepsell, T., Reifler, B., Van Belle, G., & Larson, E. (1990). The association between aluminum-coating products and Alzheimer's disease. *Journal of Clinical Epidemiology, 43,* 35–44.

Green, G. R., Linsk, N. L., & Pinkson, E. M. (1986). Modification of verbal behavior of the mentally impaired elderly by their spouses. *Journal of Applied Behavior Analysis, 19,* 329–336.

Greene, R. & Ferraro, E. (1996, November). *Adult day care services in New Jersey.* Paper presented at the annual meeting of the Gerontological Society of America, Washington, DC.

Grisso, T. (1994). Clinical assessments for legal competence of older adults. In M. Storandt & G. R. VandenBos (Eds.), *Neuropsychological assessment of dementia and depression in older adults: A clinician's guide* (pp. 119–140). Washington, DC: American Psychological Association.

Gurian, B., & Miner, J. H. (1991). Clinical presentation of anxiety in the elderly. In C. Salzman & B. Lebowitz. (Eds.), *Anxiety in the elderly* (pp. 31–46). New York: Springer.

Gurland, B. J., Copeland, J., Kuriansky, J., Kelleher, M. J., Sharpe, L., & Dean, L. (1983). *The mind and mood of aging.* New York: Haworth.

Gurland, B. J., & Cross, P. S. (1982). Epidemiology of psychopathology in old age. *Psychiatric Clinics of North America, 5,* 11–26.

Gurland, B., Wilder, D., Cross, P., Lantigua, R., Teresi, J., Barrett, V., Stern, Y., & Mayeux, R. (1995). Relative rates of dementia by multiple case definitions, over two prevalence periods, in three sociocultural groups. *American Journal of Geriatric Psychiatry, 3,* 6–20.

Gustafson, L., Brun, A., & Passant, U. (1992). Frontal lobe degeneration of non-Alzheimer type. *Baillieres Clinical Neurology, 1,* 559–582.

Haan, N., Millsap, R., & Harka, E. (1986). As time goes by: Change and stability in personality over fifty years. *Psychology and Aging, 1,* 220–232.

Haley, J. (1976). *Problem-solving therapy.* San Francisco: Jossey-Bass.

Haley, W. E. (1983). A family-behavioral approach to the treatment of the cognitively impaired elderly. *Gerontologist, 23,* 18–20.

Haley, W. E. (1996). The medical context of psychotherapy with the elderly. In S. H. Zarit & B. Knight (Eds.), *A guide to psychotherapy and aging* (pp. 221–240). Washington, DC: American Psychological Association.

Hänninen, T., Hallikainen, M., Koivisto, K., Helkala, E. L., Reinikainen, K. J., Soininen, H., Mykkänen, L., Laakso, M., Pyörälä, K., & Riekkinen, P. J. (1995). A follow-up study of age-associated memory impairment: Neuropsychological predictors of dementia. *Journal of the American Geriatrics Society, 43,* 1007–1015.

Harding, C. M., Brooks, G. W., Ashikaga, T., Strauss, J. S., & Breier, A. (1987). The Vermont Longitudinal Study of Persons with Severe Mental Illness: I. Methodology, study sample and overall status 32 years later. *American Journal of Psychiatry, 144,* 18–26.

Hardy, John. (1993). Genetic mistakes point the way for Alzheimer's Disease. *Journal of the National Institutes of Health Research, 5,* 46–49.

Hasher, L., & Zacks, R. T. (1979). Automatic and effortful processes in memory. *Journal of Experimental Psychology: General, 108,* 350–388.

Harvey, R. J., & Rossor, M. N. (1995). Does early-onset Alzheimer disease constitute a distinct subtype? The contribution of molecular genetics. *Alzheimer Disease and Associated Disorders, 9*(Suppl. 1), S7–S13.

Hayden, C. M. & Camp, C. J. (1995). Spaced-retrieval: A memory intervention for dementia in Parkinson's disease. *Clinical Gerontologist, 16*, 80–82.

Heaton, R., Paulsen, J., McAdams, L. A., Kuck, J., Zisook, S., Braff, D., Harris, J., & Jeste, D. V. (1994). Neuropsychological deficits in schizophrenia. *Archives of General Psychiatry, 51*, 469–476.

Heikkinen, M. E., & Lönnqvist, J. K. (1995). Recent life events in elderly suicide: A nationwide study in Finland. *International Psychogeriatrics, 7*, 287–300.

Helson, R., & Moane, G. (1987). Personality change in women from college to midlife. *Journal of Personality and Social Psychology, 53*, 176–186.

Henderson, V. W., Paganini-Hill, A., Emanuel C. K., Dunn, M. E., & Buckwalter, J. G. (1994). Estrogen replacement therapy in older women: Comparisons between Alzheimer's disease cases and nondemented control subjects. *Neurology, 51*, 896–900.

Herr, J. J., & Weakland, J. H. (1979). *Counseling elders and their families.* New York: Springer.

Hill, R. D., Sheikh, J. I., & Yesavage, J. A. (1988). Pretraining enhances mnemonic training in elderly adults. *Experimental Aging Research, 14*, 207–211.

Himmelfarb, S., & Murrell, S. A. (1984). The prevalence and correlates of anxiety symptoms in older adults. *Journal of Psychology, 116*, 159–167.

Hinchliffe, A. C., Hyman, I. L., Blizard, B., & Livingston, G. (1995). Behavioural complications of dementia—Can they be treated? *International Journal of Geriatric Psychiatry, 10*, 839–847.

Hinrichsen, G. A. (1992). Recovery and relapse from major depressive disorder in the elderly. *American Journal of Psychiatry, 149*, 1575–1579.

Hinrichsen, G. A., & Hernandez, N. A. (1993). Factors associated with recovery from and relapse into major depressive disorder in the elderly. *American Journal of Psychiatry, 150*, 1820–1825.

Hinrichsen, G. A., & Zweig, R. A. (1994). Family issues in late-life depression. *Journal of Long Term Home Health Care, 13*, 4–15.

Hodges, J. R. (1994). Pick's disease. In A. Burns & R. Levy (Eds.), *Dementia* (pp. 739–749). London: Chapman & Hall.

Hofland, B. F. (1995). Resident autonomy in long-term care: Paradoxes and challenges. In L. M. Gamroth, J. Semradek, & E. M. Tornquist (Eds.), *Enhancing autonomy in long-term care: Concepts and strategies* (pp. 15–33). New York: Springer.

Holland, J. C., & Tross, S. (1985). The psychosocial and neuropsychiatric sequelae of the acquired immunodeficiency syndrome and related disorders. *Annals of Internal Medicine, 103*, 760–764.

Holmes, C. (1997). Apolipoprotein E: Implications and applications. In C. Holmes & R. Howard (Eds.), *Advances in old age psychiatry: Chromosomes to community care* (pp. 30–42). Bristol, PA: Wrightson Biomedical.

Holmes, D., Splaine, M., Teresi, J., Ory, M., Barret, V., Monaco, C., & Ramirez, M. (1994). What makes special care special: Concept mapping as a definitional tool. *Alzheimer's Disease and Associated Disorders, 8*, S41–S59.

Homma, A., & Hasegawa, K. (1989). Recent developments in gerontopsychiatric research on age-associated dementia in Japan. *International Psychogeriatrics, 1,* 31–49.

Horn, J. L. (1982). The theory of fluid and crystallized intelligence in relation to concepts of cognitive psychology and aging in adulthood. In F. I. M. Craik & S. Trehub (Eds.), *Aging and cognitive processes* (pp. 237–278). New York: Plenum Press.

Horn, J. L., & Cattell, R. B. (1967). Age differences in fluid and crystallized intelligence. *Acta Psychologica, 26,* 107–129.

Horowitz, A., Reinhardt, J. P., McInerney, R., & Balisteri, E. (1994, November). *Psychosocial adaptation to age-related vision loss over time.* Paper presented at the annual meeting of the Gerontological Society of America, Atlanta, GA.

Hughes, C. P., Berg, L., Danziger, W. L., Coben, L. A., & Martin, R. L. (1982). A new clinical scale for the staging of dementia. *British Journal of Psychiatry, 140,* 566–572.

Hultsch, D. (1971). Adult age differences in free classification and free recall. *Developmental Psychology, 4,* 338–342.

Hunt, L., Morris, J. C., Edwards, D., & Wilson, B. S. (1993). Driving performance in persons with mild senile dementia of the Alzheimer type. *Journal of the American Geriatrics Society, 41,* 747–753.

Hussian, R. A. (1986). Severe behavioral problems. In L. Teri & P. M. Lewinsohn (Eds.), *Geropsychological assessment and treatment* (pp. 121–143). New York: Springer.

Hussian, R. A., & Davis, R. L. (1985). *Responsive care: Behavioral interventions with elderly persons.* Champaign, IL: Research Press.

Inouye, S. K., & Charpentier, P. A. (1996). Precipitating factors for delirium in hospitalized elderly persons. Predictive model and interrelationship with baseline vulnerability. *Journal of the American Medical Association, 275,* 852–857.

Inouye, S. K., vanDyck, C. H., Alessi, C. A., Balkin, S., Siegal, A. P., & Horwitz, R. I., (1990). Clarifying confusion: The confusion assessment method. *Annals of Internal Medicine, 113,* 941–948.

Ivnik, R. J., Malec, J. F., Smith, G. E., Tangalos, E. G., Peterson, R. C., Kokmen, E., & Kurland, L. T. (1992a). Mayo's older Americans normative studies: Updated AVLT norms for ages 56–97. *Clinical Neuropsycholgist, 6,* 83–104.

Ivnik, R. J., Malec, J. F., Smith, G. E., Tangalos, E. G., Petersen, R. C. Kokmen, E., & Kurland, L. T. (1992b). Mayo's older Americans normative studies: WAIS-R norms for ages 56 to 97. *Clinical Neuropsychologist, 6,* 1–30.

Ivnik, R. J., Malec, J. F., Smith, G. E., Tangalos, E. G., Petersen, R. C. Kokmen, E., & Kurland, L. T. (1992c). Mayo's older Americans normative studies: WMS-R norms for ages 56 to 94. *Clinical Neuropsychologist, 6,* 49–82.

Ivnik, R. J., Smith, G. E., Malec, J. F., Kokmen, E., & Tangalos, E. G. (1994). Mayo cognitive factor scales: Distinguishing normal and clinical samples by profile variability. *Neuropsychology, 8,* 203–209.

Jackson, S. W. (1969). Galen on mental disorders. *Journal of the History of the Behavioral Sciences, 5,* 365.

Jacobs, D., Troster, A. I., Butters, N., Salmon, D. P., & Cermak, L. S. (1990). Intrusion errors on the Visual Reproduction test of the Wechsler Memory Scale and the Wechsler Memory Scale—Revised: An analysis of demented and amnesic patients. *Clinical Neuropsychology, 4,* 177–191.

Jacobs, J. W., Bernhard, M. R., Delgado, A., & Strain, J. L. (1977). Screening for organic mental syndromes in the medically ill. *Annals of Internal Medicine, 86,* 40–46.

Jeste, D. V., & Wyatt, R. J. (1987). Aging and tardive dyskinesia. In N. E. Miller & G. D. Cohen (Eds.), *Schizophrenia and aging: Schizophrenia, paranoia and schizophreniform disorders in later life* (pp. 275–286). New York: Guilford Press.

Jette, A. M. (1996). Disability trends and transitions. In R. H. Binstock & L. K. George (Eds.), *Handbook of aging and the social sciences* (pp. 94–114). San Diego: Academic Press.

Johansson, B. (1988–1989). *The MIR—Memory-in-Reality Test.* Stockholm: Psykologiförlaget AB.

Johansson, B., Allen-Burge, R., & Zarit, S. H. (1997). Self-reports on memory functioning in a longitudinal study of the oldest old: Relation to current, prospective, and retrospective performance. *Journal of Gerontology: Psychological Sciences, 52B,* P139–P146.

Johansson, B., & Zarit, S. H. (1991). Dementia and cognitive impairment in the oldest old: A comparison of two rating methods. *International Psychogeriatrics, 3,* 29–38.

Johansson, B., & Zarit, S. H. (1995). Prevalence and incidence of dementia in the oldest old: A study of a population based sample of 84–90 year olds in Sweden. *International Journal of Geriatric Psychiatry, 10,* 359–366.

Johansson, B., & Zarit, S. H. (1997). Early cognitive markers of the incidence of dementia and mortality: A longitudinal population-based study of the oldest old. *International Journal of Geriatric Psychiatry, 12,* 53–59.

Johansson, B., Zarit, S. H., & Berg, S. (1992). Changes in cognitive functioning of the oldest old. *Journals of Gerontology: Psychological Sciences, 47,* P75–P80.

Judd, L. L., Rapaport, M. H., Paulus, M. P., & Brown, J. L. (1994). Subsyndromal symptomatic depression: A new mood disorder. *Journal of Clinical Psychiatry, 55*(4, Suppl.), 18–28.

Jung, C. G. (1933). *Modern man in search of a soul.* New York: Harcourt Brace Jovanovich.

Kahn, R. L. (1975). The mental health system and the future aged. *Gerontologist, 15*(1, Pt. 2), 24–31.

Kahn, R. L., & Fink, M. (1959). Personality factors in behavioral response to electroshock therapy. *Journal of Neuropsychiatry, 1,* 45–49.

Kahn, R. L., Goldfarb, A. I., Pollack, M., & Peck, A. (1960). Brief objective measures for the determination of mental status in the aged. *American Journal of Psychiatry, 117,* 326–328.

Kahn, R. L., & Miller, N. E. (1978). Assessment of altered brain function in the aged. In M. Storandt, I. C. Siegler, & M. F. Elias (Eds.), *The clinical psychology of aging* (pp. 43–69). New York: Plenum Press.

Kahn, R. L., Pollack, M., & Goldfarb, A. I. (1961). Factors related to individual differences in mental status of institutionalized aged. In P. Hoch & J. Zubin, (Eds.), *Psychopathology of aging* (pp. 104–113). New York: Grune & Stratton.

Kahn, R. L., Zarit, S. H., Hilbert, N. M., & Niederehe, G. A. (1975). Memory complaint and impairment in the aged: The effect of depression and altered brain function. *Archives of General Psychiatry, 32,* 1569–1573.

Kamboh, M., Sanghera, D., Ferrell, R., & DeKosky, S. (1995). APOE*4-associated Alzheimer's disease risk is modified by alpha-1-antichymotrypsin polymorphism. *Nature Genetics, 10,* 486–488.

Kane, R. A., & Wilson, K. B. (1993). *Assisted living in the United States: A new paradigm for residential care for frail older persons?* Washington, DC: American Association of Retired Persons.

Kaplan, E., Goodglass, H., & Weintraub, S. (1983). *Boston Naming Test.* Philadelphia: Lea & Febiger.

Kapp, M. B. (1996). Alternatives to guardianship: Enhanced autonomy for diminished capacity. In M. Smyer, K. W. Schaie, & M. B. Kapp (Eds.), *Older adults' decision-making and the law* (pp. 182–201). New York: Springer.

Kaszniak, A. W. (1986). The neuropsychology of dementia. In I. Grant & K. M. Adams (Eds.), *Neuropsychological assessment of neuropsychiatric disorders* (pp. 172–220). New York: Oxford University Press.

Kaszniak, A. W. (1987). Neuropsychological consultation to geriatricians: Issues in the assessment of memory complaints. *Clinical Neuropsychologist, 1,* 35–46.

Kaszniak, A. W. (1990). Psychological assessment of the aging individual. In J. E. Birren & K. W. Schaie (Eds.), *Handbook of the psychology of aging* (3rd ed., pp. 427–445). New York: Academic Press.

Kaszniak, A. W. (1996). Techniques and instruments for assessment of the elderly. In S. H. Zarit & B. G. Knight (Eds.), *A guide to psychotherapy and aging* (pp. 163–219). Washington, DC: American Psychological Association.

Kaszniak, A. W., Keyl, P., & Albert, M. (1991). Dementia and the older driver. *Human Factors, 33,* 527–537.

Kaszniak, A. W., & DiTraglia Christenson, G. (1994). Differential diagnosis of dementia and depression. In M. Storandt & G. R. VandenBos (Eds.), *Neuropsychological assessment of dementia and depression in older adults: A clinician's guide* (pp. 81–118). Washington, DC: Amercan Psycholgical Association.

Katz, I. R., Parmalee, P., & Brubaker, K. (1991). Toxic and metabolic encephalopathies in long-term care patients. *International Psychogeriatrics, 3,* 337–348.

Katz, S., Ford, A., Moskowitz, R., Jackson, B., & Jaffee, M. (1963). Studies of illness in the aged: The Index of ADL, a standardized measure of biological and psychosocial function. *Journal of the American Medical Association, 185,* 94–99.

Kawas, C., Metter, E. J., Resnick, S., Zonderman, A., Bacal, C. Lingle, D. D., Morrison, A., Corrada, M., & Brookmeyer, R. (1997). 16-year study is further evidence that estrogen replacement may be protective against Alzheimer's disease. *Neurology, 48,* 1517–1521.

Kay, D. W. K. (1995). The epidemiology of age-related neurological disease and dementia. *Reviews of Clinical Gerontology, 5,* 39–56.

Kay, D. W. K., Cooper, A. F., Garside, R. F., & Roth, M. (1976). The differentiation of paranoid from affective psychoses by patients' premorbid characteristics. *British Journal of Psychiatry,129,* 207–215.

Kay, D. W. K., Henderson, A. S., Scott, R., Wilson, J., Rickwood, D., & Grayson, D. A. (1985). Dementia and depression among the elderly living in the Hobart community: The effect of the diagnostic criteria on the prevalence rates. *Psychological Medicine, 15,* 771–788.

Kemper, P., & Murtaugh, C. M. (1991). Lifetime use of nursing home care. *New England Journal of Medicine, 324,* 595–629.

Kiecolt-Glaser, J. K., Dura, J. R., Speicher, C. E., Trask, O. J., & Glaser, R. (1991). Spousal caregivers of dementia victims: Longitudinal changes in immunity and health. *Psychosomatic Medicine, 53,* 345–362.

Kiloh, L. G. (1961). Pseudo-dementia. *Acta Psychiatrica Scandinavica, 37,* 336–351.

Kinsella, K., & Taeuber, C. M. (1993). *An aging world II* (International Population Reports Publication No. P95/92–3). Washington, DC: U. S. Department of Commerce.

Kirby, M., & Lawlor, B. A. (1995). Biologic markers and neurochemical correlates of agitation and psychosis in dementia. *Journal of Geriatric Psychiatry and Neurology 8*(Suppl. 1), S2–S7.

Klatka, L. A., Louis, E. D., & Schiffer, R. B., (1996). Psychiatric features in diffuse Lewy body disease: A clinicopathologic study using Alzheimer's disease and Parkinson's disease comparison groups. *Neurology, 47,* 1148–1152.

Klerman, G. L., Weissman, M. M., Rounsaville, B. J., & Chevron, E. (1984). *Interpersonal psychotherapy of depression.* New York: Basic Books.

Kliegl, R. Smith, J., & Baltes, P. B. (1989). Testing the limits and the study of adult age differences in cognitive plasticity of a mnemonic skill. *Developmental Psychology, 25,* 247–256.

Knapp, M. J., Knopman, D., Solomon, P., Pendlebury, W., Davis, C., & Gracon, S. A. (1994). 30-week randomized controlled trial of high-dose tacrine in patients with Alzheimer's disease. *Journal of the American Medical Association, 271,* 985–991.

Knight, B. G. (1986). *Psychotherapy with older adults.* Beverly Hills, CA: Sage.

Knight, B. G. (1989). *Outreach with the elderly: Community education, assessment and therapy.* New York: New York University Press.

Knight, B. G. (1992). *Older adults in psychotherapy: Case histories.* Newbury Park, CA: Sage.

Knight, B. G., Teri, L., Wohlford, P., & Santos, J. (1995). *Mental health services for older adults: Implications for training and practice in geropsychology.* Washington, DC: American Psychological Association.

Kocsis, J. H., Zisook, S., Davidson, J., Shelton, R., Yonkers, K., Hellerstein, D. J., Rosenbaum, J., & Halbreich, U. (1997). Double-blind comparison of sertraline, imipramine, and placebo in the treatment of dysthymia: Psychosocial outcomes. *American Journal of Psychiatry, 154,* 390–395.

Koenig, H. G., & Blazer, D. G. (1992). Mood disorders and suicide. In J. E. Birren, R. B. Sloane, G. D. Cohen, N. R. Hooyman, B. D. Lebowitz, M. Wykle, & D. E. Deutchman (Eds.), *Handbook of mental health and aging* (2nd ed., pp. 380–400). New York: Academic Press.

Kokmen, E., Beard, C. M., Offord, K. P., & Kurland, L. T. (1989). Prevalence of medically diagnosed dementia in a defined United States population: Rochester, Minnesota, January 1, 1975. *Neurology, 39,* 773–776.

Kosaka, K., Tsuchiya, K., & Yoshimura, M. (1988). Lewy body disease with and without dementia: A clinicopathological study of 35 cases. *Clinical Neuropathology, 7,* 299–305.

Kraepelin, E. (1971). *Dementia praecox and paraphrenia* (R. M. Barclay, Trans.). Huntington, NY: Krieger. (Original work published 1919)

Kramer, B. A. (1987). Electroconvulsive therapy use in geriatric depression. *Journal of Nervous and Mental Disease, 175,* 233–235.

Lachman, J. L., & Lachman, R. (1980). Age and actualization of knowledge. In L. W. Poon, J. L. Fozard, L. S. Cermak, D. Arenberg, & L. W. Thompson (Eds.), *New directions in memory and aging* (pp. 313–343). Hillsdale, NJ: Erlbaum.

Lachman, M. E. (1989). Personality and aging at the crossroads: Beyond stability and change. In K. W. Schaie & C. Schooler (Eds.), *Social structure and aging: Psychological processes* (pp. 167–189). Hillsdale, NJ: Erlbaum.

Lai, F., & Williams, R. S. (1989). A prospective study of Alzheimer's disease in Down's syndrome. *Archives of Neurology, 46,* 849–853.

Lansbury, P. T., Jr., Costa, P. R., Griffiths, J. M., Simon, E. J., Auger, M., Halverson, K. J., Kocisko, C. A., Hendsch, Z. S., Ashburn, T. T., Spencer, R. G., Tidor, B., & Griffin, R. G. (1995). Structural model for the beta-amyloid fibril based on interstrand alignment of an antiparallel-sheet comprising a C-terminal peptide. *Nature Structural Biology, 2,* 990–998.

Larson, E. B., Reifler, B. V., Featherstone, H. J., & English, D. R. (1984). Dementia in elderly outpatients: A prospective study. *Annals of Internal Medicine, 100,* 417–423.

La Rue, A., D'Elia, L. F., Clark, E. O., Spar, J. E., Jarvik, L. F. (1986). Clinical tests of memory in dementia, depression and healthy aging. *Journal of Psychology and Aging, 1,* 69–77.

Lawton, M. P. (1986). *Environment and aging.* Albany, NY: Center for the Study of Aging.

Lawton, M. P., & Brody, E. (1969). Assessment of older people: Self-maintaining and instrumental activities of daily living. *Gerontologist, 9,* 179–186.

Lawton, M. P., & Nahemow, L. (1973). Ecology and the aging process. In C. Eisdorfer & M. P. Lawton (Eds.), *The psychology of adult development and aging* (pp. 619–674). Washington, DC: American Psychological Association.

Lebowitz, B. D., Light, E., & Bailey, F. (1987). Mental health center services for the elderly: The impact of coordination with Area Agencies on Aging. *Gerontologist, 27,* 699–702.

Lee, V. M.-Y., Balin, B. J., Otvos, L., Jr., & Trojanowski, J. Q. (1991). A68: A major subunit of paired helical filaments and derivatized forms of normal tau. *Science, 251,* 675–678.

Leuchter, A. F. (1994). Brain structural and functional correlates of late-life depression. In L. S. Schneider, C. F. Reynolds, B. D. Lebowitz, & A. J. Friedhoff (Eds.), *Diagnosis and treatment of depression in late life* (pp. 117–130). Washington, DC: American Psychiatric Press.

Leverenz, J., & Sumi, S. M. (1986). Parkinson's disease in patients with Alzheimer's disease. *Archives of Neurology, 43,* 662–664.

Levinson, D. J. (1986). A conception of adult development. *American Psychologist, 41,* 3–13.

Levkoff, S., Cleary, P., Liptzin, B., & Evans, D. A. (1991). Epidemiology of delirium: An overview of research issues and findings. *International Psychogeriatrics, 3,* 149–167.

Levkoff, S., Liptzin, B., Cleary, P., Reilly, C. H., & Evans, D. (1991). Review of research instruments and techniques used to detect delirium. *International Psychogeriatrics, 3,* 253–271.

Levy-Lahad, E., Wijsman, E. M., Nemens, E., Anderson, L., Goodard, K. A., Weber, J. T., Bird, T. D., & Schellenberg, G. D. (1995). A familial Alzheimer's disease locus on chromosome 1. *Science, 269,* 970–973.

Lewinsohn, P. M. (1975). The behavioral study and treatment of depression. In M. Hersen, R. M. Eisler, & P. M. Miller, (Eds.), *Progress in behavior modification.* (pp. 19–64). New York: Academic Press.

Lewinsohn, P. M., Antonuccio, D. O., Steinmetz, J. L., & Teri, L. (1984). *The coping and depression course: A psychoeducational intervention for unipolar depression*. Eugene, OR: Castalia.

Lewinsohn, P. M., Biglan, A., & Zeiss, A. M. (1976). Behavioral treatment of depression. In P. O. Davidson (Ed.), *The behavioral management of anxiety, depression and pain* (pp. 91–146). New York: Brunner/Mazel.

Lewinsohn, P. M., Fenn, D. S., Stanton, A. K., & Franklin, J. (1986). Relation of age at onset to duration of episode in unipolar depression. *Psychology and Aging, 1,* 63–68.

Lewinsohn, P. M., Hoberman, H. M., & Rosenbaum, M. (1988). A prospective study of risk factors for unipolar depression. *Journal of Abnormal Psychology, 97,* 251–264.

Lewinsohn, P. M., & Libet, L. (1972) Pleasant events, activity schedules and depression. *Journal of Abnormal Psychology, 79,* 291–295.

Lewinsohn, P. M., & MacPhillamy, D. (1974). The relationship between age and engagement in pleasant activities. *Journal of Gerontology, 29,* 290–294.

Lewinsohn, P. M., Muñoz, R. F., Youngren, M. A., & Zeiss, A. M. (1992). *Control your depression* (rev. ed.). New York: Simon & Schuster.

Lewinsohn, P. M., Rohde, P., Seeley, J. R., & Fischer, S. A. (1991). Age and depression: Unique and shared effects. *Psychology and Aging, 6,* 247–260.

Lezak, M. D. (1995). *Neuropsychological assessment* (3rd ed.). New York: Oxford University Press.

Liberto, J. G., & Oslin, D. W. (1997). Early versus late onset of alcoholism in the elderly. In A. M. Gurnack (Ed.), *Older adults' misuse of alcohol, medicines, and other drugs* (pp. 94–112). New York: Springer.

Light, L. L. (1990). Interactions between memory and language in old age. In J. E. Birren & K. W. Schaie (Eds.), *Handbook of the psychology of aging* (3rd ed., pp. 275–290). New York: Academic Press.

Linde, K., Ramirez, G., Mulrow, C. D., Pauls, A., Weidenhammer, W., & Melchart, D. (1996). St. John's wort for depression—An overview and meta-analysis of randomised clinical trials. *British Medical Journal, 313,* 253–258.

Lindesay, J., Briggs, K., & Murphy, E. (1989). The Guy's/Age Concern Survey: Prevalence rates of cognitive impairment, depression and anxiety in an urban elderly community. *British Journal of Psychiatry, 155,* 317–329.

Linehan, M. M. (1993). *Cognitive-behavioral treatment of borderline personality disorder.* New York: Guilford Press.

Lipowski, Z. J. (1990). *Delirium: Acute confusional states*. New York: Oxford University Press.

Liu, H., Lin, K., Teng, E., Wang, S., Fuh, J., Guo, N., Chou, P., Hu, H., & Chiang, B. (1995). Prevalence and subtypes of dementia in Taiwan: A community survey of 5297 individuals. *Journal of the American Geriatrics Society, 43,* 144–149.

Liu, U., Stern., Y., Chun, M. R., Jacobs, D. M., Yau, P., & Goldman, J. E. (1977). Pathological correlates of extrapyramidal signs in Alzheimer's disease. *Annals of Neurology, 41,* 368–374.

Livingston, G., Hawkins, A., Graham, N., Blizard, B., & Mann, A. (1990). The Gospel Oak Study: Prevalence rates of dementia, depression and activity limitation among elderly residents in inner London. *Psychological Medicine, 20,* 137–146.

Loeb, P. (1983). *Validity of the Community Competence Scale with the elderly.* Unpublished doctoral dissertation, Saint Louis University, Saint Louis, MO.

Loevinger, J. (1976). *Ego development: Conception and theory.* San Francisco: Jossey-Bass.

Logsdon, R. G., & Teri, L. (1995). Depression in Alzheimer's disease patients: Caregivers as surrogate reporters. *Journal of American Geriatrics Society, 43,* 150–155.

Lohr, J. B., Jeste, D. V., Harris, M. J., & Salzman, C. (1992). Treatment of disordered behavior. In C. Salzman (Ed.), *Clinical geriatric psychopharmacology* (pp. 79–114). Baltimore: Williams & Wilkins.

Lopera, F., Ardilla A., Martinez, A., Madrigal, L., Arango-Viana, J. C., Lemere, C. A., Arango-Lasprilla, J. C., Hincapié, L., Arcos-Burgos, M., Ossa, J. E., Behrens, I. M., Norton, J., Lendon, C., Goate, A. M., Ruiz-Linares, A. R., Rosselli, M., & Kosik, K. S. (1997). Clinical features of early-onset Alzheimer disease in a large kindred with an E280A Presenilin-1 mutatation. *Journal of the American Medical Association, 277,* 793–799.

Loranger, A. W., & Levine, P. M. (1978). Age at onset of bipolar affective illness. *Archives of General Psychiatry, 35,* 1345–1348.

Lowenstein, D. A., Amigo, E., Duara, R., Guterman, A., Hurwitz, D., Berkowitz, N., Wilkie, F. Weinberg, G., Black, B. M., Gittleman, B., & Eisdorfer, C. (1989). A new scale for the assessment of functional status in Alzheimer's disease and related disorders. *Journal of Gerontology, 44,* 114–121.

Lund, D. A., Hill, R. D., Caserta, M. S., & Wright, S. D. (1995). Video Respite™: An innovative resource for family, professional caregivers, and persons with dementia. *Gerontologist, 35,* 683–687.

Luxenberg, J. S., Haxby, J. V., Creasey, H., Sundaram, M., & Rapoport, S. I. (1987). Rate of ventricular enlargement in dementia of the Alzheimer type correlates with rate of neuropsychological deterioration. *Neurology, 37,* 1135–1140.

Mace, N., & Rabins, P. V. (1991). *The thirty-six hour day* (2nd ed.). Baltimore: Johns Hopkins University Press.

MacKnight, C., & Rockwood, K. (1996). Bovine spongiform encephalopathy and Creutzfeldt–Jakob disease: Implications for physicians. *Canadian Medical Association Journal, 155,* 529–536.

Macmillan, D. (1967). Problems of a geriatric mental health service. *British Journal of Psychiatry, 113,* 175–181.

Mahurin, R. K., DeBettignies, B. H., & Pirozzolo, F. J. (1991). Structured assessment of indpendent living skills: Preliminary report of a performance measure of functional abilities in dementia. *Journal of Gerontology: Psychological Sciences, 46,* P58–P66.

Maletta, G. (1990). The concept of "reversible" dementia: How nonreliable terminology may impair effective treatment. *Journal of the American Geriatrics Society, 38,* 136–140.

Malmberg, B., Sundström, G., & Zarit, S. H. (1995). Evaluation des modes d'habitat et maladie d'Alzheimer en Suède. In P. Vellas, J. L. Albarede, & P. J. Garry (Eds.), *L'année gérontologique* (Vol. 9, pp. 226–227). Paris: Serdi.

Malmberg, B., & Zarit, S. H. (1993). Group homes for dementia patients: An innovative model in Sweden. *Gerontologist, 31,* 682–686.

MaloneBeach, E. E., & Zarit, S. H. (1995). Dimensions of social support and social conflict as predictors of caregiver depression. *International Psychogeriatrics, 7,* 25–38.

MaloneBeach, E. E., Zarit, S. H., & Spore, D. L. (1992). Caregivers' perceptions of case management and community-based services: Barriers to service use. *Journal of Applied Gerontology, 11,* 146–159.

Mangion, D. M., Platt, J. S., & Syam, V. (1992). Alcohol and acute medical admission of elderly people. *Age and Ageing, 21,* 362–367.

Mann, D. A. (1997). Frontal lobe dementia. In C. Holmes & R. Howard (Eds.), *Advances in old age psychiatry: Chromosomes to community care* (pp. 64–78). Bristol, PA: Wrightson Biomedical.

Marsiske, M., & Willis, S. L. (1995). Dimensionality of everyday problem solving in older adults. *Psychology and Aging, 10,* 269–283.

Maslow, K. (1994). Current knowledge about special care units: Findings of a study by the U.S. Office of Technology Assessment. *Alzheimer's Disease and Associated Disorders, 8,* S14–S40.

Massman, P. J., Delis, D. C., Butters, N., Dupont, R. M., & Gillin, J. C. (1992). The subcortical dysfunction hypothesis of memory deficits in depression: Neuropsychological validation in subgroup patients. *Journal of Clinical and Experimental Neuropsychology, 14,* 687–706.

Masur, D. M., Fuld, P. A., Blau, A. D., Thal, L. J., Levin, H. S., & Aronson, M. K. (1989). Distinguishing normal and demented elderly with the selective reminding test. *Journal of Clinical and Experimental Neuropsychology, 11,* 615–630.

Matarazzo, J. D. (1972). *Wechsler's measurement and appraisal of adult intelligence* (5th ed.). Baltimore: Williams & Wilkins.

Mattis, S. (1976). Mental status examination for organic mental syndrome in the elderly patient. In L. Bellack & T. B. Karasu (Eds.), *Geriatric psychiatry* (pp. 77–121). New York: Grune & Stratton.

Mattis, S. (1989). *Dementia rating scale.* Odessa, FL: Psychological Assessment Resources.

McArthur, J. C., Hoover, D. R., Bacellar, H., Miller, E. N., Cohen, B. A., Becker, J. T., Graham, N. M., McArthur, J. H., Selnes, O. A., Jacobson, L. P., Visscher, B. K., Concha, M., & Saah, A. (1993). Dementia in AIDS patients: Incidence and risk factors. Multicenter AIDS cohort study. *Neurology, 43,* 2245–2252.

McConnell, S., & Beitler, D. (1991). The Older Americans Act after 25 years: An overview. *Generations, 15*(3), 5–10.

McCrae, R. R., & Costa, P. T., Jr. (1984). *Emerging lives, enduring dispositions.* Boston: Little, Brown.

McIntosh, J. L., Santos, J. F., Hubbard, R. W., & Overholser, J. C. (1994). *Elder suicide: Research, theory and treatment.* Washington, DC: American Psychological Association.

McKeith, I. G. (1997). Dementia with Lewy bodies. In C. Holmes & R. Howard (Eds.), *Advances in old age psychiatry: Chromosomes to community care* (pp. 52–63). Bristol, PA: Wrightson Biomedical.

McKenzie, J. E., Roberts, G. W., & Royston, M. C. (1996). Comparative investigation of neurofibrillary damage in the temporal lobe in Alzheimer's disease, Down's syndrome and dementia pugilistica. *Neurodegeneration, 5,* 259–264.

McKhann, G., Drachman, D., Folstein, M. F., Katzman, R., Price, D., & Stadlan, E. M.

(1984). Clinical diagnosis of Alzheimer's disease: Report of the NINCDS–ADR-DA work group under the auspices of Department of Health and Human Services Task Force on Alzheimer's Disease. *Neurology, 34,* 939–944.

McNulty, J. A., & Caird, W. (1966). Memory loss with age: Retrieval or storage? *Psychological Reports, 19,* 229–230.

Meeks, S., Carstensen, L. L., Stafford, P. B., Brenner, L. L., Weathers, F., Welch, R., & Oltmanns, T. F. (1990). Mental health needs of the chronically mentally ill elderly. *Psychology and Aging, 5,* 163–171.

Meyer, B. J. F., Young, C. J., & Bartlett, B. J. (1989). *Memory improved: Reading and memory enhancement across the life span through strategic text structures.* Hillsdale, NJ: Erlbaum.

Meyers, B. S., & Greenberg, R. (1986). Late-life delusional depression. *Journal of Affective Disorders, 11,* 133–137.

Meyers, B. S., & Mei-tal, V. (1985–1986). Empirical study on an inpatient psychogeriatric unit: Biological treatment in patients with depressive illness. *International Journal of Psychiatry in Medicine, 15,* 111–124.

Miller, M. D., & Silberman, R. I. (1996). Using interpersonal psychotherapy with depressed elders. In S. H. Zarit & B. G. Knight (Eds.), *A guide to psychotherapy and aging* (pp. 83–100). New York: American Psychological Association.

Mishara, B. L., & Kastenbaum, R. (1980). *Alcohol and old age.* New York: Grune & Stratton.

Mittelman, M. S., Ferris, S. H., Shulman, E., Steinberg, G., Ambinder, A., Mackell, J., & Cohen, J. (1995). A comprehensive support program: Effect on depression in spouse-caregivers of AD patients. *Gerontologist, 35,* 792–802.

Molloy, D. W., Alemayehu, E., & Roberts, R. (1991). Reliability of a standardized mini-mental state examination compared with the traditional mini-mental state examination. *American Journal of Psychiatry, 148,* 102–105.

Moody, H. R. (1992). A critical view of ethical dilemmas in dementia. In R. H. Binstock, S. G. Post, & P. J. Whitehouse (Eds.), *Dementia and aging: Ethics, values and policy choices* (pp. 86–100). Baltimore: Johns Hopkins University Press.

Moore, K. A., Danks, J. H., Ditto, P. H., Druley, J. A., Townsend, A., & Smucker, W. D. (1994). Elderly outpatients' understanding of a physician-initiated advance directive discussion. *Archives of Family Medicine, 3,* 1057–1063.

Morgan, D. G. (1992). Neurochemical changes with aging: Predisposition towards age-related mental disorders. In J. E. Birren, R. B. Sloan, & G. D. Cohen (Eds.), *Handbook of mental health and aging* (2nd ed., pp. 175–200). San Diego: Academic Press.

Morgan, L. A., Eckert, J. K., & Lyon, S. M. (1995). *Small board-and-care homes: residential care in transition.* Baltimore: Johns Hopkins University Press.

Morris, J. C., Heyman, A., Mohs, R. C., Hughes, J. P., Van Belle, G., Fillenbaum, G., Mellits, E. D., & Clark, C. (1989). The consortium to establish a registry for Alzheimer's disease (CERAD). *Neurology, 39,* 1159–1165.

Morris, J. C., McKeel, D. W., Jr., Storandt, M., Rubin, E. H., Price, J. L, Grant, E. A., Ball, M. J., & Berg, L. (1991). Very mild Alzheimer's disease: Informant-based clinical, psychometric, and patholgic distinction from normal aging. *Neurology, 41,* 469–478.

Morris, J. C., Mohs, R. C., Rogers, H., Fillenbaum, G., & Heyman, A. (1988). Consortium to establish a registry for Alzheimer's disease (CERAD) clinical and neuropsychological assessment of Alzheimer's disease. *Psychopharmacology Bulletin, 24,* 641–652.

Morrison, J. (1997). *When psychological problems mark medical disorders: A guide for psychotherapists.* New York: Guilford Press.

Mortimer, J. A. (1988). Epidemiology of dementia—International comparisons. In J. Brody & G. Maddox (Eds.), *Epidemiology and aging* (pp. 151–164). New York: Springer.

Mortimer, J. A., French, L. R., Hutton, J. T., & Schuman, L. M. (1985). Head injury as a risk factor for Alzheimer's disease. *Neurology, 35,* 264–267.

Mortimer, J. A., & Hutton, J. T. (1985). Epidemiology and etiology of Alzheimer's disease. In J. T. Hutton & A. D. Kenney (Eds.), *Senile dementia of the Alzheimer type* (pp. 177–196). New York: Liss.

Mościcki, E. K. (1995). Epidemiology of suicide. *International Psychogeriatrics, 7,* 137–148.

Mossey, J. M., Knott, K., & Craik, R. (1990). The effects of persistent depressive symptoms on hip fracture recovery. *Journal of Gerontology, 45,* M163–M168.

Mossey, J. M., Knott, K. A., Higgins, M. & Talerico, K. (1996). Effectiveness of a psychosocial intervention, interpersonal counseling, for subdysthymic depression in medically ill elderly. *Journal of Gerontology, 51A*(4), M172–M178.

Mowry, B. J., & Burvill, P. W. (1988). A study of mild dementia in the community using a wide range of diagnostic criteria. *British Journal of Psychiatry, 153,* 328–334.

Murden, R. A., McRae, T. D, Kaner, S., & Bucknam, M. E. (1991). Mini-Mental State Exam scores vary with education in blacks and whites. *Journal of the American Geriatrics Society, 39,* 149–155.

Murphy, E. (1994). The course and outcome of depression in late life. In L. S. Schneider, C. F. Reynolds, B. D. Lebowitz, & A. J. Friedhoff (Eds.), *Diagnosis and treatment of depression in late life* (pp. 81–98). Washington, DC: American Psychiatric Press.

National Center for Cost Containment. (1993). *Geropsychology assessment resource guide.* Milwaukee: Department of Veterans Affairs.

National Center for Health Statistics. (1993). Advance report for health statistics, 1991. *Monthly Vital Statistics Report, 42*(2, Suppl.). Hyattsville, MD: Public Health Service.

National Institute of Aging Task Force. (1980). Senility reconsidered. *Journal of the American Medical Association, 244,* 259–263.

National Institutes of Health. (1987). Differential diagnosis of dementing diseases. *Consensus Development Conference Statement, 6,* 6–9.

Neary, D. (1990). Dementia of frontal lobe type. *Journal of the American Geriatrics Society, 38,* 71–72.

Nelson, H. E. (1976). A modified card sorting test sensitive to frontal lobe defects. *Cortex, 12,* 313–324.

Neugarten, B. L. (1974). Age groups in American society and the rise of the young-old. *Annals of the American Academy of Political and Social Science, 415,* 187–198.

Newmann, J. P., Engel, R. J., & Jensen, J. E. (1991). Changes in depressive-symptom experiences among older women. *Psychology and Aging, 6,* 212–222.

Niederehe, G., & Yoder, C. (1989). Metamemory perceptions in depressions of young and older adults. *Journal of Nervous and Mental Disease, 177*, 4–14.

Nilsson, L. V., & Persson, G. (1984). Prevalence of mental disorders in an urban sample examined at 70, 75, and 79 years of age. *Acta Psychiatrica Scandinavica, 69*, 519–527.

Nuland, S. B. (1993). *How we die: Reflections on life's final chapter.* New York: Knopf.

Ober, B. A., Dronkers, N. F., Koss, E., Delis, D. C., & Friedland, R. P. (1986). Retrieval from semantic memory in Alzheimer-type dementia. *Journal of Clinical and Experimental Neuropsychology, 8*, 75–92.

Odenheimer, G. L., Beaudet, M., Jette, A. M., Albert, M. S., Grande, L., & Minaker, K. L. (1994). Performance-based driving evaluation of the elderly driver: Safety, reliability, and validity. *Journal of Gerontology, 49*, M153–M159.

Okun, M. A., & Elias, C. S. (1977). Cautiousness in adulthood as a function of age and payoff structure. *Journal of Gerontology, 32*, 451–455.

Orne, M. T., & Wender, P. H. (1968). Anticipatory socialization for psychotherapy. *American Journal of Psychiatry, 124*, 1201–1212.

Osterrieth, P. A. (1944). Le test de copie d'une figure complexe. *Archives de Psychologie, 30*, 206–356. (Translated by Corwin, J. & Bylsma, F. W. (1993). *Clinical Neuropsychologist, 7*, 9–15.)

Ott, A., Breteler, M. M., van Harskamp, F., Claus, J. J., van der Cammen, T. J., Grobbee, D. E., & Hofman, A. (1995). Prevalence of Alzheimer's disease and vascular dementia: Association with education. The Rotterdam Study. *British Medical Journal, 310*, 970–973.

Ouslander, J. G., Schnelle, J. F., Uman, G., Fingold, S., Nigam, J. G., Tuico, E., & Bates-Jensen, B. (1995). Predictors of successful prompted voiding among incontinent nursing home residents. *Journal of the American Medical Association, 273*, 1366–1370.

Parkinson, S. R., & Perey, A. (1980). Aging, digit span, and the stimulus suffix effect. *Journal of Gerontology, 35*, 736–742.

Parks, R. W., Zec, R. F., & Wilson, R. S. (Eds.). (1993). *Neuropsychology of Alzheimer's disease and other dementias.* New York: Oxford University Press.

Parmalee, P. A., Katz, I. R., & Lawton, M. P. (1992). Incidence of depression in long-term care settings. *Journal of Gerontology, 47*, M189–M196.

Parmalee, P. A., & Lawton, M. P. (1990). The design of special environments for the aged. In J. E. Birren & K. W. Schaie (Eds.), *Handbook of the psychology of aging* (3rd ed., pp. 464–488). San Diego: Academic Press.

Paykel, E. S. (1974). Recent life events and clinical depression. In E. K. E. Gunderson & R. H. Rahe (Eds.), *Life stress and illness* (pp. 134–163). Springfield, IL: Thomas.

Paykel, E. S. (1979). Life events and early environment. In E. S. Paykel (Ed.), *Handbook of affective disorders* (pp. 146–161). New York: Guilford Press.

Peisah, C., Sachdev, P., & Brodaty, H. (1993). Vascular dementia. *International Review of Psychiatry, 5*, 381–395.

Penn, R. D., Martin, E. M., Wilson, R. S., Fox, J. H., & Savoy, S. M. (1988). Intraventricular bethanechol infusion for Alzheimer's disease: Results of double-blind and escalating-dose trials. *Neurology, 38*, 219–222.

Perlin, S., & Kahn, R. L. (1968). A mental health center in a general hospital. In L. J. Duhl & R. L. Leopold (Eds.), *Mental health and urban social policy: A casebook of community action* (pp. 185–212). San Francisco: Jossey-Bass.

Perlmutter, M. (1978). What is memory aging the aging of? *Developmental Psychology, 14,* 330–345.

Perry, E. K., Tomlinson, B. E., Blessed, G., Gergmann, K., Gibson, P. H., & Perry, R. H. (1978). Correlation of cholinergic abnormalities with senile plaques and mental test scores in senile dementia. *British Medical Journal, 2,* 1457–1459.

Pfeiffer, E. (1975). A short portable mental status questionnaire for the assessment of organic brain deficit in elderly patients. *Journal of the American Geriatrics Society, 23,* 433–439.

Pinkston, E. M., & Linsk, N. L. (1984). Behavioral family intervention with the impaired elderly. *Gerontologist, 24,* 576–583.

Pirozzolo, F. J., Hansch, E. C., Mortimer, J. A., Webster, D. D., & Kuskowski, M. A. (1982). Dementia in Parkinson Disease: A neuropsychological analysis. *Brain and Cognition, 1,* 71–83.

Plomin, R., Pedersen, N. L., McClearn, G. E., Nesselroade, J. R., & Bergeman, C. S. (1988). EAS temperaments during the last half of the life span: Twins reared apart and twins reared together. *Psychology and Aging, 3,* 43–50.

Pompei, P., Foreman, M., Rudberg, M. A., Inouye, S. K., Braund, V., & Cassel, C. K. (1994). Delirium in hospitalized older persons: Outcomes and predictors. *Journal of the American Geriatrics Society, 42,* 809–815.

Poon, L. W., Rubin, D. C., & Wilson, B. A. (Eds.) (1989). *Everyday cognition in adulthood and old age.* New York: Cambridge University Press.

Popkin, S. J., Gallagher, D., Thompson, L. W., & Moore, M. (1982). Memory complaint and performance in normal and depressed older adults. *Experimental Aging Research, 8,* 141–145.

Post, F. (1966). *Persistent persecutory states in the elderly.* New York: Pergamon Press.

Post, F. (1973). Paranoid disorders in the elderly. *Postgraduate Medicine, 53,* 52–56.

Post, F. (1980). Paranoid, schizophrenia-like and schizophrenic states in the aged. In J. E. Birren and R. B. Sloane (Eds.), *Handbook of mental health and aging* (2nd ed., pp. 591–615). Englewood Cliffs, NJ: Prentice-Hall.

Post, S. G., Whitehouse, P. J., Binstock, R. H., Bird, T. D., Eckert, S. K., Farrer, L. A., Fleck, L. M., Atwood, D. G., Juengst, E. T., Karlinsky, H., Miles, S., Murray, T. H., Quaid, K. A., Relkin, N. R., Roses, A. D., St. George-Hyslop, P. H., Sachs, G. A., Steinbock, B., Truschke, E. F., & Zinn, A. B. (1997). The clinical introduction of genetic testing for Alzheimer disease: An ethical perspective. *Journal of the American Medical Association, 277,* 832–836.

Préville, M., Susman, E., Zarit, S. H., Smyer, M., Bosworth, H. B., & Reid, J. D. (1996). A measurement model of cortisol reactivity of healthy older adults. *Journal of Gerontology: Psychological Sciences, 51B,* P64–P69.

Pruchno, R., & Kleban, M. H. (1993). Caring for an institutionalized parent: The role of coping strategies. *Psychology and Aging, 8,* 18–25.

Quayhagen, M. P., & Quayhagen, M. (1989). Differential effects of family-based strategies on Alzheimer's disease. *Gerontologist, 29,* 150–155.

Rabins, P. V. (1992). Schizophrenia and psychotic states. In J. E. Birren, R. B. Sloane, G. D. Cohen, N. R. Hooyman, B. D. Lebowitz, M. Wykle, & D. E. Deutchman (Eds.), *Handbook of mental health and aging* (2nd ed., pp. 464–475). New York: Academic Press.

Rabins, P. V., Merchant, A., & Nestadt, G. (1984). Criteria for diagnosing reversible dementia caused by depression. *British Journal of Psychiatry, 144,* 488–492.

Rabins, P., McHugh, P. R., Pauker, S., & Thomas, J. (1987). The clinical features of late onset schizophrenia. In N. E. Miller & G. D. Cohen (Eds.), *Schizophrenia and aging: Schizophrenia, paranoia, and schizophreniform disorders in later life* (pp. 235–238). New York: Guilford Press.

Radloff, L. (1977). The CES-D Scale: A self-report depression scale for research in the general population. *Applied Psychological Measurement, 1,* 385–401.

Raj, B. A., & Sheehan, D. V. (1988). Medical evaluation of the anxious patient. *Psychiatric Annals, 18,* 176–181.

Raschko, R. (1985). Systems integration at the program level: Aging and mental health. *Gerontologist, 25,* 460–463.

Raschko, R. (1992). Spokane community mental health center elderly services. In E. Light & B. D. Lebowitz (Eds.), *The elderly with chronic mental illness.* (pp. 232–244). New York: Springer.

Raskind, M. A., Carta, A., & Bravi, D. (1995). Is early-onset Alzheimer disease a distinct subgroup within the Alzheimer disease population? *Alzheimer's Disease and Associated Disorders, 9* (Suppl. 1), S2–6.

Raskind, M. A. & Peskind, E. R. (1992). Alzheimer's disease and other dementing disorders in J. E. Birren, R. B. Sloane, & G. D. Cohen (Eds.), *Handbook of mental health and aging* (2nd ed., pp. 478–515). San Diego: Academic Press.

Regestein, Q. R. (1992). Treatment of insomnia in the elderly. In C. Salzman (Ed.), *Clinical geriatric psychopharmacology* (2nd ed., pp. 236–254). Baltimore: Williams & Wilkins.

Regier, D. A., Boyd, J. H., Burke, J. D. Jr., Rae, D. S., Myers, J. K., Kraemer, M., Robins, L. N., George, L. K., Karno, M., & Locke, B. Z. (1988). One-month prevalence of mental disorders in the United States. *Archives of General Psychiatry, 45,* 977–986.

Reifler, B. V., Larson, E., & Hanley, R. (1982). Coexistence of cognitive impairment and depression in geriatric outpatients. *American Journal of Psychiatry, 139,* 623–626.

Reifler, B. V., Larson, E., Teri, L., & Poulsen, M. (1986). Dementia of the Alzheimer's type and depression. *Journal of the American Geriatrics Society, 34,* 855–859.

Reifler, B. V., Teri, L., Raskind, M., Veith, R., Barnes, R., White, E., & McLean, P. (1989). Double-blind trial of imipramine in Alzheimer's disease patients with and without depression. *American Journal of Psychiatry, 146,* 45–49.

Reisberg, B., Ferris, S. H., de Leon, M. J., & Crook, T. (1982). The Global Deterioration Scale for the assessment of primary degenerative dementia. *American Journal of Psychiatry, 139,* 1136–1139.

Reitan, R. M. (1958). Validity of the Trail Making Test as an indication of organic brain damage. *Percipital and Motor Skills, 8,* 271–276.

Reitan, R. M. (1969). *Manual for the administration of neuropsychological test batteries for adults and children.* Indianapolis: Author.

Reynolds, C. F., Frank, E., Perel, J. M., Mazumdar, & S., Kupfer, D. J. (1995). Maintenance therapies for late-life recurrent major depression: Research and review circa 1995. *International Psychogeriatrics, 7,* 27–40.

Rhoden, N. K. (1988). Litigating life and death. *Harvard Law Review, 102,* 375–446.

Roach, G. W., Kanchuger, M., Mangano, C. M., Newman, M., Nussmeier, N., Wolman, R., Aggarwal, A., Marschall, R., Graham, S. H., Ley, C., Ozanne, G., & Mangano, D. T. (1996). Adverse cerebral outcomes after coronary bypass surgery: Multicenter Study of Perioperative Ischemia Research Group and the

Ischemia Research and Education Foundation Investigators. *New England Journal of Medicine, 335,* 1857–1863

Robinson, L. A., Berman, J. S., & Neimeyer, R. A. (1990). Psychotherapy for the treatment of depression: A comprehensive review of controlled outcome research. *Psychological Bulletin, 108,* 30–49.

Rockwood, K., Goodman, J., Flynn, M., & Stolee, P. (1996). Cross-validation of the delirium rating scale in older patients. *Journal of the American Geriatrics Society, 44,* 839–842.

Rodin, J. (1986). Aging and health: Effects of the sense of control. *Science, 233,* 1271–1276.

Rogers, C. R. (1951). *Client-centered therapy: Its current practice, implications, and theory.* Boston: Houghton Mifflin.

Rogers, R. G., Rogers, A., & Belanger, A. (1989). Active life among the elderly in the United States: Multistate life-table estimates and population projections. *Milbank Quarterly, 67,* 370–411.

Román, G. C. (1987). Senile dementia of the Binswanger type: A vascular form of dementia in the elderly. *Journal of the American Medical Association, 258,* 1782–1788.

Román, G. C., Tatemichi, T. K., Erkinjuntti, T., Cummings, J. L., Masedeu, J. C., Garcia, J. H., Amaducci, L., Orgogozo, J. M., Brun, A., Hofman, A., Moody, D. M., O'Brien, M. D., Yamaguchi, T., Grafman, J., Drayer, B. P., Bennett, D. A., Fisher, M., Ogata, J., Kokmen, E., Bermejo, F., Wolf, P. A., Gorelick, P. B., Bick, K. L., Pajeau, A. K., Bell, M. A., DeCarli, C., Culebras, A., Korczyin, A. D., Bogouslavsky, J., Hartmann, A., & Scheinberg, P. (1993). Vascular dementia: Diagnostic criteria for research studies. Report of the NINDS-AIREN International Workshop. *Neurology, 43,* 250–260.

Ross, C. A., Peyser, C. E., Shapiro, I., & Folstein, M. F. (1991). Delirium: Phenotypic and etiologic subtypes. *International Psychogeriatrics, 3,* 135–145.

Roth, M. (1955). The natural history of mental disorder in old age. *Journal of Mental Science, 101,* 281–289.

Roth, M. (1987). Late paraphrenia: Phenomenology and etiological factors and their bearing upon problems of the schizophrenic family of disorders. In N. E. Miller & G. D. Cohen (Eds.), *Schizophrenia and aging: Schizophrenia, paranoia, and schizophreniform disorders in later life* (pp. 217–234). New York: Guilford Press.

Roth, M. (1991). Clinical perspectives. *International Psychogeriatrics, 3,* 309–317.

Roth, M., & Myers, D. H. (1975). The diagnosis of dementia. *British Journal of Psychiatry, 9* (Special Publication), 87–99.

Rovner, B. W., Kafonek, S., Filipp, L., Lucas, M. J., & Folstein, M. F. (1986). Prevalence of mental illness in a community nursing home. *American Journal of Psychiatry, 143,* 1446–1449.

Royall, D. R., Mahurin, R. K., Cornell, J., & Gray, K. (1993). Bedside assessment of dementia type using the Qualitative Evaluation of Dementia (QED). *Neuropsychiatry, Neuropsychology and Behavioral Neurology, 6,* 235–244.

Royall, D. R., Mahurin, R. K., & Gray, K. F. (1992). Bedside assessment of executive cognitive impairment: The executive interview. *Journal of the American Geriatrics Society, 40,* 1221–1226.

Ryan, J. J., Paolo, A. M., & Brungardt, T. M. (1990). Standardization of the Wechsler Adult Intelligence Scale-Revised for persons 75 years and older. *Psychological Assessment, 2,* 404–411.

Sabatino, C. P. (1996). Competency: Refining our legal fictions. In M. A. Smyer, K. W. Schaie, & M. B. Kapp (Eds.), *Older adults' decision-making and the law* (pp. 1–28). New York: Springer.

Sackheim, H. A. (1992). The cognitive effects of electroconvulsive therapy. In W. H. Moos, E. R. Gamzu, & L. J. Thal (Eds.), *Cognitive disorders: Pathophysiology and treatment* (pp. 183–228). New York: Dekker.

Sackheim, H. A. (1994). Use of electroconvulsive therapy in late-life depression. In L. S. Schneider, C. F. Reynolds, B. D. Lebowitz, & A. J. Friedhoff (Eds.), *Diagnosis and treatment of depression in late life* (pp. 259–278). Washington, DC: American Psychiatric Press.

Sadavoy, J., & Fogel, B. (1992). Personality disorders in old age. In J. E. Birren, R. B. Sloane, G. D. Cohen, N. R. Hooyman, B. D. Lebowitz, M. Wykle, & D. E. Deutchman (Eds.), *Handbook of mental health and aging* (2nd ed., pp. 433–463). New York: Academic Press.

Sakauye, K. M., Camp, C. J., & Ford, P. A. (1993). Effects of buspirone on agitation associated with dementia. *American Journal of Geriatric Psychiatry, 1,* 82–84.

Salmon, D. P., Thal, L. J., Butters, N., & Heindel, W. C. (1990). Longitudinal evaluation of dementia of the Alzheimer type: A comparison of 3 standardized mental status examinations. *Neurology, 40,* 1225–1230.

Salthouse, T. A. (1984). Effects of age and skill in typing. *Journal of Experimental Psychology: General, 113,* 345–371.

Salthouse, T. A. (1990). Cognitive competence and expertise in aging. In J. E. Birren & K. W. Schaie (Eds.), *Handbook of the psychology of aging* (3rd ed., pp. 310–391). New York: Academic Press.

Salthouse, T. A. (1994a). The nature of the influence of speed on adult age differences in cognition. *Developmental Psychology, 30,* 240–259.

Salthouse, T. A. (1994b). The aging of working memory. *Neuropsychology, 8,* 535–543.

Salthouse, T. A., & Babcock, R. L. (1991). Decomposing adult age differences in working memory. *Developmental Psychology, 27,* 763–776.

Salthouse, T. A., Babcock, R. L., & Shaw, R. J. (1991). Effects of adult age on structural and operational capacities in working memory. *Psychology and Aging,7,* 118–127.

Salzman, C. (1993). Pharmacologic treatment of depression in the elderly. *Journal of Clinical Psychiatry, 54*(2, Suppl.), 23–27.

Salzman, C. (1992). Treatment of anxiety. In C. Salzman (Ed.), *Clinical geriatric psychopharmacology* (2nd ed., pp. 189–212). Baltimore: Williams & Wilkins.

Salzman, C. S. (1994). Pharmacological treatment of depression in elderly patients. In L. S. Schneider, C. F. Reynolds, B. D. Lebowitz, & A. J. Friedhoff (Eds.), *Diagnosis and treatment of depression in late life* (pp. 181–206). Washington, DC: American Psychiatric Press.

Samuels, J. F., Nestadt, G., Romanoski, A. J., Folstein, M. F., & McHugh, P. R. (1994). DSM-III personality disorders in the community. *American Journal of Psychiatry, 151,* 1055–1062.

Sano, M., Ernesto, C., Thomas, R. G., Klauber, M. R., Schafer, K., Grundman, M., Woodbury, P., Growdon, J., Cotman, C. W., Pfeiffer, E., Schneider, L. S., & Thal, L. J. (1997). A controlled trial of selegiline, alpha-tocopherol, or both as treatment for Alzheimer's disease. *New England Journal of Medicine, 336,* 1216–1222.

Schaie, K. W. (1967). Age changes and age differences. *Gerontologist, 7*, 128–132.

Schaie, K. W. (1983). The Seattle Longitudinal Study: A twenty-one year exploration of psychometric intelligence in adulthood. In K. W. Schaie (Ed.), *Longitudinal studies of adult psychological development* (pp. 64–135). New York: Guilford Press.

Schaie, K. W. (1985). *Manual for the Schaie–Thurstone Adult Mental Abilities Test (STAMAT)*. Palo Alto, CA: Consulting Psychologists Press.

Schaie, K. W. (1989). Individual differences in rate of cognitive change in adulthood. In V. L. Bengston & K. W. Schaie (Eds.), *The course of later life: Research and reflections* (pp. 68–83). New York: Springer.

Schaie, K. W. (1990). Intellectual development in adulthood. In J. E. Birren & K. W. Schaie (Eds.), *Handbook of the psychology of aging* (3rd ed., pp. 291–309). New York: Academic Press.

Schaie, K. W. (1995). Intellectual development in adulthood. In J. E. Birren & K. W. Schaie (Eds.), *Handbook of the psychology of aging* (4th ed., pp. 266–286). San Diego: Academic Press.

Schaie, K. W. (1996). *Intellectual development in adulthood: The Seattle Longitudinal Study*. Cambridge: Cambridge University Press.

Schaie, K. W., & Hertzog, C. (1986). Toward a comprehensive model of adult intellectual development: Contributions of the Seattle Longitudinal Study. In R. J. Sternberg (Ed.), *Advances in human intelligence* (Vol. 3, pp. 79–118). Hillsdale, NJ: Erlbaum.

Schaie, K. W., & Labouvie-Vief, G. (1974). Generational versus ontogenetic components of change in adult cognitive behavior: A fourteen-year cross-sequential study. *Developmental Psychology, 10*, 305–320.

Schaie, K. W., & Willis, S. L. (1986). Can intellectual decline in the elderly be reversed? *Developmental Psychology, 22*, 223–232.

Schaie, K. W., & Willis, S. L. (1996). *Adult development and aging* (4th ed.). New York: HarperCollins.

Scharlach, A. E. (1994). Caregiving and employment: Competing or complementary roles? *Gerontologist, 34*, 378–385.

Scheibel, A. B. (1995). Structural and functional changes in the aging brain. In J. E. Birren & K. W. Schaie (Eds.), *Handbook of the psychology of aging* (4th ed., pp. 105–128). San Diego: Academic Press.

Schellenberg, G. D., Bird, T. D., Wijsman, E. M., Orr, H. T., Anderson, L., Nemens, E., White, J. A., Bonnycastle, L., Weber, J. L., Alonso, M. E., Potter, H., Heston, L. L., & Martin, G. M. (1992). Genetic linkage evidence for a familial Alzheimer's disease locus on chromosome 14. *Science, 258*, 668–671.

Schmidt, M. L., Lee, V. M., Forman, M., Chiu, T. S., & Trojanowski, J. Q. (1997). Monoclonal antibodies to a 100-kd protein reveal abundant Aβ-negative plaques throughout gray matter of Alzheimer's disease brains. *American Journal of Pathology, 151*,1, 69–80.

Schmidt, M. L., Martin, J. A., Lee, V. M., & Trojanowski, J. Q. (1996). Convergence of Lewy bodies and neurofibrillary tangles in amygdala neurons of Alzheimer's disease and Lewy body disorders. *Acta Neuropathologica, 91*, 475–481.

Schmidt, R., Fazekas, F., Offenbacher, H., Dusek, T., Zach, E., Reinhart, B., Grieshofer, P., Freidl, W., Eber, B., Schumacher, M., Koch, M., & Lechner, H. (1993). Neuropsychologic correlates of MRI white matter hyperintensities: A study of 150 normal volunteers. *Neurology, 43*, 2490–2494.

Schneider, L. S. (1996). Meta-analysis of controlled pharmacologic trials. *International Psychogeriatrics, 8,* 375–380.

Schneider, L. S., Farlow, M. R., Henderson, V. W., & Pogoda, J. M. (1996). Effects of estrogen replacement therapy on response to tacrine in patients with Alzheimer's disease. *Neurology, 46,* 1580–1584.

Schneider, L. S., & Olin, J. T. (1995). Efficacy of acute treatment for geriatric depression. *International Psychogeriatrics, 7,* 7–26.

Schneider, L. S., Pollock, V. E., & Lyness, S. A. (1990). A meta-analysis of controlled trials of neuroleptic treatment in dementia. *Journal of the American Geriatrics Society, 38,* 553–563.

Schnelle, J. F., Newman, D. R., & Fogarty, T. (1990). Management of patient continence in long-term care nursing facilities. *Gerontologist, 30,* 373–376.

Schnelle, J. F., Traughber, B., Sowell, V. A., Newman, D. R., Petrill, C. O., & Ory, M. (1989). Prompted voiding treatment of urinary incontinence in nursing home patients: A behavior management approach for nursing home staff. *Journal of the American Geriatrics Society, 31,* 1051–1057.

Schofield, P. W., Tang, M., Marder, K., Bell, K., Dooneief, G., Chun, M., Sano, M., Stern, Y., & Mayeux, R. (1997). Alzheimer's disease after remote head injury: An incidence study. *Journal of Neurology, Neurosurgery and Psychiatry, 62,* 119–124.

Schonfield, D. (1974). Translations in gerontology—From lab to life: Utilizing information. *American Psychologist, 29,* 796–801.

Schonfield, D., & Robertson, E. A. (1986). Memory storage and aging. *Canadian Journal of Psychology, 20,* 228–236.

Schulz, R., & Brenner, G. (1977). Relocation of the aged: A review and theoretical analysis. *Journal of Gerontology, 32,* 323–332.

Schulz, R., O'Brien, A. T., Bookwala, J., Fleissner, K. (1995). Psychiatric and physical morbidity effects of dementia caregiving: Prevalence, correlates, and causes. *Gerontologist, 35,* 771–791.

Schulz, R., Williamson, G. M., Morycz, R., & Beigel, D. E. (1993). Changes in depression among men and women caring for an Alzheimer's patient. In S. H. Zarit, L. I. Pearlin, & K. W. Schaie (Eds.), *Caregiving systems: Informal and formal helpers* (pp. 119–140). Hillsdale, NJ: Erlbaum.

Scogin, F., Jamison, C., & Gochneaur, K. (1989). Comparative efficacy of cognitive and behavioral bibliotherapy for mildly and moderately depressed older adults. *Journal of Consulting and Clinical Psychology, 57,* 403–407.

Scogin, F., & McElreath, L. (1994). Efficacy of psychosocial treatments for geriatric depression: A quantitative review. *Journal of Consulting and Clinical Psychology, 62,* 69–74.

Scogin, F., Rickard, H. C., Keith, S., Wilson, J., & McElreath, L. (1992). Progressive and imaginal relaxation training for elderly persons with subjective anxiety. *Psychology and Aging, 7,* 419–424.

Seligman, M. (1975). *Helplessness: On depression, development and death.* San Francisco: Freeman.

Seligman, M. (1991). *Learned optimism.* New York: Knopf.

Seltzer, M. M. (1992). Aging in persons with developmental disabilities. In J. E. Birren, R. B. Sloane, & G. D. Cohen (Eds.), *Handbook of mental health and aging* (2nd ed., pp. 583–602). San Diego: Academic Press.

Semple, S. J. (1992). Conflict in Alzheimer's caregiving families: Its dimensions and consequences. *Gerontologist, 32,* 648–655.

Shea, D., Streit, A., & Smyer, M. (1994). Use of specialist mental health services by nursing home residents. *Health Services Research, 29,* 169–185.

Shibayama, H., Kasahara, Y., & Kobayashi, H. (1986). Prevalence of dementia in a Japanese elderly population. *Acta Psychiatrica Scandinavica, 74,* 144–151.

Shuchter, S. R., Downs, N., & Zisook, S. (1996). *Biologically informed psychotherapy for depression.* New York: Guilford Press.

Siegler, I. C. (1983). Psychological aspects of the Duke Longitudinal Studies. In K. W. Schaie (Ed.), *Longitudinal studies of adult psychological development* (pp. 136–190). New York: Guilford Press.

Siegler, I. C., George, L. K., & Okun, M. A. (1979). Cross-sequential analysis of adult personality. *Developmental Psychology, 15,* 350–351.

Skoog, I. (1994). Risk factors for vascular dementia: A review. *Dementia, 5,* 137–144.

Skoog, I., Nilsson, L., Palmertz, B., Andreasson, L. A., & Svanborg, A. (1993). A population-based study of dementia in 85-year-olds. *New England Journal of Medicine, 328,* 153–158.

Sloane, P. D., & Mathew, L. J. (1991). *Dementia units in long-term care.* Baltimore: Johns Hopkins University Press.

Smith, A. D. (1996). Memory. In J. E. Birren & K. W. Schaie (Eds.), *Handbook of the psychology of aging* (4th ed., pp. 236–250). San Diego: Academic Press.

Smith, G. E., Ivnik, R. J., Malec, J. F., Kokmen, E., Tangalos, E., & Petersen, R. C. (1994). Psychometric properties of the Mattis Dementia Rating Scale. *Assessment, 1,* 123–131.

Smith, G. E., Ivnik, R. J., Malec, J. F., Kokmen, E., Tangalos, E. G., & Kurland, L. T. (1992). Mayo's older Americans normative studies (MOANS): Factor structure of a core battery. *Psychological Assessment, 4,* 382–390.

Smith, G. E., Ivnik, R. J., Malec, J. F., Petersen, R. C., Kokmen, E., & Tangalos, E. G. (1994). Mayo cognitive factor scales: Derivation of a short battery and norms for factor scores. *Neuropsychology, 8,* 194–202.

Smyer, M. A. (1989). Nursing homes as a setting for psychological practice. *American Psychologist, 44,* 1307–1314.

Smyer, M. A., Cohn, M. D., & Brannon, D. (1988). *Mental health consultation in nursing homes.* New York: New York University Press.

Smyer, M. A., Zarit, S. H., & Qualls, S. H. (1990). Psychological intervention with aging individuals. In J. E. Birren & K. W. Schaie (Eds.), *Handbook of the psychology of aging* (3rd ed., pp. 375–403). San Diego: Academic Press.

Snowdon, D. A., Greiner, L. H., Mortimer, J. A., Riley, K. P., Greiner, P. A., & Markesbery, W. R. (1997). Brain infarction and the clinical expression of Alzheimer disease: The Nun Study. *Journal of the American Medical Association, 277,* 813–817.

Spayd, C., & Smyer, M. A. (1996). Psychological interventions in nursing homes. In S. H. Zarit & B. G. Knight (Eds.), *A guide to psychotherapy and aging* (pp. 241–268). Washington, DC: American Psychological Association.

Spillman, B. C., & Kemper, P. (1995). Lifetime patterns of payment for nursing home care. *Medical Care, 33,* 280–296.

Spreen, D., & Strauss, E. (1991). *A compendium of neuropsychological tests.* New York: Oxford University Press.

Squire, L. R. (1974). Remote memory as affected by aging. *Neuropsychologia, 12,* 429–435.

St. George-Hyslop, P. H., Haines, J. L., Farrer, L. A., Polinsky, R., Van Broeckhoven, C., Goate, A., McLachlan D. R. C., Orr, H., Bruni, A. C., Sorbi, S., Rainero, I., Foncin, J.-F., Pollen, D., Cantu, J.-M., Tupler, R., Voskresenskaya, N., Mayeux, R., Growdon, J., Fried, V. A., Myers, R. H., Nee, L., Backhovens, H., Martin, J.-J., Rossor, M., Owens, M. J., Mullan, M., Percy, M. E., Karlinsky, H., Rich, S., Heston, L., Montesi, M., Mortilla, M., Nacmias, N., Gusella, J. F., Hardy, J. A., & other members of the FAD Collaborative Study group. (1990). Genetic linkage studies suggest that Alzheimer's disease is not a single homogeneous disorder. *Nature, 347,* 194–197.

St. George-Hyslop, P. H., Tanzi, R. E., Polinsky, R. J., Haines, J. L., Nee, L., Watkins, P. C., Myers, R. H., Feldman, R. G., Pollen, D., Drachman, D., Growdon, J., Bruni, A., Foncin, J., Salmon, D., Frommelt, P., Amaducci, L., Sorbi, S., Piacentini, S., Stewart, G. D., Hobbs, W. J., Conneally, P. M., & Gusella, J. F. (1987). The genetic defect causing familial Alzheimer's disease maps on chromosome 21. *Science, 235,* 885–890.

Staudinger, U. M., Marsiske, M., & Baltes, P. B. (1995). Resilience and reserve capacity in later adulthood: Potentials and limits of development across the life span. In D. Cicchetti & D. J. Cohen (Eds.), *Developmental psychopathology: Vol. 2. Risk, disorder, and adaptation* (pp. 801–847). New York: Wiley.

Steiner, V., & Zarit, S. H. (1995, November). *Ratings of the program environment as predictors of caregiver satisfaction with adult day care.* Paper presented at the annual meeting of the Gerontological Society of America, Los Angeles, CA.

Stephenson, J. (1997). Researchers find evidence of a new gene for late-onset Alzheimer disease. *Journal of the American Medical Association, 277,* 775.

Stern, Y., Alexander, G. E., Prohovnik, I., & Mayeux, R. (1992). Inverse relationship between education and parietotemporal perfusion deficit in Alzheimer's disease. *Journal of the American Neurological Association, 32,* 371–375.

Stern, Y., Gurland, B., Tatemichi, T., Tang, M., Wilder, D., & Mayeux, R. (1994). Influence of education and occupation on the incidence of Alzheimer's Disease. *Journal of the American Medical Association, 271,* 1004–1010.

Stokes, G. (1996). Challenging behaviour in dementia: A psychological approach. In R. T. Woods (Ed.), *Handbook of the clinical psychology of ageing* (pp. 601–628). New York: Wiley.

Stone, R., Cafferata, G. L., & Sangl, J. (1987). Caregivers of the frail elderly: A national profile. *Gerontologist, 27,* 616–626.

Storandt, M. (1977). Age, ability level and method of administering and scoring the WAIS. *Journal of Gerontology, 32,* 175–178.

Storandt, M. (1990). Bender–Gestalt test performance in senile dementia of the Alzheimer type. *Psychology and Aging, 5,* 604–606.

Storandt, M., Botwinick, J., Danziger, W. L., Berg, L., & Hughes, C. P. (1984). Psychometric differentiation of mild senile dementia of the Alzheimer type. *Archives of Neurology, 41,* 497–499.

Storandt, M., & Hill, R. D. (1989). Very mild senile dementia of the Alzheimer type. *Archives of Neurology, 46,* 383–386.

Storandt, M., & VandenBos, G. R. (1994). *Neuropsychological assessment of dementia and depression in older adults: A clinician's guide*. Washington, DC: American Psychological Association.

Strauss, J. S. (1987). Schizophrenia and aging: Meeting point of diagnosis and conceptual questions. In N. E. Miller & G. D. Cohen (Eds.), *Schizophrenia and aging: Schizophrenia, paranoia, and schizophreniform disorders in later life* (pp. 3–8). New York: Guilford Press.

Strassburger, T. L., Lee, H. C., Daly, E. M., Szczepanik, J., Krasuski, J. S., Mentis, M. J., Salerno, J. A., DeCarli, C., Schapiro, M. B., & Alexander, G. E. (1997). Interactive effects of age and hypertension on volumes of brain structures. *Stroke, 28,* 1410–1417.

Sulkava, R., Wikstrom, J., Aromaa, A., Raitasalo, R., Lehtinen, V., Licph, K. L., & Palo, J. (1985). Prevalence of severe dementia in Finland. *Neurology, 35,* 1025–1029.

Sultzer, D., Levin, H. S., Mahler, M. E., High, W. M., & Cummings, J. L. (1993). A comparison of psychiatric symptoms in vascular dementia and Alzheimer's disease. *American Journal of Psychiatry, 15,* 1806–1812.

Sunderland, T., Lawlor, B. A., Martinez, R., & Molchan, S. (1991). Anxiety in the elderly: Neurobiological and clinical interface. In C. Salzman & B. Lebowitz (Eds.), *Anxiety in the elderly* (pp. 105–130). New York: Springer.

Task Force on Benzodiazepine Dependency. (1990). *Benzodiazepine dependence, toxicity and abuse* (Task Force Report of the American Psychiatric Association). Washington, DC: American Psychiatric Association.

Teng, E. L., & Chui, H. C. (1987). The modified Mini-Mental State (3MS) examination. *Journal of Clinical Psychiatry, 48,* 314–318.

Teri, L. (1994). Behavioral treatment of depression in patients with dementia. *Alzheimer Disease and Associated Disorders, 8,* 66–74.

Teri, L., Hughes, J., & Larson, E. (1990). Cognitive deterioration in Alzheimer's disease: Behavioral and health factors. *Journal of Gerontology, 45,* 58–63.

Teri, L., & Lewinsohn, P. M. (1982). Modification of the pleasant and unpleasant events schedules for use with the elderly. *Journal of Consulting and Clinical Psychology, 50,* 444–445.

Teri, L., & Logsdon, R. G. (1991). Identifying pleasant activities for Alzheimer's disease patients: The pleasant events schedule—AD. *Gerontologist, 31,* 124–127.

Teri, L., Logsdon, R. G., Uomoto, J., & McCurry, S. M. (1997). Behavioral treatment of depression in dementia patients: A controlled clinical trial. *Journal of Gerontology: Psychological Sciences, 52B,* P159–P166.

Teri, L., & Truax, P. (1994). Assessment of depression in dementia patients: Association of caregiver mood with depression ratings. *Gerontologist, 34,* 213–234.

Teri, L., Truax, P., Logsdon, R., Uomoto, J., Zarit, S., & Vitaliano, P. P. (1992). Assessment of behavioral problems in dementia: The revised memory and behavior problems checklist. *Psychology and Aging, 7,* 622–631.

Teri, L., & Wagner, A. (1992). Alzheimer's disease and depression. *Journal of Consulting and Clinical Psychology, 60,* 379–391.

Terry, R. D., & Katzman, R. (1983). Senile dementia of the Alzheimer's type. *Annals of Neurology, 14,* 153–176.

Thomasma, D. C. (1992). Mercy killing of elderly people with dementia: A counterproposal. In R. H. Binstock, S. G. Post, & P. J. Whitehouse (Eds.), *Dementia and aging: Ethics, values and policy choices* (pp. 101–117). Baltimore: Johns Hopkins University Press.

Thompson, J. W., & Blaine, J. D. (1987). Use of ECT in the United States in 1975 and 1980. *American Journal of Psychiatry, 144,* 557–562.

Thompson, L. W., Gallagher, D., & Breckenridge, J. (1987). Comparative effectiveness of psychotherapies for depressed elders. *Journal of Consulting and Clinical Psychology, 55,* 385–390.

Thompson, L. W., Gallagher, D., Nies, G., & Epstein, D. (1983). Evaluation of the effectiveness of professionals and nonprofessionals as instructors of "coping with depression" classes for elders. *Gerontologist, 23,* 390–396.

Thurstone, L. L., & Thurstone, T. G. (1949). *Examiner manual for the SRA Primary Abilities Test.* Chicago: Science Research Associates.

Tombaugh, T. N., & McIntyre, N. J. (1992). The Mini-Mental State Examination: A comprehensive review. *Journal of the American Geriatrics Society, 40,* 922–935.

Tomlinson, B. E., Blessed, G., & Roth, M. (1970). Observations on the brains of demented old people. *Journal of Neurological Science, 11,* 207–242.

Toseland, R. W. (1990). *Group work with older adults.* New York: New York University Press.

Toseland, R. W., Rossiter, C. M., Peak, T., & Smith, G. C. (1990). Comparative effectiveness of individual and group interventions to support family caregivers. *Social Work, 35,* 209–217.

Treas, J. (1995). Older Americans in the 1990s and beyond. *Population Bulletin, 50*(2), 1–45.

Trzepacz, P. T., & Dew, M. A. (1995). Further analyses of the delirium rating scale. *General Hospital Psychiatry, 17,* 75–79.

Tsuang, M. T. (1986). Predictors of poor and good outcome in schizophrenia. In L. Erlenmeyer-Kimling & N. E. Miller (Eds.), *Life-span research on the prediction of psychopathology* (pp. 195–203). Hillsdale NJ: Erlbaum.

Tune, L. E. (1991). Postoperative delirium. *International Psychogeriatrics, 3,* 325–332.

Tune, L. E., & Folstein, M. F. (1986). Post-operative delirium. *Advances in Psychosomatic Medicine, 15,* 51–68.

Tuokko, H., Hadjistavropoulos, T., Miller, J. A., & Beattie, B. L. (1992). The clock test: A sensitive measure to differentiate normal elderly from those with Alzheimer disease. *Journal of the American Geriatrics Society, 40,* 579–584.

Tuokko, H., Kristjansson, E., & Miller, J. (1995). Neuropsychological detection of dementia: An overview of the neuropsychological component of the Canadian Study of Health and Aging. *Journal of Clinical and Experimental Neuropsychology, 17,* 352–373.

Tuokko, H., Tallman, K., Beattie, B. L., Cooper, P., & Weir, J. (1995). An examination of driving records in a dementia clinic. *Journals of Gerontology: Social Sciences, 50B,* S173–S181.

Tyrer, P. (1995). Are personality disorders well classified in DSM-IV? In W. J. Livesley (Ed.), *The DSM-IV personality disorders* (pp. 29–44). New York: Guilford Press.

Tyrer, P., & Seivewright, H. (1988). Studies of outcome. In P. Tyrer (Ed.), *Personality disorders: Diagnosis, management and course* (pp. 119–136). London: Wright.

Uhlmann, R. F., & Larson, E. B. (1991). Effect of education on the Mini-Mental State Examination as a screening test for dementia. *Journal of the American Geriatrics Society, 39,* 876–880.

U.S. Bureau of the Census. (1992a). *Growth of America's oldest-old population* (Profiles of America's elderly No. 2). Washington, DC: U.S. Government Printing Office.

U.S. Bureau of the Census. (1992b). *Sixty-five plus in America* (Current Population Reports, Special Studies, Series No. P23–178). Washington, DC: U.S. Government Printing Office.

Vaillant, G. E., & Vaillant, C. O. (1990). Natural history of male psychological health: XII. A 45-year study of predictors of successful aging. *American Journal of Psychiatry, 147,* 31–37.

Van Gorp, W. G., Satz, P., Kiersch, M. E., & Henry, R. (1986). Normative data on the Boston Naming Test for a group of normal older adults. *Journal of Clinical and Experimental Neuropsychology, 8,* 702–705.

Verbrugge, L. M. (1984). Longer life but worsening health? Trends in health and mortality of middle-aged and older persons. *Milbank Memorial Fund Quarterly/Health and Society, 62,* 474–519.

Wahlund, L. O. (1994). Brain imaging and vascular dementia. *Dementia, 5,* 193–196.

Walsh, D., Till, R. E., & Williams, M. V. (1978). Age differences in peripheral perceptual processing: A monoptic backward masking investigation. *Journal of Experimental Psychology: Human Perception and Performance, 4,* 232–243.

Watson, Y. I., Arfken, C. L., & Birge, S. J. (1993). Clock competition: An objective screening test for dementia. *Journal of the American Geriatric Society, 41,* 1235–1240.

Wattis, H., & Church, M. (1986). *Practical psychiatry of old age.* New York: New York University Press.

Wechsler, D. (1958). *The measurement and appraisal of adult intelligence.* Baltimore: Williams & Wilkins.

Wechsler, D. (1987). *Wechsler Memory Scale—Revised.* San Antonio: Psychological Corporation.

Wechsler, D. (1997a). *WAIS-III: Administration and scoring manual.* San Antonio: Psychological Corporation.

Wechsler, D. (1997b). *Wechsler Memory Scale* (3rd ed.). San Antonio: Psychological Corporation.

Weinstein, E. A., & Kahn, R. L. (1955). *Denial of illness: Symbolic and physiological aspects.* Springfield, IL: Thomas.

Weissman, M. M., Leaf, P. J., Tischler, G. L., Blazer, D. G., Karno, M., Bruce, M. L., & Florio, L. P. (1988). Affective disorders in five United States communities. *Psychological Medicine, 18,* 141–153.

Weissman, M. M., & Myers, J. K. (1978). Affective disorders in a U. S. urban community. *Archives of General Psychiatry, 35,* 1304–1311.

Wells, C. (1979). Pseudodementia. *American Journal of Psychiatry, 136,* 895–900.

Welsh, K., Butters, N., Hughes, J., Mohs, R., & Heyman, A. (1991). Detection of abnormal memory decline in mild cases of Alzheimer's disease using CERAD neuropsychological measures. *Archives of Neurology, 48,* 278–281.

Whelihan, W. M., Lesher, E. L., Kleban, M. H., & Granick, S. (1984). Mental status and memory assessment as predictors of dementia. *Journal of Gerontology, 39,* 572–576.

White, L., Petrovitch, H., Ross, W., Masaki, K. H., Abbott, R. D., Teng, E. L., Rodriguez, B. L., Blanchette, P. L., Havlik, R. J., Wergowske, G., Chiu, D., Foley, D.

J., Murdaugh, C., & Curb, J. D. (1996). Prevalence of dementia in older Japanese-American men in Hawaii: The Honolulu–Asia Aging Study. *Journal of the American Medical Association, 276,* 955–960.

White, P. D. (1992). Essays in the aftermath of Cruzan. *Journal of Medicine and Philosophy, 17,* 563–571.

Whitehead, A. (1970). *In the service of old age: The welfare of psychogeriatric patients.* Baltimore: Penguin.

Whitlatch, C. J., & Zarit, S. H. (1988). Sexual dysfunction in an aged married couple: A case study of a behavioral intervention. *Clinical Gerontologist, 8,* 43–62.

Whitlatch, C. J., Zarit, S. H., & von Eye, A. (1991). Efficacy of interventions with caregivers: A reanalysis. *Gerontologist, 31,* 9–14.

Whitlatch, C. J., Zarit, S. H., Goodwin, P. E., & von Eye, A. (1995). Influence of the success of psychoeducational interventions on the course of family care. *Clinical Gerontologist, 16,* 17–30.

Widiger, T. A., & Sanderson C. J. (1995). Toward a dimensional model of personality disorders. In W. J. Livesley (Ed.), *The DSM-IV personality disorders* (pp. 433–458). New York: Guilford Press.

Wiener, J. M. (1990). Which way for long-term care financing? *Generations, 10*(2) 4–9.

Wiener, J. M. (1996). Managed care and long-term care: The integration of financing and services. *Generations, 20*(2), 47–52.

Williamson, G. M., & Schulz, R. (1993). Coping with specific stressors in Alzheimer's disease caregiving. *Gerontologist, 33,* 747–755.

Willis, S. L., (1996). Assessing everyday competence in the cognitively challenged elderly. In M. Smyer, K. W. Schaie, & M. B. Kapp (Eds.), *Older adults' decision-making and the law* (pp. 87–127). New York: Springer.

Willis, S. L., Blieszner, R., & Baltes, P. B. (1981). Intellectual training research in aging: Modification of performance on the fluid ability of figural relations. *Journal of Educational Psychology, 73,* 41–50.

Willis, S. L., & Marsiske, M. (1993). *Manual for the Everyday Problems Test.* University Park: Pennsylvania State University Press.

Willis, S. L., & Nesselroade, C. S. (1990). Long-term effects of fluid ability training in old-old age. *Developmental Psychology, 26,* 905–910.

Wilson, R. S., Kaszniak, A. W., Bacon, L. D., Fox, J. H., & Kelly, M. P. (1982). Facial recognition in dementia. *Cortex, 18,* 329–336.

Wisocki, P. A. (Ed.). (1991). *Handbook of clinical behavior therapy with the elderly client.* New York: Plenum Press.

Witte, K. L., Freund, J. S., & Brown-Whistler, S. (1993). Age differences in free recall and category clustering. *Experimental Aging Research, 19,* 15–28.

Woodruff, D. S., & Birren, J. E. (1972). Age changes and cohort differences in personality. *Developmental Psychology, 6,* 252–259.

Woods, R. T. (1996). Psychological "therapies" in dementia. In R. T. Woods (Ed.), *Handbook of the clinical psychology of ageing* (pp. 575–600). New York: Wiley.

Wright, L., Clipp, E., & George, L. (1993). Health consequences of caregiver stress. *Medicine, Exercise, Nutrition and Health, 2,* 181–195.

Yale, R. (1989). Support groups for newly diagnosed Alzheimer's clients. *Clinical Gerontologist, 8,* 86–89.

Yale, R. (1991). *A guide to facilitating support groups for newly diagnosed Alzheimer's patients.* San Francisco: Alzheimer's Association, Greater San Francisco Chapter.

Yesavage, J. A. (1983). Imagery pretraining and memory training in the elderly. *Gerontology, 29,* 271–275

Yesavage, J. A., & Jacob, R. (1984). Effects of relaxation and mnemonics on memory, attention and anxiety in the elderly. *Experimental Aging Research, 10,* 211–214.

Young, J. E. (1994). *Cognitive therapy for personality disorders: A schema-focused approach* (rev. ed.). Sarasota, FL: Professional Resource Exchange.

Zarit, J. M., & Zarit, S. H. (1996). Ethical considerations in the treatment of older adults. In S. H. Zarit & B. G. Knight (Eds.), *A guide to psychotherapy and aging.* Washington, DC: American Psychological Association.

Zarit, S. H. (1996). Clinical interventions for family caregiving. In S. H. Zarit & B. G. Knight (Eds.), *A guide to psychotherapy and aging* (pp. 139–162). Washington, DC: American Psychological Association.

Zarit, S. H., Eiler, J., & Hassinger, M. (1985). Clinical assessment. In J. E. Birren & K. W. Schaie (Eds.), *The handbook of the psychology of aging* (2nd ed., pp. 725–754). New York: Van Nostrand Reinhold.

Zarit, S. H., Johansson, B., & Malmberg, B. (1995). Changes in functional competency in the oldest old: A longitudinal study. *Journal of Aging and Health, 7,* 3–23.

Zarit, S. H., Miller, N. E., & Kahn, R. L. (1978). Brain function, intellectual impairment and education in the aged. *Journal of the American Geriatrics Society, 26,* 58–67.

Zarit, S. H., Orr, N. K., & Zarit, J. M. (1985). *The hidden victims of Alzheimer's disease: Families under stress.* New York: New York University Press.

Zarit, S. H., Stephens, M. A. P., Townsend, A., & Greene, R. (in press). Stress reduction for family caregivers: Effects of day care use. *Journal of Gerontology: Social Sciences.*

Zarit, S. H., Todd, P. A., & Zarit, J. M. (1986). Subjective burden of husbands and wives as caregivers: A longitudinal study. *Gerontologist, 26,* 260–270.

Zarit, S. H., & Whitlatch, C. J. (1992). Institutional placement: Phases of the transition. *Gerontologist, 32,* 665–672.

Zarit, S. H., & Zarit, J. M. (1982). Families under stress: Interventions for caregivers of senile dementia patients. *Psychotherapy: Theory, Research and Practice, 19,* 461–471.

Zarit, S. H., Zarit, J. M., & Reever, K. E. (1982). Memory training for severe memory loss: Effects on senile dementia patients and their families. *Gerontologist, 22,* 373–377.

Zarit, S. H., & Zarit, J. M., & Rosenberg-Thompson, S. (1990). A special treatment unit for Alzheimer's disease: Medical, behavioral, and environmental features. *Clinical Gerontologist, 9,* 47–63.

Zeiss, A. M., & Steffen, A. (1996a). Interdisciplinary health care teams: The basic unit of geriatric care. In L. L. Carstensen, B. A. Edelstein, & L. Dornbrand (Eds.), *The handbook of clinical gerontology* (pp. 423–467). London: Sage.

Zeiss, A. M., & Steffen, A. (1996b). Behavioral and cognitive treatments: Social learning in older adults. In S. H. Zarit & B. G. Knight (Eds.), *A guide to psychotherapy and aging* (pp. 35–60). New York: American Psychological Association.

Zelinski, E. M., & Gilewski, M. J. (1988). Assessment of memory complaints by rating scales and questionnaires. *Psychopharmacology Bulletin, 24,* 523–529.

Zelinski, E. M., Gilewski, M. J., & Anthony-Bergstone, C. R. (1990). Memory functioning questionnaire: Concurrent validity with memory performance and self-reported memory failures. *Psychology and Aging, 5,* 388–399.

Zepelin, H., Wolfe, C. S., & Kleinplatz, F. (1981). Evaluation of a yearlong reality orientation program. *Journal of Gerontology, 36,* 70–77.

Zgola, J. M. (1987). *Doing things: A guide to programming activities for persons with Alzheimer's disease and related disorders.* Baltimore: Johns Hopkins University Press.

Zisook, S., Shuchter, S. R., Sledge, P. A., Paulus, M., & Judd, L. L. (1994). The spectrum of depressive phenomena after spousal bereavement. *Journal of Clinical Psychiatry, 55*(Suppl.), 29–36.

Zweig, R. A., & Hinrichsen, G. A. (1993). Factors associated with suicide attempts by depressed older adults: A prospective study. *American Journal of Psychiatry, 150,* 1687–1692.

Index